Central Auditory Processing Disorders

Central Auditory Processing Disorders
Problems of Speech, Language, and Learning

Edited by
Elaine Z. Lasky, Ph.D.
Professor
Department of Speech and Hearing
Cleveland State University
Cleveland, Ohio

and
Jack Katz, Ph.D.
Professor and Chairman
Department of Communicative Disorders and Sciences
State University of New York at Buffalo
Amherst, New York

5341 Industrial Oaks Boulevard
Austin, Texas 78735

Library of Congress Cataloging in Publication Data
Main entry under title:

Central auditory processing disorders.

Includes index.
1. Hearing disorders in children. 2. Auditory perception in children.
3. Speech disorders in children. 4. Language disorders in children.
5. Learning disabilities. I. Lasky, Elaine Z. II. Katz, Jack.
[DNLM: 1. Language disorders – In infancy and childhood. 2. Learning disorders – In infancy and childhood. 3. Speech disorders – In infancy and chil-
hood. 4. Perceptual disorders – In infancy and childhood. WV 272 C3975]
RF291.5.C45C446   1983   618.92'855   82-24725

ISBN 0-89079-117-1
(previously 0-8391-1802-3)

5341 Industrial Oaks Boulevard
Austin, Texas 78735

10   9   8   7   6   5   4   3   2   86   87   88   89

Contents

Contributors

Celia Bassich, M.A.
Research Speech Pathologist
Communicative Disorders Program
National Institute of Neurological
  and Communicative Disorders
  and Stroke
Building 36, Room 4A-23
9000 Rockville Pike
Bethesda, Maryland 20205

Gerald L. Brown, M.D.
Staff Investigator
Unit on Childhood Mental Illness
Biological Psychiatry Branch
National Institute of
  Mental Health
Building 10, Room 3N-310
9000 Rockville Pike
Bethesda, Maryland 20205

Katharine G. Butler, Ph.D.
Director
Special Education and
  Rehabilitation
Syracuse University
805 S. Crouse Avenue
Syracuse, New York 13210

Patricia Byrne, Ed.D.
Chief Learning Therapist
Hearing, Speech and
  Learning Center
Delaware County Memorial
  Hospital
501 N. Lansdowne Avenue
Drexel Hill, Pennsylvania 19026

L. Clarke Cox, Ph.D.
Associate Professor
Department of Speech and Hearing
Cleveland State University
East 22nd and Euclid Avenue
Cleveland, Ohio 44115

Edward A. Cudahy, Ph.D.
Associate Professor
Communicative Disorders
Syracuse University
805 S. Crouse Avenue
Syracuse, New York 13210

Charlotte Dempsey, M.A.
Private Practitioner
1138 West Chester Pike
West Chester, Pennsylvania 19380

Judith F. Duchan, Ph.D.
Associate Professor
Department of Communicative
  Disorders and Sciences
State University of New York
  at Buffalo
4226 Ridge Lea Road
Amherst, New York 14226

Rebecca E. Eilers, Ph.D.
Associate Professor of Pediatrics
  and Psychology
Language Project
Mailman Center for Child
  Development
University of Miami
Miami, Florida 33101

Philmore J. Hart, M.S.
Architect
Lecturer, John Carroll University
3080 Essex Road
Cleveland Heights, Ohio 44118

Mark Hoffman, Ph.D.
Clinical Psychologist
Hearing, Speech and
  Learning Center
Delaware County Memorial
  Hospital
501 N. Lansdowne Avenue
Drexel Hill, Pennsylvania 19026

Pamela E. Hook, Ph.D.
Consultant
Language and Learning
5524 Huisache
Houston, Texas 77081

Jack Katz, Ph.D.
Professor and Chairman
Department of Communicative
  Disorders and Sciences
State University of New York
  at Buffalo
4226 Ridge Lea Road
Amherst, New York 14226

Marcel Kinsbourne, M.D.
Director
Behavioral Neurology Department
Eunice Kennedy Shriver Center
  for Mental Retardation
200 Trapelo Road
Waltham, Massachusetts 02254

Elaine Z. Lasky, Ph.D.
Professor
Department of Speech and Hearing
Cleveland State University
East 22nd and Euclid Avenue
Cleveland, Ohio 44115

Lanny Lester, Ed.M.
Department of Psychology
  of Reading
Temple University
1801 N. Broad Street
Philadelphia, Pennsylvania 19122

Christy L. Ludlow, Ph.D.
Research Speech Pathologist
Communicative Disorders Program
National Institute of Neurological
  and Communicative Disorders
  and Stroke
Federal Building, Room 1C-13
7550 Wisconsin Avenue
Bethesda, Maryland 20205

Noel D. Matkin, Ph.D.
Professor of Audiology
University of Arizona
Tucson, Arizona 85721

Dennis L. Molfese, Ph.D.
Professor of Psychology
Southern Illinois University
Carbondale, Illinois 62901

Victoria J. Molfese, Ph.D.
Associate Professor of Psychology
Southern Illinois University
Carbondale, Illinois 62901

D. Kimbrough Oller, Ph.D.
Associate Professor of Pediatrics
  and Psychology
Language Project
Mailman Center for Child
  Development
University of Miami
Miami, Florida 33101

Elizabeth Protti, M.S.
Chief of Audiology
Administrator of Services
Hearing, Speech and
  Learning Center
Delaware County Memorial
  Hospital
501 N. Lansdowne Avenue
Drexel Hill, Pennsylvania 19026

Douglas B. Webster, Ph.D.
Departments of Otorhinolaryngol-
  ogy and Anatomy
Kresge Hearing Research Labora-
  tory of the South
Louisiana State University
  Medical Center
New Orleans, Louisiana 70119

Maxine L. Young, M.S.
Senior Audiologist
Hearing, Speech and
  Learning Center
Delaware County Memorial
  Hospital
501 N. Lansdowne Avenue
Drexel Hill, Pennsylvania 19026

Preface

The processing of auditory information is a complex task that most of us are able to accomplish with little effort. Occasionally, however, we find children who seem to have problems processing auditory information. In response to frustrations reported by those who work or live with these children, there has been an increase in the number of national conferences and workshops, convention papers, books, and journal articles devoted to issues related to central auditory processing (CAP).

As editors, we conceived this book to bring together ideas and discussions of researchers and clinicians representing different specialties but all concerned with some aspect of CAP. Our intent is to provide readable summaries of current, ongoing work for both students and professionals in various fields. Selection of the authors for this book was based on their knowledge and experience in the area of CAP. It should be clear that, as editors, we did not seek people because they adhered to either of our orientations. We believe that students and professionals will find the diversity of opinions and approaches a rewarding, if occasionally frustrating, experience. We did!

Elaine Z. Lasky
Jack Katz

To our families,
whose support has been
considerable and continuous

Central Auditory Processing Disorders

Section **I**

Philosophical
Issues

Chapter **1**

Perspectives on Central Auditory Processing

Elaine Z. Lasky and *Jack Katz*

Over the past few years there has been a gradual increase in interest and study of central auditory processing (CAP). Speech-language clinicians, audiologists, teachers, physicians, psychologists, and other professionals who work directly with children are seeking help from researchers and theoreticians. Students and practitioners want information explaining the factors involved in CAP, the assessment of both normal CAP and disorders in CAP, possible remedial approaches, and evaluation of these procedures. Answers are needed to such questions as: What is CAP? What happens if there is a problem in processing auditory information? How does CAP relate to language, speech, and learning problems? How can CAP be measured? Can one diagnose problems in CAP? What can be done for those who are deficient in CAP abilities? What kinds of research are being carried out to define CAP?

The responses to these questions are not simple. They frequently reflect divergent points of view. Virtually everyone would agree that: a) the issue is a complex one, b) there is a great deal that requires study and elaboration, and c) we are generating many important questions and few clear-cut answers.

We began this project with agreement on a few essential issues: Auditory signals received by the peripheral mechanism proceed through an extensive and complicated neural network from the cochlear nuclei in the brainstem to areas in the cortex. These signals are received, interpreted, and utilized (i.e., information is extracted from these impulses). Some children with speech, language, and learning problems seem to have difficulty with processing auditory signals.

Although there are conflicting points of view, many professionals who work closely with children in educational or therapeutic settings recognize that there are youngsters with CAP problems. There has been a lack of precision in specifying and communicating the effects of the CAP difficulty. Definitions used at times may be vague. They reflect, in part, the fact that there is much we do not know. The editors believe that this book will broaden the reader's perspective and sensitivity regarding what is involved in CAP. We think it will help in both understanding and dealing with children who have difficulties in CAP.

WHAT IS CENTRAL AUDITORY PROCESSING?

The operational definitions of CAP often differ. The least restrictive definition can allow us greatest flexibility and permit greatest learning. We, therefore, consider CAP to be the manipulation and utilization of sound signals by the central nervous system—what we do with what we hear. CAP involves a range of activities from the awareness of the presence of a sound to analysis of linguistic information. The actual processing of a sound occurs when it strikes the pinna or enters the ear canal, but CAP begins at the level of the cochlear nuclei in the brainstem. The ascending auditory system directs the auditory information through a complex array of nuclei, sections of nuclei, layers of these sections, and various cells within these layers. The results from these processes reach Heschl's gyrus of the temporal lobe via the auditory radiations. At this point the information is scattered to many parts of the brain. A complex efferent system serves higher centers in affecting and controlling lower levels.

Different professional perspectives have led to different approaches, emphases, and treatment protocols. Audiologists often stress central functions that are most closely related to peripheral hearing. They discuss the brainstem and temporal lobe functions that correspond with their work in site-of-lesion testing. Often procedures for evaluating adults with suspected central auditory nervous system (CANS) lesions are utilized or adapted for children who are thought to have CAP disorders.

The concerns of speech-language pathologists have suggested, in part, that difficulty in CAP may be an etiologic factor for some children exhibiting language difficulties or articulation problems. In concert with reading specialists, classroom teachers, and teachers of the learning-disabled, some clinicians propose that problems in CAP may be important in the learning disabilities of some children. Often academic problems of children that are confusing to the children and to their parents, teachers, and clinicians seem to stem from difficulties in listening and understanding auditory information. Clinicians and educators have attempted to analyze and break down listening-learning tasks into subskills to explain the problems. Procedures to assess and remediate specific auditory disabilities have been suggested.

Until recently, interchanges regarding these issues among audiologists, speech-language pathologists, regular classroom teachers, and specialized teachers were few. We believe we are now seeing an increasing interest in promoting discussion across professional lines.

This text provides an exchange of information as to the state of the art. It allows the reader to: 1) sample types of research that are being used to study how humans process auditory information, 2) sample different clinical procedures used for evaluation and remediation of children with CAP problems, and 3) gain an awareness of procedures used by professionals in related fields for children with CAP problems.

In the first section, different professional issues are raised that have had a bearing on the direction of intervention programs for children with CAP problems. Work with these children has been influenced by the various theoretical positions, data presented, and philosophical viewpoints. The current directions will be more logical and readily comprehended if some consideration is given to the historiography of the parameters and approaches to CAP.

Elaine Lasky in Chapter 2 uses data describing CAP in the literature of various professional disciplines to discuss issues such as the variability of the unit of perception, the types of approaches that have been utilized to analyze CAP, and the presumptions underlying current procedures to evaluate and remediate CAP. The focus then shifts to factors that affect the processing of the auditory signal in the classroom and the clinic.

Judith Duchan and Jack Katz in Chapter 3 deal with an issue that has recently divided not only the speech-language pathologist from the audiologist but workers within these disciplines as well: Are learning-disabled children poor auditory processors or are they language-impaired? Both positions are presented, followed by the suggestion that a synthesis of these views is possible and necessary. A dynamic model is presented to portray the relative emphases on signal versus higher-order processing under different task conditions.

In the second section the discussions concentrate on normal physical and physiologic bases of CAP as well as some of the problems related to difficulties in CAP. Marcel Kinsbourne in Chapter 4 delineates two alternatives for a pediatrician. One represents a limited involvement, and the other indicates what may be done if broader involvement is desired. He briefly explains the etiology of learning disability, the factors that may affect a developing child, how they are examined, and the possible consequences on a child's attending and processing behaviors.

Dennis Molfese and Victoria Molfese review in Chapter 5 the methods used to study cerebral asymmetry in response to different types of stimuli presented to infants and children. Does the left hemisphere respond differently than the right? Does the response pattern change with age? The results of auditory processing are reflected by cortical response patterns to linguistic and to nonlinguistic stimuli. Developmental changes in cortical response patterns are discussed, as are implications for speech and language processing.

Do infants perceive differences in speech sounds? How is an infant's psychophysical response judged? In Chapter 6 Rebecca Eilers and D. Kimbrough Oller outline methods used to study speech perception in infants and young children. They summarize and interpret results from a developmental perspective. Gaps or contradictions in the data are discussed, and data obtained from normal children are compared with data from children with handicaps.

To help in understanding the complexity of the central auditory nervous system, Elizabeth Protti reviews the anatomy of brainstem auditory pathways in Chapter 7. Normal and pathologic functional correlates of these auditory pathways are discussed, and types of stimuli requiring higher-level processing are indicated. Protti contrasts the processing required with objective versus subjective testing procedures in an effort to assess the integrity of the pathways.

Is there a relationship between some types of language disorder and CAP? Maxine Young provides evidence in Chapter 8 relating neurologic maturation and acquisition of language. She reviews neuropsychologic research and hypothesizes an association between language disorders and impaired lateralization of function of the two hemispheres. CAP problems that seem to involve the right hemisphere are discussed.

Children labeled as learning-disabled do not represent a single entity. Christy Ludlow, Edward Cudahy, Celia Bassich, and Gerald Brown report on results of their evaluation procedures with subtypes of learning-disabled boys (Chapter 9). They present findings comparing hyperactive boys without language or learning disabilities, hyperactive boys with reading disability but no language disability, and language-disabled boys who are not hyperactive.

Does a conductive loss affect development of higher-order functions? Are there any long-term effects of sensory hearing losses? In Chapter 10 Douglas Webster reviews studies on humans and animals and documents evidence that decreased hearing sensitivity of the peripheral mechanism affects the CNS. Depending on age, there appear to be serious implications, particularly with regard to language acquisition and CAP. Webster explains the existence of this functional/ structural interdependence between peripheral and central auditory pathways.

In the third section of the book, procedures are delineated which are used diagnostically to identify the problem and provide direction for remediation. Intervention procedures to facilitate CAP are discussed.

A variety of tests are used to evaluate CAP. In Chapter 11 Charlotte Dempsey describes some of the more frequently used tests. She discusses factors that affect selection of the child, purpose of testing, type of stimuli utilized, equipment needed, and variables that may influence test performance and interpretation. Results are interpreted with implications as to the child's listening and learning in the classroom.

Audiologist Noel Matkin and reading-education specialist Pamela Hook point out different professional approaches utilized with children with CAP (Chapter 12). The evaluation procedures of the audiologist are compared with those of the language/learning specialist in terms of predictive or diagnostic values. Whether specific auditory abilities are prerequisites to or correlates of the development of language comprehension is investigated.

The eclectic approach of Elaine Lasky and Clarke Cox in Chapter 13 stresses helping children to comprehend, integrate, and remember auditory information. Emphasis is placed on use of materials and tasks that are representative of those with which the children have greatest difficulty: those used in the classroom.

Jack Katz in Chapter 14 discusses phonemic synthesis and related procedures used over the past 50 years to evaluate and remediate auditory processing disorders associated with problems of articulation, language, spelling, and reading. Emphasis is on recent investigations of effects of auditory therapy in developing phonemic synthesis skills and its influence on other auditory skills and articulation disorders. A. R. Luria's work provides a basis for a theoretical framework to explain these findings.

Katharine Butler in Chapter 15 introduces new approaches to the study of selective attention, cognition, and memory and the possible effects of problems on auditory language processing. Although these areas are interrelated and mutually dependent, Butler argues that evaluation of language processing should include specific procedures to assess attention, cognition, and memory. Intervention strategies can be developed to improve performance in these areas.

The fourth section discusses the other professional support services needed by many children with CAP problems. Mark Hoffman writes in Chapter 16 about the emotional disorders that may be observed among children with CAP difficulties. His explanation of intervention procedures includes therapeutic techniques with family members and guidelines for working directly with the child. The case histories presented provide examples of children's behaviors and their responses to therapy.

Teachers and others concerned with the psychoeducational functioning of children need to identify children who should be referred to the audiologist because of possible CAP disorder. Patricia Byrne and Lanny Lester discuss in Chapter 17 the performance on tests of intelligence, learning aptitude, achievement, and laterality of a group of children with CAP disorders. A psychoeducational battery is recommended that includes procedures for assessing and comparing strengths and weaknesses in sensory modalities.

The physical environment of the classroom may have a greater effect on children with CAP disorders than on other youngsters. In Chapter 18 Philmore Hart explains that acoustical properties of school and classroom construction may particularly affect the learning of these children. Alterations are suggested to enhance and support learning and listening.

We hope the reader will gain a greater understanding of various facets of the auditory system:

1. As we learn about the auditory system, we recognize its complexity, flexibility, and efficiency.
2. Extensive interaction is seen between the preprogrammed development of the auditory system and the influencing factors from the not-so-programmed environment.
3. A breadth of evaluation procedures help in the study of the auditory processes in the normal child and in those youngsters with special problems. Procedures are geared to numerous levels of this system from the peripheral mechanism up through the areas that involve complex analysis and integration.
4. Based on both research and conjecture we see auditory processes are related to learning and communication. All of the relationships that must be relevant have not been precisely defined. We must

await new developments and contributions from research in various professional disciplines.

5. Evaluation cannot be considered the sum and substance of our contribution to children with CAP disorders. Support, guidance, direct therapy, and other forms of management should be the goal.

6. Speech-language pathology and audiology cannot expect to work alone. The family, school, physician, and many other specialists have a large part to play if a child is to be helped to reach his or her most productive and satisfying level.

Chapter 2

Parameters Affecting Auditory Processing

Elaine Z. Lasky

Information is presented verbally in preschool, elementary, and secondary school classrooms, in clinics, and in homes. The listener receives that information auditorily and must process it. Processing information includes an awareness that a signal exists and a recognition that the signal carries meaning to be interpreted, comprehended, accepted or rejected, responded to, and perhaps remembered. Some children experience difficulties in processing auditory information for communication and learning. This chapter reviews research relevant to central auditory processing and discusses variables that affect CAP. These variables involve the signal and its presentation, the environment, response task required, and the strategies an individual brings to the task. The focus is not on children who have peripheral hearing impairments or who have failed to develop language or communication skills. Rather, it is on children who exhibit difficulties when they begin to use language for learning. These children often have language disorders, learning disabilities, dyslexia, or CAP difficulties. They are not a homogeneous group. Their problems may involve attending, following directions, and remembering and using auditory information.

The relationships among perceptual, linguistic, and cognitive processes are not clear-cut. One needs, then, to be global and systematic in evaluating performance of the listener/learner.

COMPONENTS CONTRIBUTING TO
PROCESSING OF AUDITORY INFORMATION

To discuss the components of CAP, current research and clinical data from several disciplines should be considered, including speech-language pathology, audiology, speech and hearing science, sociolinguistics, neurology, neuropsychology, developmental and cognitive psychology, learning disability, and education (Tower, 1979). We must relate these data to our traditional approaches for children whose behaviors suggest problems in CAP.

A first consideration is: Are there discrete auditory components? A traditional approach suggests there is a discrete sequence of skills that the listener performs to process auditory information. The skills are purported to involve discriminating, sequencing, and remembering segments of speech presented auditorily, as well as other skills such as auditory analysis or segmentation, synthesis, and selective attention. Programs exist to train these skills in children with language and/or learning problems.

The literature, however, is conflicting with regard to the designation of separate and discrete CAP skills that can be evaluated and taught in order to improve processing the auditory signal. Proponents have argued the value of training of skills for persons with CAP difficulties (Barr, 1976; Katz, Chapter 14, this volume; Rampp, 1980). Opponents argue that one or more specific skills cannot be isolated as discrete factors in CAP, and little data exist supporting any gain in language or learning abilities from training these skills (Rees, 1973; Sanders, 1977; Willeford & Billger, 1978). Let us consider part of the underlying rationale of evaluating and training auditory skills.

Some programs point to CAP difficulties as impairments in identifying, discriminating, or sequencing phonemes, which are the smallest classes of distinguishable speech sounds (e.g., /p/, /b/, /s/). Others implicate syllables, whereas still others emphasize words or phrases. Is there a single, invariable unit in speech processing? Is the critical unit of perception the phoneme? the syllable? the word? the phrase? or even the sentence? Each of these linguistic units may contribute important perceptual information. Teachers and users of alphabetic notations often assume that the key unit is the phoneme (Foss & Hakes, 1978). Data from speech perception research in both adults and infants provide evidence supporting this assumption. Eimas (1979), however, indicated that adjacent phonemes and the entire linguistic context affect categorization of the acoustic signal, and that a complete explanation of the process of extracting meaning cannot focus on one single pattern or unit. Massaro (1975) presented data implicating the vowel at times and the syllable at times, whereas Freund (1975) and Helliage (1975) argued for the phrase. What is perceptually real, according to McNeill and Lindig (1973), is what one attends to; this is usually the *meaning* of the utterance. The subordinate levels are consciously considered only under special (or difficult) circumstances. One interpretation suggests that through a series of consecutive analyses the acoustic signal is broken into a stream of small units which are fed up to a language processor (bottom-up, data-driven). Another position argues that language processing is primarily affected by knowledge of the language and what to expect from the signal (top-down, knowledge interprets signal). Both positions are discussed further in Chapters 3 and 15.

CAP, however, seems to have a flexible and variable basis. "Phonemes, syllables, words, morphemes, phrases, and linguistic constituents may all act as functional segments under appropriate circumstances" (Neisser, 1967, p. 183), and language difficulty, as Cutting and Pisoni (1978) have suggested, is not likely to be due to a malfunction in only one stage of processing. The speech signal is so redundant that if the listener has some knowledge of what to expect, and if even a small part of the signal is intact, meaning can be derived.

Although studies have consistently reported that children with language disorders have difficulty in the sequencing or temporal ordering of speech sounds, particularly with rapidly presented stimuli (Lowe & Campbell, 1965; Stark & Tallal, 1981; Tallal & Piercy, 1974; Tallal & Newcombe, 1978), this must be interpreted cautiously. The phoneme embedded in a speech signal is very different from the phoneme in isolation (Shearme & Holmes, 1962). Judging the time of occurrence of two isolated phonemes is totally different from retrieving information from context-dependent and redundant running speech "where there is no one-to-one correlation between the acoustic events and perceived phonemes" (Zaidel, 1979, p. 57). Tallal (1978) also summarized reports of cases in which children could not sequence phonemes but did comprehend language. These arguments urge caution in the evaluation and training of discrete skills and emphasize that the critical unit is not simple or invariant but depends on the task.

AN ECLECTIC APPROACH TO EVALUATING PROCESSING OF AUDITORY INFORMATION

Audiologists are standardizing and expanding batteries of procedures to evaluate the central auditory nervous system (CANS). Originally used to determine site of lesion, these procedures are now in use to evaluate aspects of processing (see Dempsey, Chapter 11, this volume). To put stress on the CANS, the linguistic signal is made more difficult by distorting or degrading it. Degrading can occur by compressing or expanding the time frame, removing or filtering certain frequencies, or presenting the signal in an atypical manner such as by switching back and forth between ears or presenting the signal with competing messages. Responses of a listener are compared to responses from a sample of normal subjects. Changes in responses are observed as the signal becomes more or less degraded, degraded in a different manner, or when competing messages are added.

The following assumptions underlie these procedures: First, both the linguistic signal and the neural pathways are redundant. To show problems in processing, the signal must be made more difficult by reducing the redundancies. Second, the normal listener utilizes a constructive process. Using knowledge of the language and certain expectations, the listener fills in parts of the signal and tolerates variability in acoustical patterns of phonemes and syllables (Stevens & House, 1972; Cole & Jakimik, 1980). Degrading the signal makes processing more difficult. The listener cannot use the same expectancies or has less time to determine what is missed. Third, whereas normal subjects do not generally have problems even with degraded signals, persons with CANS dysfunction may show patterns of difficulty. If a person usually operates with a degraded signal, externally degrading the signal should amplify any difficulty and help determine the type of problem and site of dysfunction.

To analyze CAP there is a need to go beyond simple tasks of repetition of a word, phrase, or sentence. Stress on the system becomes apparent with the need to listen and learn, process longer constructions with difficult concepts, or perform more difficult tasks. We must evaluate peripheral sensitivity and then systematically evaluate the integrity of the neural pathways, and we must analyze the performance of listeners in tasks simulating those on which they break down outside the clinic. What increases stress or processing load for a child? What problems culminate in a child's being labeled an "auditory processing problem"?

To evaluate CAP and the factors affecting comprehension, remembering, and using information, we consider variables in the *signal* and its *presentation*, the *environment*, the *response* required, and the *strategies* an individual uses (SPERS). Let us first examine objective data from electrophysiologic studies relating changes in CAP due to difficulty of the signal, the task, and the physical condition of the listener.

ELECTROPHYSIOLOGIC STUDIES OF CAP

For research and clinical purposes, CAP may be observed through recorded electrical potentials from neural activity (see Chapters 5 and 7, this volume). Neural activity is identified by time of appearance (latency) or amplitude of electrical potentials. Electrical activity following auditory stimulation is classified as an early, middle, or late response according to its latency (2–10 msec, 10–50 msec, or 50–500 msec, respectively).

The early response represents neural activity elicited from cranial nerve VIII and auditory brainstem structures. The auditory brainstem response (ABR) reflects the integrity of the initial portion of the CANS. To elicit ABR, nonlinguistic stimuli of very brief duration (transients) are used. (Although speech stimuli are also highly transient, it is not valid to assume that ABR abnormalities in response to nonspeech stimuli reflect abnormal functioning associated with speech stimuli.)

Middle and later neural responses are elicited by different types of stimuli and tasks. Unlike the ABR, later responses are contingent to varying degrees on cognition and are affected by several factors. Donchin and McCarthy (1979) reviewed studies showing that latency (timing of the response relative to the stimulus) and amplitude of a neural response reflect the task the subject is doing. Middle and especially later neural responses are event-related potentials (ERP) and are evoked by the processing demands of the task. When subjects are presented with frequent tones at one frequency (e.g., 1000 Hz), termed the frequent event, and told to expect and count tones at a different frequency (e.g., 1500 Hz), termed the rare event, their neural responses, ERP, following the rare event show a large positive (P) deflection about 340 msec after the stimulus. The rare event is made to occur randomly with varying probabilities. The response, labeled P300, following the rare event is not observed following the frequent event; it only occurs after the rare event *if* the subject is monitoring it. A similar P300 response is noted when the frequent event is repetition of a name, such as "David, David, David . . .," and the rare event is "Nancy." If the task is made more difficult, with the rare tone harder to discriminate, for example, a rare tone of the same frequency but slightly different intensity (such as 3 dB), latency is longer. That is, a longer time is required to process and make a decision. A frequent event of different male names ("David, Eric, Neil . . .") contrasted with a harder task of discerning a female name ("Nancy") as the rare event shows a still longer latency for P300. The more difficult tasks seem to require longer processing time (Squires, 1981). We relate this later to experiments in cognitive psychology which demonstrate longer reaction times occurring with more difficult processing tasks.

Aging affects latency. Latency decreases through infancy and early childhood to the middle teens. Latency then increases progressively through the decades (Squires, 1981; Squires et al., 1980). We observe this behaviorally: response time is longer with increasingly older age groups. Squires (1981) reported pilot studies indicating that fatigue and health states affect latency of the P300 response. One resident physician showed shorter latency and faster reaction time after 8-10 hr of sleep than after being on call for up to 24 hr. During periods of exacerbation in multiple sclerosis, latency increased for one patient; during remission, instances of decreased latency were noted. ERP in alcoholic patients reflected longer processing time, with longer latencies for P300 than in controls. Similar results were obtained for neurologic patients with dementia. Neurologic patients without dementia performed essentially as did their normal age-mates (Squires et al., 1980). These data support a rationale that factors within the signal and its presentation, the response task, and the individual affect performance. Let us proceed to discuss these and other variables in the environment that may affect CAP.

THE SIGNAL AND ITS PRESENTATION AFFECT PROCESSING

Linguistic Factors

The language signal can be described in terms of phonology, pragmatics, syntax, and semantics. Although separated for study and evaluation, these components are interactive and interdependent. In this section these components, their complexity, and their effects on the processing of information are discussed. Syntactic complexity, semantic difficulty, rate, redundancy, and contextual cues in the presentation are emphasized as critical.

Phonologic Segmental Features   The normal listener is mostly unaware of receiving and interpreting the segmental features of phonology, or the rapidly changing sound patterns of consonants and vowels that comprise the raw data of speech. One focuses on individual phonemes only if one needs to, if the signal is distorted or the speaker is difficult to understand (Perfetti, 1979). Mature listeners know that the speech signal is composed of phonologic segments that blend into syllables, and that syllables make up words. Fewer than half of a sample of 4-year-old children with normal language development, however, could learn to determine the number of syllables in a word (e.g., tell=1, telling =2; telephone=3; see Cutting & Pisoni, 1978; Liberman et al., 1974). Difficulties in syllabification, phonologic segmentation, and sequencing thus for some children may reflect immaturity in a developing process rather than a CAP problem.

Phonologic Suprasegmental Cues and Pragmatics   Suprasegmental phonologic features include such features as stress, rate, and loudness. These cues not only indicate the emotions and intentions of the speaker, but also indicate phrase and sentence boundaries, content words, and given or presupposed information (information assumed to be known by both speaker and listener). Stress signals new information or focus for the listener. Changing the emphasis from word to word in the sentence "Pamela took Eric home" changes the interpretation. Different patterns alter the meaning and what is supposedly new to a listener.

Suprasegmental cues also provide, in part, contextual or pragmatic information as to the speaker's intentions. Is the speaker joking? being sarcastic? frightened? angry? Pragmatics refers to social rules of using language in any situation: Who talks or listens to whom? How does one talk or interpret what is said? Humor, sarcasm, and emotions are signaled by intonation patterns.

Difficulties occur when listeners misinterpret the speaker's intentions or when the presuppositions held by speaker and listener do not match. Inability to interpret suprasegmental cues and other pragmatic signals is frequently observed in children referred for CAP problems. They often fail to pick out sarcasm or recognize even an obvious joke. Failure to interpret these cues may be socially devastating for a child. Processing of suprasegmental cues is not generally evaluated, but perhaps should be considered.

Syntax   Syntax refers to the form, structure, and word order of a sentence. Syntax increases in complexity through the addition, deletion, or change in order of morphemes, words, modifiers, phrases, embedded sentences, or conjoined sentences. The transformational generative grammar model measures syntactic complexity by the number of transformations involved (see, for example, Jacobs & Rosenbaum, 1968). All transformations do not add or add equally to syntactic complexity, but in general, comprehension by children and adults is negatively affected, both in speed and accuracy, by increasing syntactic complexity (Gough, 1965; Savin & Perchonock, 1965; Slobin, 1966). As syntactic complexity is increased, processing time increases and accuracy of comprehension decreases (Lasky & Chapandy, 1976).

Semantics   Semantics refers to information about word meaning. When a child acquires the meaning of a word, he or she may acquire a partial rather than a full conventional adult meaning (Clark, 1973). The child, however, does not know he or she may not have the full meaning and may miscomprehend the word. When asked, "Who knows what a scale is?" one child responded that she knew, "That's where mommy measures her feet every day." What the child knows about "scale" (or any word) affects how she processes a sentence containing it.

If both syntactic complexity and semantic knowledge affect comprehension, then their interaction is critical for comprehending and using language. Consider your own processing of the following sentence: "Under these conditions, best-fitting linear, quadratic, cubic functions are most readily associated with r levels of an independent variable" (Winer, 1962, p. 354). The semantic load may result in some readers skipping parts of the sentence or not understanding it. Many members of an audience soon stop listening if complex, unfamiliar sentences are presented. With more familiar concepts or with simplified syntax, listeners usually attend. They may also understand enough to ask a question or for a repetition.

Some children find materials presented in a classroom as syntactically and semantically complex at their level as some readers found the example sentence above. The semantic load for the child with a language, CAP, or learning disorder may be sufficiently difficult that that child cannot listen or attend. Performance in listening tasks by first-grade children can be helped by a) simplifying the syntax for presenting instruction, and b) directly teaching the semantic concepts before incorporating them in the lessons (Lasky & Chapandy, 1976).

Materials for assessing CAP by audiologists and language processing by speech-language pathologists contain relatively simple syntactic structures and semantic concepts. Auditory processing should be evaluated with material as complex and challenging syntactically and semantically as that used in classrooms.

Other Variables Affecting Comprehension of the Signal

Contextual Cues   Contextual cues influence perception and facilitate comprehension (Moates & Schumacher, 1980). They trigger a listener's expectations and affect interpretations of words, sentences, and prose. Performance is better for words presented in sentence contexts (70% correct) than as single words (40% correct; Miller, 1962). Subjects shown a picture cueing the context of a paragraph prior to reading it recalled twice as much or more than subjects receiving no cues or partial cues, or receiving cues after the reading (Bransford & Johnson, 1973). In a classic study, Bransford and Johnson (1972) presented this passage:

> The procedure is actually quite simple. First, you arrange things into different groups depending on their makeup. Of course, one pile may be suffi-

cient depending on how much there is to do. If you have to go somewhere else due to lack of facilities that is the next step, otherwise, you are pretty well set. It is important not to overdo any particular endeavor. That is, it is better to do too few things at once than too many . . . (p. 722).

Subjects who were cued with the words "washing clothes" before reading the paragraph comprehended it more easily than those not given the cue. An outline given prior to a lecture facilitates processing by setting a context. Text materials, particularly for lower grades, use pictorial cues and topic headings to facilitate comprehension. Other cues helping comprehension include statements of theme and instructions to listeners (Moates & Schumacher, 1980). Evaluating CAP with isolated words or third-order approximations of sentences provides some information regarding the subject's behaviors. Other data can be gained by analyzing performance when contextual cues are available. Do cues improve performance?

Rate of Presentation Comprehension of speech by learning-disabled children, aphasic children, and aphasic adults is increased when a slower rate of speech is used (Lasky, Weidner, & Johnson, 1976; Peck, 1977; McCroskey & Thompson, 1973; Weidner & Lasky, 1976). Presentation can be slowed through expanding each word; however, inserting pauses is more effective (Lasky et al., 1976). A pause inserted between the noun phrase and the verb phrase of a sentence, between the verb and the following noun phrase, or before and after an embedded sentence helps a listener chunk information and permits additional time for processing. Normal and learning-disabled first-grade level children and language-disordered children in the clinic showed improved comprehension when new material was slowed by adding interphrase pause times of 0.75 to 1 sec. Interspersing pauses between major constituents improves comprehension of complicated material by college students.

Repetition Exact repetition of a complex, critical, or novel point enables listeners to hear it again and enhances comprehension. If the idea is complicated, listeners at many levels report the redundancy helpful. By presenting the stimulus phrase twice, performance on the Test of Auditory Comprehension of Language (Carrow, 1973) was significantly improved (Haynes & McCallion, 1981).

Intensity and Location Research is limited regarding the effects of intensity and location of the signal source for the child with CAP difficulties. Increasing signal intensity decreases reaction time up to a point (Massaro, 1975). Clinical evidence indicates that comprehension is enhanced for some children, with intensity increased by talking louder or by amplification. For some children, close proximity to the signal source facilitates comprehension. This may help the child focus attention and may also enhance the ratio of signal to background noise.

This section has stressed some factors in the signal and its presentation that affect processing: suprasegmental cues, syntactic complexity plus semantic complexity, rate, redundancy, and contextual cues. Emphasis has been on including materials for evaluation that are as complex as those that children must process in classrooms.

THE ENVIRONMENT AFFECTS AUDITORY PROCESSING

A specialist evaluating CAP probably tests a child in a one-on-one environment, generally in a quiet, controlled setting and at least in part under earphones. If the evaluation is performed in an audiologic test suite, ambient or background noise is controlled, as are other facets of the environment. The child can respond to the test stimuli immediately. Usually the only observer is the tester, so the child need have no concern about reactions from a social peer group. In a classroom, the lesson, instructions, and work required are done in a group setting. Variables in that environment can influence CAP.

Competing Auditory Stimuli

Auditory stimuli in classrooms include stimuli presented by the teacher and stimuli from the students, stimuli that are relevant and stimuli that are nonrelevant to the learning task. Through perceptual focusing and directing attention, the child tunes in selected stimuli and resists competing stimuli. To learn, the child must maintain attention on relevant stimuli and disregard competing ones. Interference from competing stimuli depends on the number of competing talkers (Miller, 1947; Hogan & Hanley, 1963), content of the messages (Carhart, Tillman, & Greetis, 1969; Speaks, Karmen, & Benitez, 1967), and difficulty of the task (Webster & Solomon, 1955, Treisman, 1964). Lasky and Tobin (1973) demonstrated that children with suspected learning disabilities performed more poorly under some competing messages of 0 and +10 dB S/N (signal intensity compared to noise intensity); linguistic competing messages were disruptive, whereas a nonlinguistic competition (white noise) was not. Children with reading problems showed difficulty recalling stimuli under competing messages (Satz, Rardin, & Ross, 1971). When we are involved with an easy and interesting task, such as listening to a story, nearby chatting does not disturb us. The same chatting may be disturbing and disruptive, however, if we are attempting a difficult task such as listening to a complicated lecture on an unfamiliar topic or learning complicated material. CAP, then, should be evaluated on a relatively difficult task accompanied by one to three competing talkers. If more than four talkers comprise the competition, the effect is like random (white) noise and is easier to disregard (Miller, 1947).

Working in a carrel limits visual distraction, but not auditory distraction. The voice of the teacher working with one child can distract the others.

Immediate Versus Delayed Response

In a classroom, a child cannot respond immediately but must raise his or her hand and wait to be called on. Time following a question may be a few seconds or more, thus requiring use of memory. Delay in response may affect performance compared to an immediate response. Recall may be poorer even when short delays are required (Bauer, 1977). What is processed and remembered is affected by time and by the strategies used to help in remembering.

Reaction from Social Peer Groups

We may remember emotions that interfered with our usual pitch levels, rate, fluency, heart rate, and adequacy of response when we were required to report in class. Our performance and our feelings about our performance were negatively affected: we could not listen, hear, and respond as well. Children, especially those experiencing academic difficulty, often relate similar or even more intense feelings. Many have poor self-images, expect to do poorly, and do perform more poorly.

Observed behavior and responses of these children are often worse and more exaggerated in group situations. These variables should be considered when evaluating the child's abilities and performance.

Subtle Modifications Due to
Interaction Between Speaker and Listener

The speaker's rate of speech, stress patterns, amount of redundancy, and other variables are often a function of listener reaction. Even presentations of standardized tests vary to some extent depending upon listener reactions and responses. Presentation of instructions and feedback on performance are influenced by size of group, size of room, and proximity of the speaker-listener. Performance by the child may in turn be differentially affected.

This section has suggested that, in evaluation of CAP, the child's performance may be different when the child is alone with one adult, in a small group, or in a larger group environment. The literature consistently emphasizes that performance may be worsened by interaction with an unfamiliar adult, foreign room environments, and testing procedures that continue until failure is evident. Performance may also differ in the different environments in which the information is presented, whether clinic, classroom, or home.

THE RESPONSE TASK AFFECTS EVALUATION OF CAP

To evaluate CAP, response tasks need to increase systematically in difficulty, ultimately reflecting the level required in home or school. Levels of task difficulty may be described in a hierarchy beginning with the easiest tasks and progressing through those that are more complex or more difficult (Bloom, 1956; Forgus & Melamed, 1976). In a perceptual hierarchy, the detection of a signal, that is, responding only to presence or absence of a signal (as in obtaining an auditory threshold), is the simplest level. More difficult task levels require more effort by the listener and range from the detection task, through gross discrimination, fine discrimination, and recognition tasks, to recall tasks and then to problem solving. Gross discrimination tasks, such as selecting one of two very different sounds, is easier than fine discrimination, such as selecting one of two similar sounds. Recognition of one item in a multiple-choice paradigm is next in this hierarchy, followed by a recall task or fill-in question in which no alternative choices are presented (Davis, Sutherland, & Judd, 1961; Massaro, 1975). It is simpler to recognize a name or fact from a short list of possible responses than to try to *recall* or generate the name or fact to fit a definition (Brown, 1976). Manipulation of the signal for problem solving and social perception are at the highest levels. These involve cognitive memory plus use of the information for induction or deduction.

Specification of level of task difficulty in comparing results of different testing procedures is stressed in current literature (Brown, 1976; Hagen, 1979; Kintsch, 1979; Massaro, 1975; Nuttin, 1976). The number correct in a yes/no test is not directly comparable to number correct in a multiple-choice procedure, because the number of alternatives increases the difficulty of a task (Kintsch, 1979). Determining whether two stimuli are the same or different is a good deal easier than telling what the stimuli are (Zurif & Caramazza, 1978). Procedures that require word or sentence repetition are lower-level tasks than those that require paraphrasing. Many tests of CAP use a recognition (multiple-choice) picture-pointing task or verbatim repeating of sentences or words. Verbatim repetition, in which subjects tend to bypass comprehension of sentence meaning, is not similar to everyday sentence processing. To ensure processing, a response should require paraphrasing (Gagné & White, 1978). Electrophysiologic studies, discussed earlier, have demonstrated that increasing task difficulty resulted in increased reaction time and increased latency. Greater task difficulty for any subject is reflected in lowered performance scores and increased reaction time (Bahrick, 1979; Jenkins, 1979; Massaro, 1975).

If a child is having difficulty listening, remembering, and using the auditory information and is referred for CAP evaluation, the tasks required should reflect the difficult demands of the client's home and classroom. To assess CAP performance, we should evaluate children with simple tasks and with progressively more complex tasks. It is important to observe if, when, and how a child begins to break down in CAP as the task requirements become more difficult for the child. Examples of specific evaluation and remedial techniques are presented in Chapter 13 of this volume.

FACTORS WITHIN THE INDIVIDUAL THAT AFFECT CAP

What characteristics or abilities may affect how the individual processes an auditory signal? What does the child bring to the task of listening and comprehending auditory information? As Jenkins (1979) has argued, everyone knows that a person's skills, abilities, knowledge, intentions, and motivations affect performance. This section briefly summarizes some of these variables that have specific relevance for CAP.

Linguistic Competence

Through exposure to the speech signal and interaction with caregivers in the environment, the child acquires some degree of competence in comprehending and producing language. Obviously the level of competence affects what the child is able to extract from the auditory information.

Meaningfulness and Familiarity of the Linguistic Signal

Meaningfulness and familiarity of words, sentences, or prose passages influence whether and how easily one perceives and comprehends them. Familiar words are learned, perceived, guessed, or read faster, with less attention and effort, and more accurately than unfamiliar words (Kintsch, 1977; Sanders, 1977). Comprehension of stories and retention of narrative material are significantly better when more familiar rather than less familiar words are used (Chapandy & Lasky, 1981; Marks, Doctorow, & Wittrock, 1974). We all know from experience and from our work how difficult it is to process and attend to meaningless or unfamiliar stimuli (Lasky, Jay, & Hanz-Ehrman, 1975).

Expectations

It was argued that a listener's perception of a message is in part dependent on sounds heard and in part self-generated from linguistic, contextual, and situational expectancies. Expectations can preset attention and improve efficiency and processing time (Keele & Neill, 1978). If the message content or situation does not fit what is expected, we may process the information inefficiently, if at all. If a child does not use an expectation set, he or she may be unsure of what to do and may demonstrate confusion.

Sociolinguistic Knowledge and Communicative Competence

A child is exposed to various verbal and nonverbal interaction patterns dependent upon family and cultural background. *What* a child hears and comprehends is influenced by his or her linguistic competence, by what has occurred in similar situations, what the child has learned to expect, his frames (vanDijk, 1977), and his schemata (Rumelhart & Ortony, 1977). An infant or a toddler is not expected to comprehend and respond to all that is said. No one says to the 5-year-old, "From now on you must listen, attend, understand, and remember everything that is said to you." This is the behavior required in school, but like other sociolinguistic rules this rule is rarely, if ever, explicitly stated (Cook-Gumperz, 1975). In schools one sees children who seem oblivious to their ambience, unaware of what their teachers expect them to be doing, and unaware of the sociolinguistic rules of the classroom.

Motivation, Interests, and Intentions

A listener's motivational state, interests, and intentions regulate and direct activity and attention (Weiner, 1976). Tasks tied to real-life interests produce greater effort and comprehension; intent to learn produces greater learning (Nuttin, 1976). Does the child comprehend any presentation adequately to become interested and motivated? Perhaps tasks should be selected that are intrinsically motivating and performance compared on these with that on standardized materials. Does the child function, attend, and remember better if the auditory signal contains names of sports figures or cartoon characters or classmates?

Some of the more common parameters have been discussed. Myriad other variables could be added, including use of strategies such as verbal mediation, rehearsal, knowing what is known, understanding questions, narrative organization, and making inferences (see Lasky & Cox, Chapter 13, this volume). The goal of this section is to urge professionals to observe and understand the relevance of such variables as linguistic and sociolinguistic competence, expectations, interests, and motivation as they affect the child and his or her listening strategies.

CONCLUSIONS

This chapter has presented various dimensions involved in the processing of auditory information. No attempt was made to separate CAP from linguistic or cognitive processing, because the child with problems in CAP often has difficulty when he or she must attend, comprehend, manipulate, interpret, and remember auditorily presented linguistic signals, generally in cognitive tasks. The processes of perception, comprehension, learning, and memory are essentially similar, interactive, and difficult to separate (Bransford et al., 1977; Jacoby & Craik, 1979). Audiologists, speech-language pathologists, and other professionals must observe how the child responds to linguistic auditory signals of increasing difficulty under conditions that make greater and greater demands and in environments in which the processing tasks may be difficult for the child. The next few chapters demonstrate more of the complexities involved in CAP, how evaluation has been traditionally approached by the audiologist, by the speech-language pathologist, and by the educator, and what are some different approaches being suggested.

REFERENCES

Bahrick, H. 1979. Broader methods and narrower theories for memory research: Comments on the papers by Eysenck and Cermak. In: L. Cermak and F. Craik (eds.), Levels of Processing in Human Memory, pp. 141–158. Lawrence Erlbaum Associates, Hillsdale, N.J.

Barr, D. F. 1976. Auditory Perceptual Disorders. Charles C Thomas, Springfield, Illinois.

Bauer, R. H. 1977. Memory processes in children with learning disabilities: Evidence of deficient rehearsal. Journal of Experimental Child Psychology 3:415–430.

Bloom, B. S. (ed.). 1956. Taxonomy of Educational Objectives Handbook I: Cognitive Domain. David McKay, New York.

Bransford, J. D., and Johnson, M. K. 1972. Contextual prerequisites for understanding: Some investigations of comprehension and recall. Journal of Verbal Learning and Verbal Behavior 11:717–726.

Bransford, J. D., and Johnson, M. K. 1973. Considerations of some problems of comprehension. In: W. G. Chase (ed.), Visual Information Processing, pp. 383–438. Academic Press, New York.

Bransford, J. D., McCarrell, N. S., Franks, J. J., and Nitsch, K. E. 1977. Toward unexplaining memory. In: R. Shaw and J. Bransford (eds.), Perceiving, Acting, and Knowing, pp. 431–466. Lawrence Erlbaum Associates, Hillsdale, N.J.

Brown, J. 1976. An analysis of recognition and recall and of problems in their comparison. In: J. Brown (ed.), Recall and Recognition, pp. 1–36. John Wiley & Sons, New York.

Carhart, R., Tillman, T. W., and Greetis, E. S. 1969. Perceptual masking in multiple sound backgrounds. Journal of the Acoustical Society of America 45:694–703.

Carrow, E. 1973. Test for Auditory Comprehension of Language. Learning Concepts, Austin, Tx.

Chapandy, A., and Lasky, E. 1981. The effect of word familiarity on children's comprehension and memory. Ohio Journal of Speech and Hearing 15:1–11.

Clark, E. V. 1973. What's in a word? On the child's acquisition of semantics of his first language. In: T. E. Moore (ed.), Cognitive Development and the Acquisition of Language, pp. 65–110. Academic Press, New York.

Cole, R. A., and Jakimik, J. 1980. A model of speech perception. In: R. A. Cole (ed.), Perception and Production of Fluent Speech, pp. 133–164. Lawrence Erlbaum Associates, Hillsdale, N.J.

Cook-Gumperz, J. 1975. The child as a practical reasoner. In: M. Sanches and B. G. Blount (eds.), Language, Thought, and Culture, pp. 137–162. Academic Press, New York.

Cutting, J. W., and Pisoni, D. B. 1978. An information processing approach to speech perception. In: J. F. Kavanagh and W. Strange (eds.), Speech and Language in the Laboratory, School, and Clinic, pp. 38–72. MIT Press, Cambridge, Mass.

Davis, R., Sutherland, N. S., and Judd, B. R. 1961. Information content in recognition and recall. Journal of Experimental Psychology 61:422–429.

Donchin, E., and McCarthy, G. 1979. Event-related brain potentials in the study of cognitive processes. In: C. L. Ludlow and M. E. Doran-Quine (eds.), The Neurological Bases of Language Disorders in Children: Methods and Directions for Research, pp. 109–128. NINCDS Monograph No. 22. National Institutes of Health, Bethesda, Md.

Eimas, P. D. 1979. On the processing of speech: Some implications for language development. In: C. L. Ludlow and M. E. Doran-Quine (eds.), The Neurological Bases of Language Disorders in Children: Methods and Directions for Research, pp. 159–171. NINCDS Monograph No. 22. National Institutes of Health, Bethesda, Md.

Forgus, R. H., and Melamed, L. E. 1976. Perception: A Cognitive-State Approach. McGraw-Hill, New York.

Foss, D. J., and Hakes, D. T. 1978. Psycholinguistics: An Introduction to the Psychology of Language. Prentice-Hall, Englewood Cliffs, N.J.

Freund, A. 1975. Word and phrase recognition in speech processing. In: D. W. Massaro (ed.), Understanding Language: An Information-Processing Analysis of Speech Perception, Reading, and Psycholinguistics, pp. 357–389. Academic Press, New York.

Gagné, R. M., and White, R. T. 1978. Memory structures and learning outcomes. Review of Educational Research 28:187–222.

Gough, P. B. 1965. Grammatical transformations and speed of understanding. Journal of Verbal Learning and Verbal Behavior 4:107–111.

Hagen, J. 1979. Development and models of memory: Comments on the papers by Brown and Naus and Halasz. In: L. Cermak and F. Craik (eds.), Levels of Processing in Human Memory, pp. 289–300. Lawrence Erlbaum Associates, Hillsdale, N.J.

Haynes, W. O., and McCallion, M. B. 1981. Language comprehension testing: The influence of three modes of test administration and cognitive tempo on the performance of preschool children. Language, Speech and Hearing Services in Schools 12:74–81.

Helliage, J. B. 1975. The role of generated abstract memory. In: D. W. Massaro (ed.), Understanding Language: An Information-Processing Analysis of

Speech Perception, Reading, and Psycholinguistics, pp. 391–424. Academic Press, New York.

Hogan, D. D., and Hanley, T. D. 1963. Some effects on listener accuracy of competing messages varied systematically in number rate and level. Journal of the Acoustical Society of America 35:293–295.

Jacobs, R. A., and Rosenbaum, P. S. 1968. English Transformational Grammar. Xerox College Publishing, Waltham, Mass.

Jacoby, L., and Craik, F. 1979. Effects of elaboration of processing at encoding and retrieval: Trace distinctiveness and recovery of initial context. In: L. Cermak and F. Craik (eds.), Levels of Processing in Human Memory, pp. 1–22. Lawrence Erlbaum Associates, Hillsdale, N.J.

Jenkins, J. J. 1979. Four points to remember: A tetrahedral model of memory experiments. In: L. Cermak and F. Craik (eds.), Levels of Processing in Human Memory, pp. 429–446. Lawrence Erlbaum Associates, Hillsdale, N.J.

Keele, S., and Neill, W. 1978. Mechanisms of attention. In: E. C. Carterette and M. P. Friedman (eds.), Handbook of Perception, V. IX Perceptual Processing, pp. 3–47. Academic Press, New York.

Kintsch, W. 1977. Memory and Cognition. John Wiley & Sons, New York.

Kintsch, W. 1979. Levels of processing language material: Discussion of the papers by Lachman and Lachman and Perfetti. In: L. Cermak and F. Craik (eds.), Levels of Processing in Human Memory, pp. 211–222. Lawrence Erlbaum Associates, Hillsdale, N.J.

Lasky, E. Z., and Chapandy, A. M. 1976. Factors affecting language comprehension. Language, Speech, and Hearing Services in Schools 7:159–168.

Lasky, E. Z., Jay, B., and Hanz-Ehrman, M. 1975. Meaningful and linguistic variables in auditory processing. Journal of Learning Disabilities 8(9):570–577.

Lasky, E. Z., and Tobin, H. 1973. Linguistic and non-linguistic competing message effects. Journal of Learning Disabilities 6:243–250.

Lasky, E., Weidner, W., and Johnson, J. 1976. Influence of linguistic complexity, rate of presentation, and interphrase pause time on auditory verbal comprehension of adult aphasic patients. Brain and Language 3:386–395.

Liberman, I. Y., Shankweiler, D., Fischer, F. W., and Carter, B. 1974. Explicit syllable and phoneme segmentation in the young child. Journal of Experimental Psychology 18:201–212.

Lowe, A. D., and Campbell, R. A. 1965. Temporal discrimination in aphasoid and normal children. Journal of Speech and Hearing Research 8:313–314.

Marks, C. B., Doctorow, M. J., and Wittrock, M. C. 1974. Word frequency and reading comprehension. Journal of Educational Research 67:259–262.

Massaro, D. W. 1975. Experimental Psychology and Information Processing. Rand McNally, Chicago.

McCroskey, R. L., and Thompson, N. W. 1973. Comprehension of rate controlled speech by children with specific learning disabilities. Journal of Learning Disabilities 6:621–627.

McNeill, D., and Lindig, K. 1973. The perceptual reality of phonemes, syllables, words, and sentences. Journal of Verbal Learning and Verbal Behavior 12:419–430.

Miller, G. A. 1947. The masking of speech. Psychological Bulletin 44:105–129.

Miller, G. A. 1962. Some psychological studies of grammar. American Psychologist 17:748–762.

Moates, D. R., and Schumacher, G. M. 1980. An Introduction to Cognitive Psychology. Wadsworth, Belmont, Calif.

Neisser, U. 1967. Cognitive Psychology. Appleton-Century-Crofts, New York.

Nuttin, J. R. 1976. Motivation and reward. In: W. K. Estes (ed.), Handbook of Learning and Cognition Processes, Volume 3, Human Learning and Motivation, pp. 247–281. Lawrence Erlbaum Associates, Hillsdale, N.J.

Peck, D. J. 1977. The effects of presentation rates on the auditory comprehension of learning-disabled children. Paper presented at the Annual Convention of the American Speech-Language-Hearing Association, Chicago, Ill.

Rampp, D. L. 1980. Auditory Processing and Learning Disabilities. Cliff Notes, Lincoln, Nebr.

Rees, N. S. 1973. Auditory processing factors in language disorders: The view from Procrustes' bed. Journal of Speech and Hearing Disorders 38:304–315.

Rumelhart, D. E., and Ortony, A. 1977. The representation of knowledge in memory. In: R. C. Anderson, R. J. Spiro, and W. E. Montague (eds.), Schooling and the Acquisition of Knowledge, pp. 93–135. Lawrence Erlbaum Associates, Hillsdale, N.J.

Sanders, D. 1977. Auditory Perception of Speech. Prentice-Hall, Englewood Cliffs, N.J.

Satz, P., Rardin, D., and Ross, J. 1971. An evaluation of a theory of specific developmental dyslexia. Child Development 42:2001–2009.

Savin, H. B., and Perchonock, E. 1965. Grammatical structure and the immediate recall of English sentences. Journal of Verbal Learning and Verbal Behavior 4:348–353.

Shearme, J. N., and Holmes, J. N. 1962. An experimental study of the classification of sounds in continuous speech according to their distribution in the formant 1-formant 2 plane. In: A. Sovijarvi and P. Aalto (eds.), Proceedings of the Fourth International Congress of Phonetic Sciences, pp. 232–240. Mouton, The Hague.

Slobin, D. I. 1966. Grammatical transformations and sentence comprehension in childhood and adulthood. Journal of Verbal Learning and Verbal Behavior 5:219–227.

Squires, K. C. 1981. Auditory brainstem response and auditory processing, learning, and language disabilities. Paper presented at the Auditory Brainstem Response Testing Workshop, June 17–18. Cleveland, Ohio.

Squires, K. C., Chippendale, T. J., Wrege, K. S., Goodin, D. S., and Starr, A. 1980. Electrophysiologic assessment of mental function in aging and dementia. In: W. Poon (ed.), Aging in the 1980's: Psychological Issues, pp. 125–134. American Psychological Association, Washington, D.C.

Speaks, C., Karmen, J. L., and Benitez, L. 1967. Effects of a competing message on synthetic sentence identification. Journal of Speech and Hearing Research 10:390–395.

Stark, E., and Tallal, P. 1981. Selection of children with specific language deficits. Journal of Speech and Hearing Disorders 46:114–122.

Stevens, K. N. 1978. The speech signal. In: J. F. Kavanagh and W. Strange (eds.), Speech and Language in the Laboratory, School and Clinic, pp. 3–27. MIT Press, Cambridge, Mass.

Stevens, K. N., and House, A. S. 1972. Speech perception. In: J. Tobias (ed.), Foundations of Modern Auditory Theory, Volume 2, pp. 1–62. Academic Press, New York.

Tallal, P. 1978. Implications of speech perceptual research for clinical populations. In: J. F. Kavanagh and W. Strange (eds.), Speech and Language in the
Laboratory, School and Clinic, pp. 73–88. MIT Press, Cambridge, Mass.

Tallal, P., and Newcombe, F. 1978. Impairment of auditory perception and
language comprehension in dysphasia. Brain and Language 5:13–24.

Tallal, P., and Piercy, M. 1974. Developmental aphasia: Rate of auditory processing and selective impairment of consonant perception. Neuropsychologia
12:83–93.

Tower, D. B. 1979. Foreword. In: C. L. Ludlow and M. E. Doran-Quine (eds.),
The Neurological Bases of Language Disorders in Children: Methods and
Directions for Research. NINCDS Monograph No. 22. National Institutes of
Health, Bethesda, Md.

Treisman, A. M. 1964. Verbal cues, language, and meaning in selective attention. American Journal of Psychology 77:211.

vanDijk, T. A. 1977. Semantic macro-structure and knowledge frames in
discourse comprehension. In: M. A. Just and P. A. Carpenter (eds.), Cognitive
Processes in Comprehension, pp. 3–32. Lawrence Erlbaum Associates,
Hillsdale, N.J.

Webster, J. C., and Solomon, L. N. 1955. Effects of response complexity upon
listening to competing messages. Journal of the Acoustical Society of America 27:1199–1203.

Weidner, W., and Lasky, E. 1976. The interaction of rate and complexity of
stimulus on the performance of adult aphasic subjects. Brain and Language
3:34–40.

Weiner, B. 1976. Motivation from the cognitive perspective. In: W. K. Estes
(ed.), Handbook of Learning and Cognitive Processes, Volume 3, Human
Learning and Motivation, pp. 283–308. Lawrence Erlbaum Associates,
Hillsdale, N.J.

Willeford, J. A., and Billger, J. M. 1978. Auditory perception in children with
learning disabilities. In: J. Katz (ed.), Handbook of Clinical Audiology,
pp. 410–425. Williams & Wilkins, Baltimore.

Winer, B. J. 1962. Statistical Principles in Experimental Design. McGraw-Hill,
New York.

Zaidel, E. 1979. The split and half-brain as models of congenital language disability. In: C. L. Ludlow and M. E. Doran-Quine (eds.), The Neurological Bases
of Language Disorders in Children: Methods and Directions For Research.
NINCDS Monograph No. 22, pp. 55–89. National Institutes of Health,
Bethesda, Md.

Zurif, E., and Caramazza, A. 1978. Comprehension, memory, and levels of
representation: A perspective from aphasia. In: J. F. Kavanagh and
W. Strange (eds.), Speech and Language in the Laboratory, School and Clinic,
pp. 377–387. MIT Press, Cambridge, Mass.

Chapter **3**

Language and Auditory Processing

Top Down Plus Bottom Up

Judith F. Duchan and *Jack Katz*

Often children with speech and language or general learning problems have been found to have concomitant auditory processing problems (Lubert, 1981), for which they are frequently referred for auditory processing evaluations. The particular tests and procedures used for such evaluations depend upon the preferences of the diagnostician and upon the patterns of symptoms the child presents. The following case history of a child captures the general flavor of an auditory processing evaluation.

A 10-year-old girl named Chris was referred to an audiologist for a hearing evaluation and an assessment of auditory perception. The youngster was referred because of severe reading and spelling difficulties as well as an articulation impairment. The teacher had indicated that Chris might be having problems with hearing or possibly with auditory processing.

The child was tested and found to have normal pure tone thresholds and tympanograms, as well as good discrimination for monosyllabic words. (Of course, the presence of a fluctuating hearing problem cannot be ruled out as a contributory factor.) The evaluation of central auditory functions was simplified because of the evidence of normal peripheral hearing. The first processing test was phonemic synthesis, a sound-blending task in which each sound in a word is presented slowly, one at a time, and the child is asked to identify the word. Chris scored below the 5th percentile, when compared with her agemates.

The second auditory processing procedure was the Staggered Spondaic Word (SSW) Test. In this task four words are presented, two to each ear. The two middle words, which are in opposite ears, compete temporarily with one another. Chris' score for the competing condition in the right ear was 1 standard deviation above the mean for her age level (significantly depressed), and the left competing score was 2 standard deviations above the mean. She also demonstrated significant response biases: First, she had 10 reversals (correct response except that the words were out of sequence). This reversal pattern is often associated with spelling and reading problems as well as with poor organizational skills (Lucker, 1981). Second, she tended to make more errors on the last two monosyllabic words than on the first two. This primacy pattern is called an order effect L/H (Katz, 1978) and is associated with inefficient decoding, which causes a child to become overloaded when listening to long complex signals (Katz, Chapter 14, this volume).

In another procedure, word discrimination scores in a quiet environment were compared to the child's performance when words were mixed with noise. Each ear was assessed separately to see whether one or both of them might show reduced functions in a noisy environment. The signal-to-noise ratio was +5 dB (speech=40 dB sensation level [SL]; noise=35 dB SL). In the right ear the drop in accuracy was from 96% in quiet to 80% in noise, and in the left ear the reduction went from 92% to 66%. The deterioration in the left ear was more than 1 standard deviation below the mean and is therefore considered significant.

Finally, a masking level difference (MLD) test was administered at 500 Hz. In this test a tone is presented to each ear in phase in the presence of noise. The individual is retested with the tone to one ear shifted 180° out of phase. Normally, children improve by about 15 dB for the out-of-phase condition, whereas learning-disabled children show far less benefit (Sweetow & Reddell, 1978). On this test Chris showed an improvement of 12 dB, which is within normal limits.

In summary, Chris demonstrated significant difficulties on certain auditory processing tasks. These difficulties can be related to or underlie the specific problems that the child is having in learning and communication and suggest therapeutic and compensatory procedures to aid her. The auditory tests indicate: 1) difficulty with phonemic synthesis (which challenges a variety of basic auditory skills); 2) difficulty on the SSW (showing difficulty with competing messages, disorganization in handling auditory information, and an inefficient processing of the ends of items); and 3) difficulty in repeating speech in a background of noise.

Children such as the one described above are often referred to speech-language pathologists because of problems with spoken or written language. As with an auditory processing evaluation, the makeup of the speech and language assessment will depend on the individual clinician. The following is a sample evaluation of a 10½-year-old third-grader who has difficulty in reading and spelling. The language evaluation was carried out to determine whether her academic difficulties might stem from a language problem, and if so, to determine the nature of the language problem.

A sample of the child's conversation with the clinician was video-recorded, transcribed, and analyzed to determine her knowledge of phonology, syntax, and semantics, and her conversational competencies. Also included in the evaluation were a test of language comprehension and an analysis of her errors in reading a passage aloud from her school reader.

Results of the assessment revealed that the child distorted /l/ and /r/ after vowels, occasionally underarticulated or glottalized stop consonants in medial and final positions, and displayed weak syllable omissions in rapid speech (e.g., "tato" for "potato"). Her speech was unintelligible at times if her listener did not know the topic.

The child tended on occasion to omit articles, contractions, auxiliaries, and inflectional morphemes, making her speech sound infantile. She seldom used embedded clauses, although she imitated and understood them in isolated sentences. When she talked about topics not pertaining to what was currently going on, she lost the sense of topic in both her own and other's discourse. This was evidenced by topic shifts in her monologues and in her failure to continue with the topic of her conversational partner. She performed at 1 standard deviation below average on a formal test of language comprehension (Clinical Evaluation of Language Functions; Semel & Wiig, 1980), and her score reflected difficulties with semantics as well as with syntax.

The sample taken of her reading revealed a topic tracking problem. Her reading of passages that included familiar words was fluent and accurate, but when asked general questions about what she read she had difficulty recalling the overall themes. She was able to answer questions about specific details, however. When presented with nonsense words she was unable to sound them out.

Finally, a sample of her writing revealed a severe spelling problem in which she omitted consonants and syllables in longer words and omitted function words and word endings. Many of her grapheme substitutions were not phonetically related to the target (for example, p for r).

In conclusion, this child had a language disorder in at least three areas relating to and perhaps underlying her problems in reading and writing. It was recommended that she receive language therapy in these three areas of difficulty: 1) phonology problems on both the phonemic and syllabic levels; 2) problems with complex syntax in both comprehension and production; and 3) problems with keeping track of topics.

Although one might never tell from the above two case descriptions, they are of the same child. The differences in the reports reflect an ongoing dispute in our field, sometimes surfacing but often existing underground, which divides clinicians as well as researchers into two distinct camps. There are some who consider auditory processing important to language and other kinds of learning, and there are others who focus on the linguistic and cognitive aspects of language processing because they feel auditory processing is either nonexistent or unimportant.

Which of these views better describes the child? We present here an outline of both the auditory processing and language processing views and argue that neither covers all relevant aspects of the child's problems and that both are at least partially right. Consider an analogy between a poor tennis player and a child who has language or academic problems. The player may be poor because of lack of knowledge of the game, and yet be endowed with sufficient vision, strength, and coordination to be a good player. Alternatively, the player may have sufficient knowledge of the rules but be poor because of weakness in more peripheral abilities such as vision, eye-hand coordination, or strength. Of course, a player may have neither the conceptual knowledge nor the physical abilities to play tennis. It is very likely that there are interactional effects. A person who lacks conceptual knowledge of tennis is more likely to choose other activities and therefore fail to develop further the skills and strengths needed for playing tennis. Conversely, the person who has physical limitations for tennis is less likely to learn the rules of the game when other choices are available. Both of the above players will be more handicapped in playing tennis than the primary deficit would indicate.

Physical inability in tennis can be compared to signal processing inabilities in learning-disabled or language-disabled children. Lack of knowledge of the rules of tennis can be seen as paralleling language-disordered children's lack of linguistic knowledge or lack of knowledge about their world. Before we go into the details of our approach to the argument, however, let us elaborate the language processing and signal processing views, presenting separately the evidence for the importance of each and why they have seemed incompatible.

THE LANGUAGE PROCESSING VIEW

Language processing proponents contend that most information about language is in the mind of the listener, and that very little can be gleaned from the acoustic signal. It follows, then, that most language processing must be done using higher-level linguistic and cognitive knowledge, applying them to the fuzzy and uninformative acoustic signal. Chomsky used this argument to refute the behavioristic view that learning takes place by stimulus-response associations (Chomsky, 1959), and he and others postulated abstract structures to explain language comprehension and production (Chomsky, 1965; Fodor, Bever, & Garrett, 1974). The suggested paucity of information in the signal is used to argue for the role of abstract processing at the phonologic as well as the semantic and syntactic information levels. Essentially the view is that language processing involves a guessing game in which the listener uses knowledge of the language and the world to make informed guesses about the speaker's message. Let us detail the sorts of evidence that lead to this top-down view of processing.

If we examine the acoustic signal, we do not find evidence of discrete phonemes. That is, the wave form lacks features that always distinguish one phoneme from another (e.g., /t/ from /d/). Instead, each contains variations of acoustic patterns depending upon the phonetic contexts of the sounds. If we were to take the syllable as the basic unit, we would also find smearing from adjacent syllables and inconsistencies in acoustic parameters. This lack of acoustic invariance in the signal has led to the postulation of theoretical constructs such as feature detectors, whereby the linguistic processor can recode the signal by filtering and reorganizing the acoustic information into usable linguistic forms such as phonemes and syllables. Thus, even at the beginning levels of processing, the influence of higher-order language categories is felt.

One aspect of this signal recoding has been called categorical perception, because continuous signals are perceived as having clear and discrete boundaries. For example, a slight variation of the acoustic cue can create a disproportional jump in perception of /b/ and /p/ sounds when that change occurs at a category boundary of /p/ and /b/. If, however, the same degree of variation in the signal occurs within either the /p/ or the /b/ category, the change is hardly perceptible. These discontinuities in perception at phoneme boundaries occur even in infants, attesting to the very early existence of categorical perception and the top-down influence on their processing of linguistic stimuli.

Processing of the acoustic signals is also heavily influenced by the lexical and semantic knowledge of the perceiver. Familiar words are perceived faster and more accurately. Indeed, the features that come to be regarded as significant to the listeners are those which serve them in making meaning distinctions between similar sounding words. For example, /r/ and /l/ phonemes are perceived as different in English because words differ in meaning when /r/ changes to /l/. This meaning distinction between /r/ and /l/ is not made in Japanese, for example.

Listeners, when they misperceive unfamiliar words as familiar ones, and when they substitute expected sounds and words for unexpected ones, are unknowingly demonstrating to us how their higher-order knowledge influences their speech perception. The fact that higher-level processing is involved in the listener's determination of the semantics and syntax of larger language units has been less contested. That is, most agree that higher-order linguistic knowledge is used in processing phrase and sentence structure. What has not been appreciated is that this process is highly abstract and that listeners do not rely on acoustic cues or word ordering for processing. Sentences that may appear on the surface to be the same syntactically are analyzed differently by listeners (for example, "John is easy to please" versus "John is eager to please"), and sentences that seem to be very different on the surface are interpreted as the same (for example, "The ball was hit by the boy" versus "The boy hit the ball"). We do not simply read across a sentence as it is heard from left to right; rather, we perceive and interpret it hierarchically through our abstract knowledge. (For a review of the literature on this topic, see Fodor, Bever, & Garrett, 1974; and Clark & Clark, 1977). Nor can we rely solely on pauses and intonation in the acoustic signal to give us cues to the units that need processing.

Given this view that we understand and perceive language through our knowledge, we can see how it feels wrong to conceive of language processing as entailing auditory discrimination, auditory memory, and auditory sequencing skills. From this view, auditory discrimination is not an ability to learn the differences between acoustically similar sound pairs, but rather it is seen as the ability to apply the correct feature detection devices to the opaque and varying cues in the signal. It is an identification problem, not one of discrimination. From this language framework, both immediate and long-term memory are not unstructured, but organized linguistically and cognitively. We remember and process what we understand and find pertinent, not what our memories can span. Finally, it is felt that the notion of auditory sequencing incorrectly assumes a left-to-right processing sequence, ignoring the abstract and hierarchical requirements of language processing skills. Because auditory processing tasks involve higher-order knowledge, it is not surprising to find studies showing a high correlation between performance on such tasks and language knowledge. Those correlations are not taken as evidence that children with language processing problems have poor auditory processing capabilities; rather, they show that the same higher-order knowledges are required for both.

THE AUDITORY PROCESSING VIEW

We who subscribe to the bottom-up view agree that it would be difficult to explain the speed and efficiency of auditory processing if we had to deal with each sound individually as if they were beads strung together. The structure of language helps us to listen and understand without having to scrutinize each sound or each word. We are able to listen more effectively by knowing where certain information is contained in the message, and by anticipating from our language and worldly knowledge what will be said. In these senses we have no argument with the language processing proponents.

What is less acceptable is the suggestion that listening is limited to these top-down modes, with little emphasis on the acoustic signal and on auditory analysis of it. The following discussion rests on logical arguments designed to show that, under certain circumstances, information from the acoustic signal must be processed through several steps and in several ways before it becomes influenced by higher-level knowledge. These arguments emphasize the importance of processing the information contained in the acoustic signal prior to its linguistic interpretation. A second set of arguments is correlational in nature, showing that the incidence of auditory processing problems is high in children with language and learning problems, and that working with them on auditory processing tasks can result in improvement of some of their higher-order learning and cognitive skills.

Language processing advocates argue that words are identified by a synthetic process wherein the listener relies heavily on context, such as the situation or syntax, for the interpretation of the signal. However, words in sentences are frequently unpredictable—for example, a person's name. Common names such as Smith and Jones might require relatively little auditory processing before we are satisfied that we do indeed know the person's name, but how would we know a name such as Jolly Smiggers without a careful analysis of the individual speech sounds? Furthermore, if we ask a person a question, we might anticipate some range of reasonable responses, but we do not know specifically what the response is until we hear it. Even when the choices are narrowed down to a pair (yes/no, stop/start, Republican/Democrat), we must still hear the word and identify it on the basis of the acoustic information that we are given.

The top-down view states that phonemes are not easily observable when one examines the acoustic signal, and concludes that phoneme is not an entity identifiable from the signal. If this were true, how would we know that a person had a speech problem, and why would we care if the problem is not detectable to the listener? Our dependency on acoustic information is quite evident when we consider the difficulties with language processing experienced by the hearing impaired, who have less access to the acoustic signal. In addition, all of us have had problems in processing language in noisy environments, when the auditory signal cannot be distinguished readily from the background. There must be something in the affected signal, variable or not, that causes these communicative difficulties.

The language processing view also argues against a linear sense of phoneme perception. We agree that phonemes overlap, both acoustically and perceptually, but if we had no sense of one sound occurring in time before the next, why would we not perceptually confuse "past" with "pats," "ski" with "seek," or "kitchen" with "chicken"? Obviously our systems are capable of these linear distinctions, and we must be using our ordering skills in both our comprehension and production of language.

Further, if language and higher-order knowledge were all that was required to process speech, how could people process nonsense syllables that have minimal linguistic content? We find that even when we strip a situation of its context, as we do when we ask listeners to identify nonsense syllables as part of an audiologic or psychologic test battery, the listeners can identify these stimulus materials with great accuracy. What they cannot do as successfully is respond correctly when acoustic information is eliminated by being masked or when the signal is distorted by filtering or time alteration.

The existence of correct sound identification is necessary in the normal development of speech and language functions. After a period of reflexive babbling, children narrow their productions to the sounds of their own native language. They babble these sounds prior to comprehension of language and before they are able to produce the sounds in meaningful linguistic units (Oller et al., 1976). Those who use the categorical perception argument to invalidate auditory perception point out that even young children have well established acoustic boundaries for various phonemes. By the same token, if the advocates of strict language processing are to explain away the influence of auditory (bottom-up) learning, they must deal with why children raised in Japan develop the different phoneme boundaries appropriate to that sound system, whereas those raised in the United States have the appropriate categories for English. It seems undeniable that the auditory stimulation of the sounds around us contribute strongly to our phonemic conceptualization. Furthermore, even if we were to agree that normal children are born with categorical perception for consonants, it remains to be explained how and why children develop auditory processing difficulties. Some proponents of the top-down view minimize the results of auditory processing studies by suggesting that there are contaminating variables. They suggest that vocabulary, IQ, and the lack of the concept of same versus different invalidate the results or at least make them suspect. Such explanations do not take into account that auditory processing deficits could influence verbal IQ test performance and language just as surely as the reverse. Their argument does not explain why words that are well within the child's vocabulary should be erred on whereas others that are equally familiar (or unfamiliar) are not, depending on the acoustic conditions or the phonetically contrasted word. A child who does not have the requisite vocabulary or conceptual knowledge should perform at a chance level regardless of task difficulty.

Most of the above has been presented to counter the arguments put forth by those holding a rigid language processing position. In addition, it would be proper to indicate how the auditory processing approach is viable in its own right. It is based on research that has shown that children with language and learning problems often show a deficit in their ability to process auditory information. Most notable is the work of Paula Tallal and her colleagues (Tallal, 1980; Tallal et al., 1980), who have shown that children with language disabilities have a deficit in processing rapid transitions in both linguistic and nonlinguistic signals. What also makes the argument for the significance of auditory processing so persuasive is that children who receive auditory processing training improve in their speech production and academic performance (see, for example, Orton, 1937; Van Riper, 1963; Chall, Roswell, & Blumenthal, 1963; Katz & Burge, 1971; Katz, Chapter 14, this volume).

THE RESOLUTION

There are several ways that the theoretical discrepancies we have been describing can be resolved. Perhaps the easiest way is for the proponents of each theory to ignore one another or presume the other to be blatantly wrong. Thus, some language processing advocates say there is no such thing as signal processing of language separable from higher-order processing (Rees, 1975, 1981), and some auditory processing advocates consider language processing as building basically on processing skills (Katz & Illmer, 1972).

A second resolution for the theorists is to contend that the theories are the same—that the terms, when used in their common sense, are equivalent or at least parallel, and that the differences between the views were merely in the terms used by each. Thus, auditory comprehension equals language comprehension, auditory processing equals language processing, and auditory discrimination equals categorical perception. This does not appear to be the case, however. Those who use one set of terms do not mean the same things as those using the other.

Because of the confrontations and communications among proponents of both views, many people can now feel comfortable in combining the top-down and bottom-up approaches in their clinical work. A third position is exemplified by the work of Butler (Chapter 15, this volume) and others (Cromer, 1981; Wiig & Semel, 1976). For example, they might assume that a child has both auditory processing and language processing problems and therefore deal with each type of problem independently. They could concern themselves with the signal side with auditory training on figure-ground skills and then try to remediate the language and cognitive problems by concept teaching or working on syntax.

Although this third view is an advanced one at this time, we foresee that further developments will permit a greater fusing of the language processing and auditory processing approaches. At the present time these amalgamated methods have not been worked out; however, Lasky and Cox, Young (Chapter 8, this volume), and others are already developing synthesized approaches. This fourth view is different from the third in that it is not simply additive but rather interactive and includes the possibility of different kinds of top-down and bottom-up processing going on, depending on the task and the processor.

Some examples will serve to illustrate our synthetic conceptualization. Let us start with a description of tasks that are highly dependent upon signal information and minimally dependent upon higher-level knowledge for their execution. We will call them signal-focused tasks. It seems logical that the least linguistic processing is used for tasks for which we have the fewest expectations. This might occur in situations where speech signals are difficult to identify, unfamiliar, and/or non-meaningful. An example of signal-focused processing occurs when we hear speech that cannot at first be understood or even segmentalized and that is held in mind in signal form until it can be interpreted. Listeners in this circumstance might use a processing strategy of recycling the signal in its close-to-original form until it can be processed further. It is this rehearsal process that exemplifies signal-focused processing.

A second example of signal-focused processing is that involved in sensory imagery. Some autistic children seem, from their delayed echoes, to be capable of exact recall of intonational and segmental aspects of sentences without any apparent understanding. This indicates an unusual ability to maintain in long-term memory the signal aspects of what they hear. Eidetic or sensory imagery is, by definition, a recollection of the signal aspects of the original experience, including irrelevant detail.

Another set of tasks that can require heavy focus on signal processing and minimal focus on higher-order processing is immediate recall tasks. One can, of course, bring to bear higher-order processing in immediate recall. However, we are imagining tasks in which higher-order processing is minimized, as in a foreign language lesson containing sentence repetitions that are devoid of meaning for the language learner. This is likely to be the case for the beginner who gives back a rendition close to the target, yet one still outside his or her own linguistic or conceptual framework.

Finally, experimenters and clinicians who want to test auditory processing often design tasks that are signal-focused. The synthetic speech studies of Tallal and her colleagues (Tallal, 1980; Tallal et al., 1980), which carefully manipulate variables in the acoustic signal and minimize linguistic content, are signal-oriented tasks.

In sum, we suggest that there are real-life as well as experimentally induced tasks that require that children focus on the signal and need not depend heavily on higher-order conceptualizations for their execution. Of course, we have been emphasizing the extreme case in which the signal is the main source of information. Most tasks involve signal processing as well as higher-order processing. For example, to attend selectively, to recognize a phonetic sequence as a linguistic entity, to process nonsense syllables, to analyze words into sound elements, or to synthesize sounds into words, the listener will draw on varying amounts of linguistic and cognitive knowledge as well as knowledge gained from acoustic and perceptual cues.

What we imagine happening in most situations is a continual fluctuation between signal and cognitive or linguistic operations in the listener. The signal must be attended to more at the points in the event that are most unpredictable and least redundant. Thus, the signal contributes more than higher-order understanding when there is some doubt about what is being said. These signal-focused portions will occur intermittently when something is unexpected, when the signal is distorted, or when new information is being presented.

What about higher-order processing tasks that require minimal signal processing? The debate between top-down and bottom-up proponents has been mainly confined to the domain of language comprehension. In that domain, the role of linguistic knowledge is strongest when listeners use their pragmatic knowledge of narratives, conversations, or how events are ordinarily organized, and when they use their knowledge of linguistic forms. For example, highly ritualized aspects of our communication such as openings of conversations would allow listeners to predict what is said and thereby listen less carefully and perhaps less often to the signal. Familiar events would draw on higher-order processing more and signal processing less by virtue of their high degree of predictability.

We have discussed three levels of tasks, those involving speech that is essentially nonmeaningful and nonpredictable; those that are more meaningful and somewhat predictable; and those that are almost totally predictable. We see these as requiring differing degrees of signal and higher-order processing, as depicted graphically in Figure 1. The

Great   Minimum

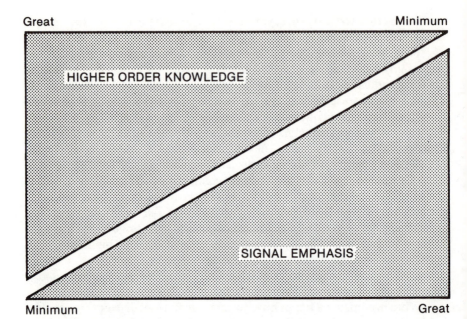

Minimum   Great

Figure 1.   Complementarity of levels of processing.

upper triangle in Figure 1 indicates relative amounts of higher-order
processing that can be brought to bear on a task. The tasks involving
the greatest amount of higher-order processing are represented at the
left of the triangle, those involving moderate amounts of higher-order
processing are depicted in the middle range, and those involving the
least are on the right. Similarly, the lower triangle portrays the amount
of signal processing brought to bear on the task, proceeding from minimal processing at the left to a maximum at the right. The triangles are
complementary in that the reliance on signal processing increases when
the listener cannot bring to bear higher-order knowledge and decreases
when higher-order knowledge is at a maximum. Thus, when presented
with highly predictable information, the listener would be processing
primarily at the left of the two triangles, with fluctuations toward more
signal reliance at points in the sentence that are less predictable.

There are different processing styles among normal listeners. Some
are more signal-oriented and others more dependent upon higher-order
knowledge. The signal emphasizers would more readily notice distortions in the signal, and would have vivid auditory imagery. Higher-
order emphasizers would pay less attention to the nuances in the signal
and instead rely more on their expectations for their processing. They
interpret distorted signals as if they were Rorschach inkblots, guessing

at what was said, whereas the signal emphasizers require more information from those acoustic blots before making their interpretations.

What then of the children with learning or communication disorders? Those who are forced to depend heavily on higher-order processes without sufficient signal processing might seem impulsive, respond in strange ways, or even seem hearing-impaired. Those who are primarily bottom-up processors, on the other hand, may miss the nuances conveyed from higher-order knowledge. They could appear to think concretely and have difficulty making higher-level abstractions.

Normal listeners differ so widely from one another that models can be used only as a general guide. Disordered children, even more than normal children, are likely to differ from one another, making a general model for them even less applicable. These children might require individual models of their overall approach to communication, taking into account their strengths, limitations, and preferences. These abilities might be sorted out by designing tasks in which the child must rely either on information provided in the signal or on higher-order knowledge, so that the responses will vary depending upon whether the child has a preference for top-down or bottom-up processing strategies.

To determine the disordered children's auditory and language competencies, tests can be used which emphasize the different aspects of processing. The results of traditional formal and informal tests can be used, such as the ones used for Chris at the beginning of this chapter. The less meaningful and relatively unpredictable messages which require limited linguistic background represent the signal-focused tasks (e.g., pure tone, speech amid noise, and phonemic synthesis). The SSW test is likely to require knowledge of yet a higher order. Finally, language tasks demand the greatest amount of higher-order processing. As it turned out, Chris did poorly on all levels, suggesting a multidimensional problem that involves higher-order knowledge as well as lower-order signal processing capabilities.

IMPLICATIONS

Recently, clinicians have begun to combine the strong and applicable features of both top-down and bottom-up approaches. The contents of this book attest to this new trend. A single specialist in speech, language, and hearing disorders seeking to help children with communication and academic disabilities must work out the pertinent information from two conflicting literatures. Although such specialists might be appropriately trained in the future, at present most programs are not geared to such a broad focus. The information provided below lists some short-term goals toward achieving a synthetic clinical approach. The clinician should:

1. Begin to think about academic and communication disorders as possibly resulting from signal as well as higher-order problems;
2. Assume an interdependence of signal and language processing skills in each individual;
3. Appreciate that certain tasks require more emphasis on one kind of processing than the other;
4. Assume that children have different approaches to communication tasks based on their unique constellation of abilities and disabilities;
5. Develop applicable remediation strategies to help children develop their top-down and/or bottom-up skills.

The long-term solution rests on researching the relationship between higher-order and signal-focused processing in both normal and abnormal groups. This information could then be applied in combined diagnostic and therapeutic approaches. The eventual application of this synthesis will be to train professionals who are able to carry out their clinical work from this perspective.

REFERENCES

Chall, J. S., Roswell, F. G., and Blumenthal, S. 1963. Auditory blending ability: A factor in success in early reading. Reading Teacher 17:113-120.
Chomsky, N. 1959. Review of Skinner's Verbal Behavior. Language 35:26-58.
Chomsky, N. 1965. Aspects of the Theory of Syntax. MIT Press, Cambridge, Mass.
Clark, H., and Clark, E. 1977. Psychology and Language. Harcourt Brace Jovanovich, New York.
Cromer, R. 1981. Reconceptualizing language acquisition and cognitive development. In: R. Schiefelbusch and D. Bricker (eds.), Early Language: Acquisition and Intervention. University Park Press, Baltimore.
Fodor, J., Bever, T., and Garrett, M. 1974. The Psychology of Language. McGraw-Hill, New York.
Katz, J. 1978. SSW Workshop Manual. Allentown Industries, Buffalo, N.Y.
Katz, J., and Burge, C. 1971. Auditory perception training for children with learning disabilities. Menorah Medical Journal 2:18-29.
Katz, J., and Illmer, R. 1972. Auditory perception in children with learning disabilities. In: J. Katz (ed.), Handbook of Clinical Audiology. Williams & Wilkins, Baltimore.
Lubert, N. 1981. Auditory perceptual impairments in children with specific language disorders: A review of the literature. Journal of Speech and Hearing Disorders 46:3-9.
Lucker, J. R. 1981. Interpreting SSW test results of learning disabled children. SSW Newsletter 3(May):1-3.

Oller, D., Wieman, L., Doyle, W., and Ross, C. 1976. Infant babbling and speech. Journal of Child Language 3:1–12.

Orton, S. T. 1937. Reading, Writing and Speech Problems in Children. Norton, New York.

Rees, N. 1975. Auditory processing factors in language disorders: The view from Procrustes' bed. Journal of Speech and Hearing Disorders 38:304–315.

Rees, N. 1981. Saying more than we know: Is auditory processing disorder a meaningful concept? In: R. Keith (ed.), Central Auditory and Language Disorders in Children. College Hill Press, Houston.

Semel, E. M., and Wiig, E. H. 1980. Clinical Evaluation of Language Functions. Charles E. Merrill, Columbus, Ohio.

Sweetow, R., and Reddell, R. 1978. Masking level differences for children with auditory perceptual problems. Journal of the American Auditory Society 4:52–56.

Tallal, P. 1980. Auditory processing disorders in children. In: P. Levinson and C. Sloan (eds.), Auditory Processing and Language. Grune & Stratton, New York.

Tallal, P., Stark, R., Kallman, C., and Mellits, D. 1980. Perceptual constancy for phonemic categories: A developmental study with normal and language impaired children. Applied Psycholinguistics 1:49–64.

Van Riper, C. 1963. Speech Correction: Principles and Methods. Prentice-Hall, Englewood Cliffs, N.J.

Wiig, E., and Semel, E. 1976. Language Disabilities in Children and Adolescents. Charles E. Merrill, Columbus, Ohio.

Section II

Physical and Physiologic Aspects of Central Auditory Processing

Chapter 4

Pediatric Aspects of Learning Disorders

Marcel Kinsbourne

WHAT TO EXPECT OF THE PEDIATRICIAN

When a child fails in school, a pediatrician is often consulted; the pediatrician may elect either to play a limited, strictly medical role, or to examine all relevant aspects of the child's development. Strictly medical concerns comprise:

1. Determining whether a medical illness (e.g., anemia, epilepsy, or brain degeneration) is simulating learning disorder;
2. Documenting abnormalities in the child's family and personal (especially prenatal and birth) history and in the physical (general and neurologic) examination that could be relevant to the problem (occasionally radiographic and electroencephalographic studies are done);
3. Managing those aspects of the child's program that involve medication;
4. Making a diagnosis (for purposes of third-party compensation or to put the child in contact with resources mandated by law).

A broader approach supplements these steps with:

5. Coordinating the crossdisciplinary assessment of the child's learning-related mental, physical, and emotional strengths and weaknesses;
6. Interpreting to and counseling the family and the child;
7. Procuring and maintaining the child's multimodal program.

When referring a child to a physician or clinic, one should specify what is wanted. A medical referral for a failing child is not a self-evident step; if all one learns from the physician is that there are signs of neurologic damage or dysfunction, one has not contributed to planning for the child. Impaired neurologic maturation is not irrelevant to children's learning; it must underlie all disabilities that are developmental. If such an impairment has occurred, its consequences are now irreversible; decisions must be based on the child's present condition, not its presumed origin—we cannot improve a child's nervous system. We can, however, offer symptomatic, supportive, and remedial help.

Any information that might assist in selecting among available treatment options is relevant. Any information that could not be put to such use in the present state of knowledge is at best tangential, usually irrelevant, and at worst detrimental and confusing.

Ruling Out Disease Simulating Learning Disability

One general guideline helps segregate the unusual case of a medical disease affecting intellect and conduct from the majority of learning-disabled children who are not sick: organic disease has a definable onset. If the child's school work or conduct at large suffers change, the possibility of progressive organic disease arises. The disease could be anemia, hypothyroidism, childhood depression, or a progressive brain-degenerative condition. When the condition has no definable onset or unexpected characteristic, simulation by disease is unlikely.

Family History A number of family histories have been documented in which dyslexia is frequently represented, particularly among males. Although the nature of the genetic transmission remains controversial, its participation *is* established. It is not clear, however, to what extent such inheritance contributes to the overall problem of selective reading and writing disability.

Hyperactivity in parents indicates a genetic risk of hyperactive offspring, as do what may be called the impulsive psychopathologies: sociopathy, alcoholism, and hysteria (Cantwell, 1978). Childhood psychopathologies are more prevalent in adopted than in natural children (Mesh, 1973). Hyperactivity is exceptionally prevalent among adoptees (Deutsch et al., 1982). It is unclear to what extent this finding is attributable to the following:

1. Teenage pregnancy, which in 1970 was associated with 88% of all nonrelative adoptions (U.S. Department of Health, Education and Welfare, 1972) and is often characterized by ill managed health care of the pregnant teenager;

2. Identification bias, or the possibility that adoptive parents have more stringent criteria for normality, and therefore bring minor behavioral deviations in their adopted children to notice;
3. Genetic transmission of the parents' impulsive temperament, perhaps connected with the unwanted pregnancy and the decision to give the child up.

Events During Pregnancy   Heavy smoking and drinking by the mother raise the risk of hyperactivity. The situation is confounded by the possibility that impulsive personality might be inheritable, and that smoking and drinking during pregnancy might be manifestations of impulsive behavior by the mother. Some offspring of drinking mothers show the "fetal alcohol syndrome," which, in addition to physical abnormalities, includes hyperactivity. Other prevalent problems, such as nutritional deficit or infection, may affect mental development adversely, but do seem to show a predilection for causing the *selective* defects that comprise learning disabilities.

Perinatal Events   The literature on long-term outcome of perinatal status is indefinite. Severe adverse perinatal events clearly raise the possibility of mental retardation. A large-scale attempt to relate these to minimal brain dysfunction (MBD) was unsuccessful in showing anything more than that low socioeconomic status is a major risk factor (Nichols & Chen, 1981).

Sex   There is a preponderance of males among attention-defective and learning-defective children. Differential treatment of boys and girls is partly responsible, because girls are more encouraged to conform, seek approval, and act prosocially. Where inadequacies of attention and learning are not severe, the problems in boys might result from developmental immaturity.

If one measures the variable incidence of behaviors relevant to attention-defective deficit (ADD) among normal children, one generally finds that girls are cited as less hyperactive, impulsive, and inattentive than boys at a given age (Swanson, Logan, & Pelham, 1982). Girls at a given age seem more advanced in developing skills presumably prerequisite to learning to read; notable among these is verbal fluency (McGuinness, 1976). If learning disability reflects the lower end of a continuum of variation, then boys would be represented in greater numbers than girls below some point near the lower end of the continuum. If, however, learning disability is conceived as more related to adverse events, such as perinatal trauma (Towbin, 1971) and postmaturity (Field et al., 1977), then the generally greater incidence of adverse pregnancy and birth-related circumstances for boys is an explanation for the sex differential.

The Neurologic Examination   The purpose of the neurologic examination is to make inferences about various aspects of nervous system
function. This is accomplished by:

1. Making inferences from the configuration of bodily parts (e.g.,
   asymmetry of skull or limbs);
2. Observing spontaneously assumed postures and movements;
3. Eliciting response to stimulation (i.e.,verbal and motoric);
4. Eliciting movements by command.

Each observation is notated against age-related expectation and classified as within or outside the normal range. The outcome can be:

1. Within the normal range for the child's age;
2. Normal for a younger child; or
3. Abnormal at any age.

Outcomes 2 and 3 are called soft signs and hard signs, respectively.
Hard signs may be severe or mild (Denckla, 1977), but in either case
represent damage to a "hardwired" area of the nervous system; therefore, there is little variation upon later development. In contrast,
damage to relatively unspecified areas may permit substantial compensation by other parts of the brain, and damage to areas not yet specified
leads to delay in their assumption of control over behavior and perhaps
a lower endpoint of efficiency.

The areas of brain responsible for cognitive functions, such as
those involved in school performance, are relatively softwired. The
neurologist will not expect to find hard signs of damage, except coinci-
dentally. Indeed, if the adverse influence is restricted to brain areas
involved in cognition, then neither hard nor soft sensorimotor signs will
be found. An extended neuropsychologic examination will reveal cognitive soft signs, indicating immaturity of particular mental operations.
Were the patient younger, such findings would be normal.

If the noxious influence overlapped areas of motor control, motor
soft signs, such as persistence of primitive reflexes, synergisms, and
associated movements, would accompany the cognitive immaturity.
As a modicum of motor control is necessary for reading and writing,
such deficits will contribute to the educational problem. Impaired eye-
hand coordination and a clumsy grip of the pen will cause illegible
script; clumsy scanning movements of the eyes, characterized according to Pavlides (1981) by an excess of regressive eye movements, will
hamper the fluent succession of fixation and saccade that characterizes
skilled reading. Clumsy articulation complicates the task of reading
aloud. In dyslexia, however, difficulties occur even with the reading of
single letters and words (where eye movements are not needed) and in
spelling orally, as well as in writing. We cannot, therefore, accept the

proposal of Mattis, French, and Rapin (1975) that articulation and graphomotor problems should be classified as a subtype of dyslexia. Such difficulties are admissible under the wider umbrella of MBD, as is a subset of children who have difficulties of retention or of processing, as described by Kinsbourne and Caplan (1979) and later in this discussion.

Compensation for damage to brain areas that subserve higher mental functions can be spectacular, if the damage is sustained early enough, and if the area in question is completely eliminated. Thus, total loss of the left hemisphere before age 1 year may be followed by a normal developmental sequence of language skills culminating in language ability well within normal range. Yet if hemispherectomy is done later or if the language area is only partly eliminated, substantial language delays may occur. The outcome seems to depend on the extent to which equipotential areas in the right hemisphere take over. After left hemisphere loss, full brainstem facilitation for verbal activity can be channeled to the right side. If however, the left hemisphere remains, although damaged (Annett, Lee, & Ounstead, 1961) or disconnected from the right (Zaidel, 1977), the right hemisphere does not have full benefit of that activation (Kinsbourne, 1981). Its pattern of functioning is suggestive of an underactivated part of the brain, able to perform automatically but not to abstract information or decontextualize its processing when under the influence of salient percepts (Zaidel, 1977).

There is evidence that the left hemisphere of right-handed individuals is predestined even before birth for the future verbal role (Kinsbourne, 1981). In spite of the supportive anatomical asymmetries between the hemispheres at birth (Witelson & Pallie, 1973; Wada, Clark, & Hamm, 1975), there is no evidence that the left hemisphere is solely hardwired for language. Attempts to prove that the isolated right hemisphere is less capable than the left with respect to certain syntactical and phonologic tasks (Dennis, 1977; Bishop, 1982), prove the reverse. Some patients who are verbally based in the right hemisphere function as well as patients with residual left hemispheres.

Zaidel (1977) has claimed that children with selective language/ reading problems should be considered to be using right hemisphere language. We accept this proposal, amended to read: Children with selective language/reading delays may have a deficit in fully addressing whichever hemisphere is responsible for language. This would explain why such children often do not manifest the expected right-side advantage for verbal materials in dichotic and visual half-field paradigms. Perceptual asymmetry indicates the uneven distribution of activation between the hemispheres (Kinsbourne, 1970). Its absence may be due to engagement of both hemispheres, or of neither. Diminished asymmetry cannot be directly related to deficient reading skill, because females show less asymmetry yet seem better in language and reading tasks than males.

Left-handedness and ambidexterity have long been suspected of a causal relationship with a variety of developmental deficits. Although genetically the system may favor right-handedness, the left-handed individual does not seem to incur any deficit in performance, even if he or she is "ill lateralized" cognitively. The left-handedness may be pathologic (Satz, 1972), caused by shift from dextral genotype to sinistral phenotype by early damage, presumably to the left motor strip. Early damage could also produce consequences along a variety of parameters of mental development.

In summary, the neurologic examination and the neurophysiologic examination for laterality relationships may uncover qualitative nervous system deficit, quantitative nervous system immaturity, or no abnormality. Qualitative deficits may be unrelated to the learning problem. Quantitative immaturities suggest, but do not prove, that the academic problem is based on a similar delay in neurologic maturation. Normality may merely indicate a cognitive deficit so restricted that it does not manifest itself through impaired performance on neurologic and laterality testing. The positive findings on examination yield only circumstantial evidence for the organic (developmental) nature of the child's problem, and negative findings justify no conclusion.

Findings from the history and examination may fuel speculation about whether the disorder is due to unfavorable genetic programming or to damage to the brain. Even if such an etiology could be established, it would serve no useful purpose. The disability is best defined by meticulous delineation of what the child can and cannot do, and how this affects the outcome of the child's efforts to achieve and to relate to others. It is on such information that treatment, including medical treatment, is based, not on presumed pathogenesis.

Choice and Management of Medication

Hyperactive behavior is properly viewed as diverging from normal behavior in degree, not in kind. The effect of stimulant drugs is to shift the child's attentional abilities toward the middle of the normal range. This symptomatic treatment relies on the brain's latent capability. The child's own behavioral control mechanisms become available for purposes of problem solving and sustained endeavor. It follows that stimulant medication must:

1. *Be given to the right child.* Not all impulsive and inattentive behavior is due to underactivated behavioral control mechanisms that will respond to drugs.

2. *Be given in the right amount.* An overdose will impair attention; however, the optimal dosage range is very wide.

3. *Be given to secure the closest approximation to continuous coverage.* By using medium-acting (8-hour) rather than short-acting (4-hour) stimulants, "drug holidays" can be avoided. This obviates baffling swings in personality and mood, and probably also helps minimize the state dependence of learning (Swanson & Kinsbourne, 1976).

4. *Be given as long as needed.* Medication should be administered as long as there is observable benefit rather than according to some arbitrarily chosen age limit. One safety factor inherent in the use of stimulant drugs is their brief action, so that one can observe and make judgements about any child on and off drugs every day of treatment. There is a remarkable lack of known long-term hazards associated with stimulant therapy.

Diagnosis

Differentiating the individual needs of learning-disabled children is essential to individualizing their educational programs. For this purpose, it is often possible to dispense altogether with diagnostic labels. Labels, however, are often necessary to meet the requirements of third parties involved in compensation. Diagnostic labeling must also be used with care to meet the stipulations of Public Law 94-142 and other legislation.

LEGISLATED EDUCATIONAL
PROVISIONS FOR THE SPECIAL NEEDS CHILD

Under Public Law 94-142, and laws passed by the states that go further, each local school system is mandated to provide for every child with special needs, including learning-disabled children, an appropriate individual education plan (IEP) that it can implement in the least restrictive setting possible. If the school system lacks the services called for in an individual case, it can pool resources with other systems or contract out to a private agency.

Many parents now dispute the IEPs planned for their children, claiming them to be inappropriate, not implementable, or both. It is the parents' legal right to reject any such IEP. The parents can then attempt to compel the system to support their child in another school that the parents feel is better able to meet the child's needs. Neurologists are increasingly asked to examine the child and testify for the parents, or to examine the records, interview school personnel, and testify for the school system. At this time the gulf between the medically based diagnostic process and the educational provisions that presumably follow is apt to become embarrassingly apparent.

The diagnosis of some such entity as dyslexia or hyperactivity, however valid, is rarely sufficient to enable one to specify in the required detail the IEP that would best suit the child. No one educational program is generally accepted as best for children of a given diagnosis. Instead, the physician should be prepared to delineate the child's specific needs, with reasons for each conclusion, and to match up the IEP's provisions against that inventory:

1. Does the IEP provide for, and can the school system deliver, individualized instruction at the child's actual achievement level?
2. Is the instructor familiar enough with selective academic problems to be able to choose intelligently among different approaches, rather than automatically implementing one unvarying program for all such children?
3. Does the IEP include provision for controlling any conduct or attitudinal disorder the child has and for safeguarding each child against disruptive behavior by any other?
4. Can the child still benefit from his or her location in a regular school by being mainstreamed in subjects outside the problem area?
5. Is there sufficient communication among teachers to ensure that each is kept apprised of the child's level of achievement, and can teaching be tailored to use the child's strengths and avoid humiliating the child?
6. Is ancillary therapy (speech, physical, or occupational) available as needed?
7. Is counseling available to support the child's self-respect and morale during his or her intense efforts to adapt, especially in the face of derogation by peers?

If the answers to these questions are affirmative, then usually no case exists for moving the child to a private school, as a private school is unquestionably a more restrictive setting in the sense of the legislation. If one or more of these ingredients cannot be provided in a public school but can be provided in a private school, then it is necessary to use judgment in balancing the educational advantage of a move against the drawback of a more restrictive setting.

In order to give a valid opinion a physician will usually need to show familiarity with educational resources (from interview or from the record) as well as with the child and the family. Above all, the physician must be thoroughly conversant with the details of the rejected IEP.

WHY A CHILD MIGHT FAIL TO LEARN

If a child fails to learn or does not behave normally in the classroom, and other reasons have been ruled out, then the child may be constitutionally different from his or her peers. A medically based defect approach postulates an underlying maldevelopment and consequent malfunction of the child's nervous system. A normative approach views the deviance as an instance, perhaps extreme, of individual difference.

Although the defect model and the difference model are alternative interpretations of reading problems, logically they can coexist. Some children might be selectively retarded in the maturation of certain school readiness skills for genetic reasons, and others due to early brain damage. Indeed, both conditions might occur in the same child. Biologic variation dictates that some children will be relatively immature with regard to any stated attribute. There is no limit (along a Gaussian function) to the degree of such relative immaturity; one can say only that the greater the discrepancy, the more rarely will it appear. When faced with an individual child, one cannot tell how rare his or her predicament is. With respect to early brain damage, a similar logic holds. Early brain damage occurs, and readiness skills cannot be invulnerable to such early damage. Of course, early damage may involve additional functions. When additional signs of brain involvement are found, the probability that an academic problem has similar antecedents is increased. The absence of such signs would make genetic diversity a more likely explanation; however, lesions can be highly selective. Brain damage unrelated to an academic problem can clearly coincide with an academic problem based on individual difference arising from genetic diversity. One cannot be certain about the origin of a problem in an individual without some objective correlate. In adult neuropsychology, two sources of help exist. One is the premorbid background of verifiable competence against which the deficit arises. The other is, usually, a demonstrable and even localizable area of brain malfunction. In the developmental case, the former help is absent, and demonstrating an area of brain dysfunction may not resolve the issue, unless there are hallmarks of qualitative abnormality (i.e., a "hard sign," such as a focus of paroxysmal discharge in the electroencephalogram). Our knowledge of electroencephalography is sufficiently incomplete to render areas of electrical "abnormalities" ambiguous with respect to either immaturity or damage. Further, there is no reason why an area of damage in the brain should not at times exist in someone whose academic problems are the consequence of an extreme of normal variation. Of course, if one could demonstrate and verify neuropathologically a stable pattern of impairment in a reading-relevant part of the brain in a sufficient sample of dyslexics, this would go far to clarify the neuropsychologic status of the disability. Efforts to date in this direction (Galaburda et al., 1978) are inconclusive.

Implicit in these contrasting perspectives are differences in the action one might choose to take. The defect model might lead to a fruitless search for a way to correct the defect—to change the brain. The difference model accepts the physiologic status quo and channels the effort toward correcting a maladaptive interaction between the child and the instructional situation. This can be achieved by a multimodal program that at times includes pharmacologic measures. Insofar as stimulant drugs help hyperactive children maintain the task-directed focus of attention, and to the extent that certain diets do so as well, brain function is improved, but the improvement lasts only as long as the treatment is continued, and the brain is not changed. In practice, however, to be effective all approaches converge on an IEP with adjunct symptomatic measures (medical, nutritional, behavioral). This program is not affected by speculations about whether the learning problem was due to genetic or brain damage factors, because the effects of these two causes on learning and attention are indistinguishable. If a brain territory is damaged early enough, the effect is simply a delay in onset and a slowed rate of acquisition of the mental ability in question, just as occurs in the genetic case. Insofar as the ability develops at all, it pursues the same developmental sequence as in intact children, although it takes longer. Knowing the origin of the difficulty does not help predict its outcome. A learning disability clearly associated with structural damage of the brain does not necessarily carry a worse prognosis than one in an apparently undamaged child. In sum, although tracing back a learning disability to its origin is of obvious research interest, in the present state of knowledge, doing this contributes nothing to the issue of prognosticating or developing treatment.

The converging effect of various factors can limit brain development and render the child selectively immature. The child uses the affected cognitive processes as would a younger normal child. This does not imply that the delay will vanish and the child will catch up to close the gap between himself or herself and unaffected peers. This may happen, or the child's development may reach a plateau at a lower level than normal. There is no known way of telling which of these will occur. The delay model does, however, help demystify the nature of the block to learning. If one tries prematurely to teach young children academic skills in a formal manner, learning disability signs will appear. Teaching a learning-disordered child correctly is like teaching a younger normal child material that the child is too young to master, at least when taught in the usual group setting in the classroom.

The delay model seems also to apply to ADD, but to a more limited extent. The lack of inhibitory control, the emotional lability, and the immature behavior do suggest a normally developing younger child, and many of these children prefer games appropriate to a younger age and the company of younger children. Young children, like ADD children, tend to act out their intentions and feelings in physical movement, rather than confine them in their minds. ADD children tend to be "sensation seekers" (Zuckerman et al., 1964), and sensation seeking is thought to vary with age. One cannot, however, assert that young children are impulsive in general or that they lack ability to concentrate. Possibly the ADD temperament represents the continuation of a particular temperamental variant identified in infants, namely, the "approach" type (Thomas et al., 1963).

More fundamentally, ADD children cannot be regarded as inexorably maturationally delayed like those children who are slow to progress through one or more developmental sequences. In favorable cases, a single dose of a psychostimulant can render the child's behavior essentially age-appropriate. If a relatively simple pharmacologic maneuver can do this, one must regard the ADD child as in a state of latent maturity, with overt maturity masked by some chemical (neurotransmitter?) imbalance, often correctable. Whether that imbalance can be aggravated, or even generated, by synthetic additives to the diet is currently being debated (Weiss, 1982).

SUBTYPES OF SELECTIVE READING DISABILITY

If there were an adequate validated model of reading acquisition, it would doubtless comprise numerous different component processes. Each process is the product of maturation along some developmental sequence. If one were able to measure each process in isolation, one could deduce from the resulting profile of component efficiency which process is the most immature and therefore most responsible for holding up reading progress. If we had such direct information, there would for practical purposes be little further to learn from the psychometric and neuropsychologic testing used today, but in fact we are nowhere near having such a model. Given this lack of basic information, it has been found useful to subdivide arbitrarily the prerequisites of reading into several components having face validity. We have gathered some normative information (Kinsbourne, 1976) and demonstrated its predictive value for reading acquisition by preschoolers (Light & Kins-

bourne, in preparation). Pending the further development and validation of measures specific to individual reading-related cognitive processes, we must content ourselves with a broader-based, indirectly
relevant typology. Such a typology relies largely on demonstrating
inferior performance on tests that do not directly involve reading but
tap ability in areas of intellect presumed in a general way to be pertinent to being able to learn to read.

There is general agreement on the need to identify the insuffi-
ciently matured cognitive process(es) in dyslexic children. Beyond that
surface consensus, however, wide differences in approach result from
different preconceptions about the nature of selective reading disability. A unitary disease model (Hinshelwood, 1917; Critchley, 1970)
specifies a supposed single brain-based process that has gone awry.
Given the variability of dyslexic symptomatology, such formulations
tend to be couched in broad terms, invoking difficulty in symbolization,
sequencing, directionality, and the like (e.g., Hermann, 1959; Orton,
1937). Even outside the medical model, Vellutino (1978) deemed it
reasonable to stipulate the type of processing most critical for normal
reading acquisition (i.e., linguistic, at the phonologic-syntactic level
and argued that one should look there for the factor that limits reading
progress in these children. Satz and Fletcher (1979) made a similar
attempt to stipulate what may be called the "performance-limiting"
function. They, like Bakker (1967), considered linguistic factors to be
critical only after the child has progressed beyond the beginning
reading stage, when visuospatial functions were thought to be more
important. This position has now been abandoned (e.g., Satz & Morris,
1980), but on empirical rather than conceptual grounds alone.

Learning to read and write must enlist many cognitive processes,
and deficient use of any one could result in performance poor enough to
constitute reading failure. Among these children there are many different error patterns, depending on which process is lacking. Only if all
dyslexics made the same pattern of errors in reading and writing could
a unitary hypothesis be upheld. Different types of reading failure can
be demonstrated by use of educational diagnostic and achievement
tests (e.g., Doehring, 1981). The problem with respect to origin is: Are
the different types of failure assumed to index different cognitive
deficits, or could they have resulted from the impact of different
teaching methods on the same deficit? We return to this confounding of
biology and experience when we consider Boder's (1973) typology.

The most radical departure from unitary models seems the most
reasonable position to take. We regard all reading-relevant processes as
vulnerable to whatever adverse influences can cause selective reading
difficulties. We can expect as many subtypes of dyslexia as there are

performance-limiting operations during reading acquisition. A further distinction should be made between 1) broad-based deficits that arise from deficient processes with wide-ranging applicability, and 2) narrowly based deficits that involve processes used almost exclusively for reading. The broad-based deficit can be identified by selectively impaired test performance outside the reading domain. The narrower-based deficit will remain unidentified in psychometric neuropsychologic test performance and at present can only be diagnosed by exclusion. It is hardly more helpful to find deficit on all the tests used than on none. Authors typically attribute such findings to the presence of a combination of syndromes in the child—the "mixed subtype." One wonders whether some degree of unrecognized mental retardation might not more economically explain this reading problem.

Definition of the learning-disabled sample is also influenced by the investigator's preconceptions. Advocates of the medical model will confine attention to severe cases with verifiable selectivity of deficit. They exclude children who are emotionally disturbed or socioeconomically disadvantaged and thus comprise a limited sample of middle-class children. Others who prefer a developmental model feel comfortable in including as many as nearly 40% of children in a regular school system in their study sample, defined solely in terms of their educational achievement scores (Satz & Morris, 1980). Indeed, Taylor, Satz, and Friel (1979) challenged the rationale of exclusionary diagnosis of dyslexia when they reported themselves unable, on a variety of tests and other parameters, to distinguish children who conformed to the criteria for dyslexics from equally impaired readers who did not qualify for this diagnosis. This finding does underline the contention that "dyslexics" cannot be assumed to be qualitatively different from other failing readers in the nature of their reading difficulty, and therefore presumably in the remediation that they require. To clarify the basic mechanisms in dyslexia, however, it is necessary to exclude cases in which reading failure could have been multiply determined. Until we have uncovered the basic cognitive deficit(s) in selective reading failure, similar deficiencies in one or more groups of readers failing for other reasons cannot be asserted or denied.

If one concedes a diversity of possible causes of broadly based selective reading failure, one would wish to scrutinize the three domains of intellect most prominently revealed by factor analysis: verbal comprehension, perceptual organization, and freedom from distractibility. Deviation quotients, or "pseudo-IQs," for each of these factors can be calculated using scaled scores from subtests of the Wechsler Intelligence Scale for Children—Revised (WISC-R) and appropriate formulas (Gutkin, 1979). The verbal comprehension deviation quotient is

1.47 (Information+Similarities+Vocabulary+Comprehension)+41.2. For perceptual organization, the formula is 1.60 (Picture Completion +Picture Arrangement+Block Design+Object Assembly)+36.0, and for freedom from distractibility it is 2.2 (Arithmetic+Digit Span+Coding)+34. Large disparities between the deviation quotients and the full-scale IQ suggest weaknesses in these areas of cognition. Although each group of investigators uses different labels, the subtypes in general conform to children selectively deficient in one of these three areas of intellect. If they were deficient in all three, they would most likely be regarded as mentally retarded.

The wide range of human cognitive skills can be subdivided into two kinds of mental operations: selection and processing. Selective operations ready the organism for the task at hand. Ongoing activity is interrupted, the body and sense organs are appropriately positioned, and the individual adopts and maintains the "mental set" called for by the task. Failure to adopt or maintain this task orientation may be due to undermotivation, failure to understand or even be aware of the task demands, or abnormality in the attentional processes themselves. The rapid fadeout of on-task concentration is inimical to learning to read, as it is to any consistent or coherent intellectual activity.

The selection deficits are usually easily distinguished from difficulties in the processing actually called for by the task. Even given satisfactory task orientation, the mental processes required for learning may be immature and not available in usable form. In contrast to the ADD children, whose ill-sustained attention gets them into trouble socially as well as academically, the children with processing problems act badly only when faced with tasks that tax the arena of their cognitive underdevelopment. Their attention may lag and they may withdraw or behave in disruptive ways symptomatic of their aversion to the task. Any attentional anomalies in disorders of processing are thus secondary and situationally specific. Although it is usually clear which children are substantially handicapped in their selective processes because of ADD, a trial of stimulant medication will usually resolve the issue in a doubtful case.

Children with processing disorders may of course be subtyped according to academic subject, but attempts have been made to go beyond this to isolate distinct underlying neurodevelopmental syndromes. The following methodologies have been employed:

1. Neuropsychologic: analogy with adult cortical symptomatology.
2. Neuropsychologic test battery data: clinical inspection.
3. Neuropsychologic test battery data: empirical analysis.
4. Analysis of prevalent error patterns in academic performance.

A neuropsychologic approach views the academic problem as a surface manifestation of a brain-based deficit or immaturity of some cognitive process; given the correct test format, this deficit could be sampled independently of reading or writing performance. One can determine which is the right test either by formulating hypotheses about the affected process and testing them or by deploying a comprehensive battery that presumably samples all relevant cognitive processes and determining empirically what syndromes emerge.

The hypothesis testing approach was used by Kinsbourne and Warrington (1963b). They drew analogies between dyslexia and two adult neuropsychologic syndromes that implicate reading and writing: aphasia and dominant parietal lobe symptomatology of the Gerstmann type.

Aphasics generally make errors in reading and writing similar to those they make in speech, although usually the reading and writing errors are more severe. Correspondingly, in a sample of dyslexic children chosen for their relatively depressed Verbal compared with Performance WISC subscale scores, Kinsbourne and Warrington (1963a) demonstrated delayed language development and a similar degree of deficit in reading and writing achievement, with relative sparing of arithmetic, and impaired performance on the Token Test, a measure of receptive language skill.

Nonaphasic patients with posterior-inferior parietal lobe lesions in the dominant hemisphere may exhibit Gerstmann's syndrome. Their difficulty is in remembering sequence. They cannot identify their fingers based on their serial position on the hand (Kinsbourne & Warrington, 1962), correctly label left and right, or recall the sequence of letters in words or the place value of digits. Kinsbourne and Warrington found similar difficulties among a group of dyslexic children sampled on the basis of a relative performance deficit on the WISC. These children also had more difficulties with writing than with reading, difficulty in copying figures, and other signs of left and possibly biparietal dysfunction.

Subsequently, work has generally endorsed this subtyping, although different tests and terminology have been used (Mattis et al., 1975; Denckla, 1977). In addition, a longitudinal study has found finger identification to be highly predictive of reading disorder (Satz & Friel, 1974). This finding would be puzzling if we did not know about Gerstmann's syndrome. Pirozzolo (1981) found that the visuospatial (Gerstmann) group manifests directional abnormalities in saccadic eye movements, with excess regressive saccades, episodic reversal of direction of scan, and inaccurate return sweep to the left side of the page. An additional graphomotor subtype has been contributed (Mattis at al., 1975).

Further efforts have been made through empirical approaches. In a series of publications, Rourke and his colleagues (Rourke & Strang, 1978, 1981; Rourke, Young, & Vlewelling, 1971) and Doehring and his colleagues (1981) have presented factors and cluster-analytic information suggesting the possibility of several subtypes in the verbal domain; whether deficits differ in kind or only in degree is not yet clear. One of Doehring's subtypes could be considered to include a visuospatial deficit. Satz and Morris (1980) also claimed a visuospatial subtype on the basis of their cluster analysis. Whether this subtype is the same as the Gerstmann subtype or a separate deficit based on right hemisphere immaturity is not known. Curiously, none of these studies acknowledge the effect of ADD in limiting progress in learning to read. As no steps seem to have been taken to exclude such children from the study sample, substantial numbers of children with this common disability were presumably included. Perhaps they largely account for the children who could not be classified (Satz & Morris, 1980).

If one accepts that children aggregate in some of the above ways, it remains unclear whether this subtyping has anything to do with CAP or learning disability. Perhaps normal readers cluster in the same way as poor readers have been found to do. In other words, although empirical studies generally use tasks that are reliable, there is no guarantee that they are valid. To relate defective test performance casually to defective reading, a further step must be taken. The pattern in deficient performance in reading should be predictable from the neuropsychologic test profile. Kinsbourne and Warrington reported such an error pattern, a relatively high incidence of letter substitution errors in spelling by their language group and order errors in their Gerstmann group (Hermann, 1959). Pirozzolo (1981) confirmed these findings.

Boder's (1973) error analysis into visual-dyseidetic and auditory-dysphonetic confusions operationalizes Myklebust's (1965) clinical intuition that some "dyslexic" children find it harder to learn through the visual modality and some find the auditory harder. This dichotomy in reading tends to reduce to whole-word and phonic approaches. In terms of cerebral functions, one might suggest correspondence with visual-sequential and language deficits, respectively (perceptual organization and verbal factors). A standardized test instrument is now available (Boder, 1981). The chief unknown factor is the contribution made by the method of prior instruction. A child might make visual ("looks alike") confusions in reading because of visual memory problems, insufficient prior instruction in whole-word approaches, weakness in (phonic) word attack, or excessive reliance on pattern memory, or the child may make visual errors not because visual memory is weak but because it is overextended to compensate for an auditory weakness. By the same logic, confusions in the auditory signal need not indicate auditory weakness, but could be due to lack of phonics instruction or compensatory overuse of the auditory channel. Clearly Boder's system is best used in conjunction with diagnostic educational tests that reveal the child's strategies in attempting to read. It would be validated as a means for subtyping, as claimed, if children so classified conformed to corresponding visual and verbal syndromes established by other means. Doehring (1981) attempted to uncover such a correspondence, but was unsuccessful.

In summary, there is reason to suppose that deficits in any of the three major domains of intellect (verbal skill, perceptual organization, and freedom from distractability) will result in reading failure. The inadequacy may not involve the whole domain, however, and perhaps there is more than one type of linguistic problem and more than one type of perceptual organization problem that may prejudice learning to read. It is generally acknowledged, except by Mattis, French, and Rapin (1975), that no test battery reveals a plausibly relevant pattern of neuropsychologic deficit in every dyslexic child. Children may exist whose deficits are so delimited that they may not impinge on performance of any tests unrelated to reading itself.

The attempt to subtype has important implications. It focuses attention on the individuality of the child's problem, if not its uniqueness. It depends on diagnosis by exclusion and from the description of the inadequacies of these children. It attempts to narrow the gap between the outcome of medical-psychologic assessment and the need for guidelines in individualizing education. This gap is at present wide, so wide that much "learning clinic assessment" is sterile in that it does not secure cooperation from teachers. Only those findings that can be operationalized as answers to questions posed by teachers and parents are useful in this field.

REFERENCES

Annett, M., Lee, D., and Ounstead, C. 1961. Intellectual disability in relation to lateralized features of the EEG. In: Hemiplegic Cerebral Palsy in Children and Adults. Little Club Clinics in Developmental Medicine 4:86–112.
Bakker, D. J. 1967. Temporal order, meaningfulness, and reading ability. Perceptual and Motor Skills 24:1927–1930.
Bishop, D. V. M. 1982. Linguistic impairment after left hemi-decortication for infantile hemiplegia: A reappraisal. Quarterly Journal of Experimental Psychology. In press.

Boder, E. 1973. Developmental dyslexia: A diagnostic approach based on three atypical reading-spelling patterns. Developmental Medicine and Child Neurology 15:663–687.

Boder, E. 1981. Reading-Spelling Pattern Test. A Diagnostic Screening Test for Subtypes of Reading Disability. Grune & Stratton, New York.

Cantwell, D. P. 1978. Hyperactivity and antisocial behavior. Child Psychiatry 2:252.

Caplan, B., and Kinsbourne, M. 1981. Cerebral laterality, preferred cognitive mode, and reading ability in normal children. Brain and Language 14:349–370.

Critchley, M. 1970. The Dyslexic Child. Charles C Thomas, Springfield, Ill.

Denckla, M. 1977. Minimal brain dysfunction in dyslexia: Beyond diagnosis by exclusion. In: M. F. Blau, I. Rapin, and M. Kinsbourne (eds.), Topics in Child Neurology, pp. 243–262. Spectrum, New York.

Dennis, M. 1977. Cerebral dominance in three forms of early brain disorder. In: M. F. Blau, I. Rapin, and M. Kinsbourne (eds.), Topics in Child Neurology. Spectrum, New York.

Deutsch, C. K., Swanson, J. M., Buell, J. H., Cantwell, D. P., Weinberg, V., and Baren, M. 1982. Overrepresentation of adoptees in children with the attention deficit disorder. Behavior Genetics 12:231–238.

Doehring, D. G., Trites, R. L., Patel, P. G., and Viedorowicz, C. A. M. 1981. Reading Disabilities: The Interaction of Reading Language and Neuropsychological Deficits. Academic Press, New York.

Field, T. M., Dabiri, M. D., Hallock, B. S. N., and Shuman, M. D. 1977. Developmental effects of prolonged pregnancy and the postmaturity syndrome. The Journal of Pediatrics 90:836–838.

Galaburda, A. M., Le May, M., Kemper, T. L., and Geschwind, N. 1978. Right-left asymmetries in the brain. Science 199:852–856.

Gutkin, T. B. 1979. The WISC-R verbal comprehension, perceptual organization and freedom from distractibility deviation quotients: Data for practitioners. Psychology in the Schools 16:359–360.

Hermann, K. 1959. Reading disability: A medical study of word blindness and related handicaps. Charles C Thomas, Springfield, Ill.

Hinshelwood, J. 1917. Congenital Word Blindness. Lewis, London.

Kinsbourne, M. 1970. The cerebral basis of lateral asymmetries in attention. Acta Psychologica 33:183–201.

Kinsbourne, M. 1976. Looking and listening strategies and beginning reading. In: T. Guthrie (ed.), Aspects of Reading Acquisition, pp. 141–161. Johns Hopkins University Press, Baltimore.

Kinsbourne, M. 1981. The development of cerebral dominance. In: S. Filskov and T. J. Boli (eds.), Handbook of Clinical Neuropsychology, pp. 399–417. John Wiley & Sons, New York.

Kinsbourne, M., and Caplan, P. J. 1979. Childrens' Learning and Attention Problems. Little, Brown, Boston.

Kinsbourne, M., and Warrington, E. K. 1962. A study of finger agnosia. Brain 85:47–66.

Kinsbourne, M., and Warrington, E. K. 1963a. Developmental factors in reading and writing backwardness. British Journal of Psychology 54:145–156.

Kinsbourne, M., and Warrington, E. 1963b. The developmental Gerstmann syndrome. Archives of Neurology 8:490–501.

Light, M., and Kinsbourne, M. Retrospective and perspective effects of a preschool individualized reading program. In preparation.

Mattis, S., French, J. H., and Rapin, I. 1975. Dyslexia in children and young adults: Three independent neuropsychological syndromes. Developmental Medicine and Child Neurology 17:150-163.

McGuinness, D. 1976. Sex differences in the organization of perception and cognition. In: B. Lloyd and J. Archer (eds.), Exploring Sex Differences. Academic Press, New York.

Mech, E. V. 1973. Adoption: A policy perspective. In: B. M. Caldwell and H. N. Ricciuti (eds.), Child Development Research, Vol. 3: Child Development and Social Policy, pp. 467-508. University of Chicago Press, Chicago.

Myklebust, H. R. 1965. Development and Disorders of Written Language: Picture Story Language Test. Grune & Stratton, New York.

Nichols, P. L., and Chen, T. 1981. Minimal Brain Dysfunction: A Prospective Study. Lawrence Erlbaum Associates, Hillsdale, N.J.

Orton, S. T. 1937. Reading, Writing and Speech Problems in Children. Norton, New York.

Pavlides, G. T. 1981. Do eye movements hold the key to dyslexia? Neuropsychologia 19:57-64.

Pirozzolo, F. 1981. The Neuropsychology of Developmental Reading Disorders. Praeger, New York.

Rourke, B. P., and Strang, J. D. 1978. Neuropsychological significance of variations in patterns of academic performance, motor, psychomotor and tactile-perceptual abilities. Journal of Pediatric Psychology 5:62-66.

Rourke, B. P., and Strang, J. D. 1981. Subtypes of reading and arithmetic disabilities. In: M. Rutter (ed.), Behavioral Syndromes of Brain Dysfunction in Children. Guilford, New York.

Rourke, B. P., Young, G. C., and Vlewelling, R. W. 1971. The relationships between WISC Verbal-Performance discrepancies and selected verbal, auditory-perceptual, visual-perceptual, and problem-solving abilities in children with learning disabilities. Journal of Clinical Psychology 27:475-479.

Satz, P. 1972. Pathological left-handedness: An explanatory model. Cortex 8:121-135.

Satz, P., and Fletcher, J. M. 1979. Early screening tests: Some uses and abuses. Journal of Learning Disabilities 12:53-60.

Satz, P., and Friel, J. 1974. Some predictive antecedents of specific learning disability: A preliminary two-year follow up. Journal of Learning Disabilities 7:437-441.

Satz, P., and Morris, R. 1980. Learning disability subtypes. A review. In: F. J. Pirozzolo and M. C. Wittrock (eds.), Neuropsychological and Cognitive Processes in Reading. Academic Press, New York.

Satz, P., and Morris, R. 1980. The search for subtype classification in learning disabled children. In: R. E. Trites (ed.), The Child at Risk. Oxford University Press, New York.

Swanson, J. M., and Kinsbourne, M. 1976. Stimulant-related dependent learning in hyperactive children. Science 192:1354-1356.

Swanson, J. M., Logan, M., and Pelham, N. 1982. The Snap Rating Scale for the Diagnosis of Attention Deficit Disorders. Unpublished manuscript, University of California at Irvine.

Taylor, H. G., Satz, P., and Friel, J. 1979. Developmental dyslexia in relation to other childhood reading disorders. Significance and utility. Reading Research Quarterly 15:84–107.

Thomas, A., Chess, S., Birch, H., Hertzig, M., and Korn, S. 1963. Behavioral Individuality in Early Childhood. New York University Press, New York.

Towbin, A. 1971. Organic causes of minimal brain dysfunction. Journal of the American Medical Association 217:1207–1214.

United States Department of Health, Education and Welfare. 1972. Adoptions in 1970, (DHEW Publication No. SRS 72-03259.) United States Department of Health, Education and Welfare, Washington, D.C.

Vellutino, F. R. 1978. Toward an understanding of dyslexia. Psychological factors in specific reading disability. In: A. Benton and D. Pearl (eds.), Dyslexia—An Appraisal of Current Knowledge. Oxford University Press, New York.

Wada, J., Clarke, R., and Hamm, A. 1975. Cerebral asymmetry in humans. Archives of Neurology 32:239–246.

Weiss, B. 1982. Food additives and environmental chemicals as sources of childhood behavior disorders. Journal of the American Academy of Child Psychiatry 21:144–152.

Witelson, S. R., and Pallie, W. 1973. Left hemisphere specialization for language in the newborn: Neuroanatomical evidence of asymmetry. Brain 9:641–646.

Zaidel, E. 1977. Unilateral auditory language comprehension on the Token Test following cerebral comissuratomy and hemispherectomy: A comparison with child language and aphasia. Neuropsychologia 15:1–18.

Zuckerman, M., Kolin, E. A., Price, L., and Zoob, I. 1964. Development of a sensation-seeking scale. Journal of Consulting Psychology 28:477–482.

Chapter **5**

Development of Symmetrical and Asymmetrical Hemispheric Responses to Speech Sounds

Electrophysiologic Correlates

Dennis L. Molfese and *Victoria J. Molfese*

For over a century it has been commonly believed that language abilities in adults are controlled by discrete mechanisms, which are lateralized to the left cerebral hemisphere. Acceptance of this belief has come with the accumulation of corroborating research findings from studies utilizing a variety of methodologies, such as dichotic listening techniques (Kimura, 1967; Shankweiler & Studdert-Kennedy, 1967), split brain procedures (Gazzaniga, 1970), clinical populations (Geschwind, 1965; Luria, 1966), anatomical procedures (Geschwind & Levitsky, 1968), as well as electroencephalogram and evoked potential recording techniques (Morrell & Salamy, 1971; Donchin, Kutas, & McCarthy, 1977; Molfese, 1979). Although research has shown evidence of differential hemisphere abilities in adults, not until 1972 were such hemisphere differences found in young infants (Molfese, 1972).

Previously, hemisphere differences were thought to develop only with the onset of productive language abilities, between 2 and 3 years of age. According to Lenneberg (1967), "at the beginning of language development both hemispheres seem to be equally involved; the dominance phenomenon seems to come about through a progressive decrease in involvement of the right hemisphere" (p. 151), and "a polarization of function between right and left takes place during childhood, displacing language entirely to the left and certain other functions predominantly to the right" (p. 153).

The first work to test systematically for the presence of early hemisphere differences was done by Molfese (1972) using auditory evoked potential response recording procedures. Such procedures consist of recording a temporally stable and reliable waveform from electrodes placed on the scalp. The evoked potential technique was chosen because, although it placed no demand on subjects to respond, the procedure reflected the subject's sensitivity to stimulation (Regan, 1972). It also provided some information concerning hemispheric responding (Morrell & Salamy, 1971; Wood, Goff, & Day, 1971). Molfese recorded auditory evoked responses (AERs) generated over the left and right scalp regions in response to a series of speech syllables (/ba/ and /dæ/), monosyllabic words (/bɔi/ and /dɔg/), a C major piano chord, and a white noise burst. Subjects were 10 infants, 1 week to 10 months old (mean of 5.8 months), 11 children 4–11 years old (mean of 6.0 years), and 10 adults 23–29 years old (mean of 25.9 years). Differences in amplitudes of the AERs between left and right hemispheres were found at each age level, even in the young infants. Larger amplitude responses to speech stimuli occurred in the left hemisphere, whereas greater amplitude responses to nonspeech stimuli occurred in the right hemisphere.

Work by other researchers has also supported hemisphere differences in infancy. Barnet, de Sotillo, and Campos (1974) investigated AERs of normal and malnourished groups of 6-month-old infants to speech stimuli (the infants' names) and nonspeech stimuli (clicks). Both groups showed greater evoked responses to the click stimuli in the right hemisphere. Only the normal infants showed greater evoked responses to the speech stimuli in the left hemisphere.

Three studies employing the dichotic listening paradigm have also examined hemisphere differences in responsiveness to speech and nonspeech stimuli in infancy. Entus (1977) reported finding hemisphere differences in groups of infants with ages of 43.3–100 days. The babies were tested using high-amplitude sucking as the behavioral response. Pairs of either speech stimuli (/ma/ and /ba/, /da/ and /ba/, /da/ and /ga/) or musical note stimuli executed on different instruments (piano and cello, piano and bassoon, and viola and bassoon) were presented through earphones while the infants sucked on a pacifier. After the continuous presentation of one stimulus of the pair for a period of time, the sucking rate decreased. When a prespecified decrement level in sucking was reached, the stimulus was changed. Entus found the rate of sucking recovered faster if the changed stimulus was a speech sound presented to the right ear or a musical sound presented to the left ear. Because the right ear is believed to project primarily to the left hemisphere and the left ear to the right hemisphere (Kimura, 1961), Entus interpreted these data as indicating that in early infancy the left hemisphere was already specialized for language and the right hemisphere for nonlanguage functions.

Although Entus's results seem to support the hypothesis of early hemisphere differences, Vargha-Khadem and Corballis' (1979) study with slightly younger infants failed to replicate the findings. This failure to replicate is important because stimuli, response criteria, and equipment identical to those used by Entus were used. Thus, the evidence for hemisphere difficulties based on high-amplitude sucking responses is equivocal.

Glanville, Best, and Levenson (1977) also used a dichotic listening paradigm to study hemispheric differences in infants, but used heart rate habituation as the response measure. The stimuli were consonant-vowel (CV) syllable pairs (set A consisted of the syllables /ba/, /da/, /ga/; set B of /pa/, /ta/, /ka/) and musical note pairs played on different instruments (set A: piano, brass, reed; set B: organ, string, flute). The sets were presented dichotically to infants 93–130 days old. For eight of the 12 infants, greater recovery from heart rate habituation occurred when novel speech stimuli were presented to the right ear (left hemisphere), whereas greater recovery occurred when novel musical stimuli were presented to the left ear (right hemisphere). Glanville et al. concluded, as did Entus, that hemisphere differences were present in early infancy and that such differences reflected ability of the left hemisphere to process language-related stimuli whereas the right hemisphere was more involved with nonlanguage materials.

Although hemisphere differences in response to speech and nonspeech stimuli have now been noted in both infant and adult populations, relatively little work has examined the nature of the cortical mechanisms responsible for the differences or identified the specific acoustic features that trigger these differences. In part, this failure has been due to the use of relatively gross stimulus features in the early studies. Most of the speech and nonspeech stimuli utilized have differed along many dimensions (e.g., differences in formant structure, number of formants, the presence or absence of frequency transitions, the shift in frequency transitions). Consequently, although the magnitude and direction of hemisphere differences were found to shift depending on the general type of stimuli presented—that is, whether speech or nonspeech—the specific stimulus characteristics responsible for the hemisphere difference have not been identified.

In spite of the attention given to demonstrating the existence of hemisphere differences, little as yet is known about how mechanisms responsible for such differences operate, what specific stimulus features they are sensitive to, or how they are utilized cognitively. Our laboratory in recent years has attempted to isolate and identify electrophysiologic correlates for various speech cues. The work outlined here has focused within the area of speech perception on stop consonant perception involving voicing contrasts and place of articulation contrasts.

VOICING CONTRASTS

Voicing contrast or voice onset time (VOT) reflects the temporal relationship between onset of laryngeal pulsing (i.e., vocal fold vibration) and consonant release (i.e., the separation of lips to release a burst of air from the vocal tract during the production of bilabial stop consonants such as /b/ and /p/). When VOT was systematically manipulated, adult listeners discriminated changes in VOT only to the extent that they could assign unique labels to these sounds (i.e., one phoneme label or another; Liberman et al., 1967). Listeners failed to discriminate between bilabial stop consonants with VOT values of 0 and +20 msec and identified both stimuli as /ba/. Subjects identified stimuli with +40 and +60 msec VOT as /pa/ and failed to discriminate between them. However, these adults did discriminate between and assign different labels to stimuli with VOT values of +20 and +40 msec. These stimuli were from different phoneme categories (/b/ versus /p/). The 20-msec difference in VOT between speech syllables was only detected when the VOT stimuli were from different phoneme categories, again such as /b/ versus /p/. Consequently, perceived changes in VOT appeared to be categorical. These findings have been consistent in adults (Lisker & Abramson, 1964; Liberman, Delattre, & Cooper, 1958) as well as in young infants with whom high-amplitude sucking procedures were used (Eimas et al., 1971; Trehub & Rabinovitch, 1972). Findings with infants as young as 1 month indicate that VOT perception is present early in life, long before the emergence of language production. This suggests that some mechanisms which subserve language functions are innately specified from birth. However, given the severe limitations of behavioral techniques such as high-amplitude sucking with infants less than 1 or 2 months of age, no behavioral studies to date have successfully shown when the mechanisms for VOT perception first appear in development.

Additional questions not addressed directly with behavioral procedures concern localization of VOT mechanisms in the cortex and how such mechanisms change as the child develops into a sophisticated language user. Because VOT is known to be an important speech cue, and speech processes have been thought to be controlled by the language-dominant hemisphere, generally the left, most scientists have concluded that VOT perception is controlled by mechanisms within the left hemisphere. This theory has, however, never been systematically addressed. A final question concerns the nature of the VOT cue itself. Is VOT processed by specialized speech mechanisms or by more basic acoustically tuned cortical mechanisms (Stevens & Klatt, 1974; Pisoni, 1977)?

Our laboratory has utilized electrophysiologic recording procedures as well as behavioral techniques to address these issues. The electrophysiologic techniques involve presentation of an auditory stimulus and recording of the brain's AERs triggered by this event. Various portions of the AERs reflect different properties of the stimulus. In the earliest electrophysiologic study on adult VOT perception, Molfese (1978) recorded AERs from the left and right temporal regions of 16 adults during a phoneme identification task. Subjects were presented with a randomly ordered series of synthesized bilabial stop consonants varied in VOT by values of 0, +20, +40, and +60 msec. After each stimulus presentation, the subjects pressed one button if they heard a /b/ and a second button if they heard a /p/. Individuals identified CVs with VOT values of 0 and +20 msec as /ba/ approximately 97% and 93% of the time, respectively, whereas CVs with VOT times of +40 and +60 msec were identified, respectively, 95% and 98% of the time as /pa/. AERs to each stimulus were recorded during the identification task and later analyzed by standard averaging techniques. Subsequent analyses involving principal components analysis and analyses of variance indicated that two early AER components recorded from electrodes placed over the right hemisphere varied systematically as a function of phoneme category of the evoking stimulus. Stimuli with VOT values of 0 and +20 msec elicited different AER waveforms from the right hemisphere sites than did the +40- and +60-msec stimuli. No differences in the AER waveforms were found between the VOT values within a phoneme category (i.e., no differences were found between the +40- and +60-msec responses). These AER patterns of responding were comparable to the behavioral responses given by these subjects during the testing session. Components of the left hemisphere responses reflected an ability to differentiate between 0- and +60-msec stimuli and to differentiate 0- and +60-msec from +20- and +40-msec stimuli. The left hemisphere seemed responsive to the boundaries of the VOT stimuli used but did not reflect the phoneme category-only discriminations shown by the right hemisphere.

Similar effects have also been found with 4-year-old children when velar stop consonants (/k/, /g/) were presented (Molfese & Hess, 1978). In this study AERs were recorded from the left and right temporal regions of 12 nursery school-age children (mean age was 4 years, 5 months) in response to a series of synthesized CV syllables which varied in VOT for the consonant (0, +20, +40, +60 msec). As with the adults, one AER component from the right hemisphere electrode site varied systematically as a function of phoneme category but could not distinguish between VOT values within a phoneme category. A second and distinct (orthogonal) AER component also discriminated between VOT values along phoneme boundaries. However, unlike that found for adults, this component was present in recording sites over both hemispheres. The group-averaged AER recorded from all the children is presented in Figure 1 along with the four components of the AER that varied as a function of stimulus parameters and scalp recording sites. The centroid or grand mean AER characterized the information and waveform characteristics common to all the AERs recorded from children in that study. It contained three major peaks, an N156 peak that reached its most negative point 156 msec after stimulus onset, a large positive wave (P312) that peaked at 312 msec following stimulus onset, and a final negative wave N444 with a peak latency of 444 msec. The four components reflected variations in peak structure from the centroid. An analysis of variance found several of the components to vary systematically as a function of VOT. These included factor 1 (with peak latencies of 198 and 342 following stimulus onset) and factor 2 (peak latencies at 120, 312, and 444 msec).

Figure 2 presents the averaged AERs for the various stimulus conditions for two preschoolers, a female (subject F-4) and a male (subject M-1). For example, factor 1 of Figure 1 affects the overall amplitude from 198 to 342 msec of the AERs in Figure 2. This includes the central region from the first large negative peak (N156) to the first large positive peak (P312). Examining this area of the AERs from both hemispheres, one notes that the overall amplitude from the N156 to the P312 component declines steadily from the 0-msec stimulus to the +60-msec stimulus. However, if the impact of factor 2 (which largely reflects the relative amplitude of the wave from P312 until N444) is observed, it is clear that this region is considerably larger for the AERs

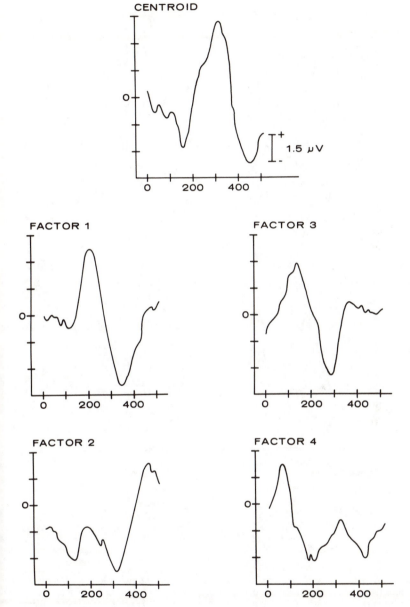

Figure 1. The centroid (grand mean) and the four factors extracted over all stimulus conditions by the varimaxed principal components analysis. The calibration marker is 1.5 μV with positive up. The time course is 498 msec.

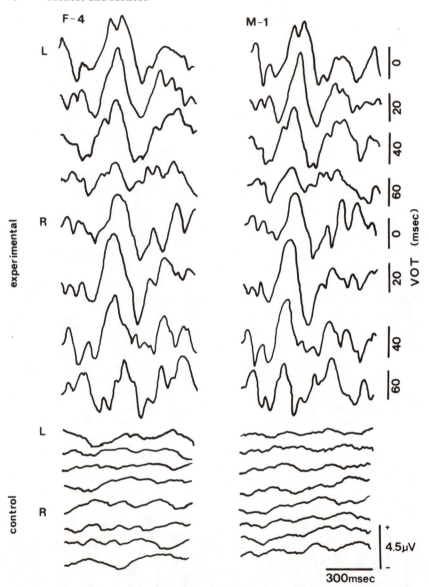

Figure 2.   Averaged brain electrical activity from two preschool children, a female (F-4) and a male (M-1), elicited in response to VOT stimuli (experimental) and during periods of no stimulus presentation (control). For both the experimental and the control conditions, the top four brain waves were recorded from the left hemisphere (L) while the second four were recorded from the right hemisphere (R). The VOT values of the evoking stimuli that elicited each brain wave are listed along the right side of the graph. The calibration marker is 4.5 μV with positive up. The waveforms began with stimulus onset and continued for 900 msec. Only the first 500 msec was used in the data analysis.

recorded over the RH for the 0-msec and +20-msec stimuli than for the +40-msec and +60-msec stimuli. This indicates that stimuli belonging to the voiced phoneme category (elicited by 0- and +20-msec stimuli) elicit one AER response, whereas stimuli from a second category, voiceless, elicited a different AER waveform. No such voiced/voiceless difference is observed at this portion of the AER waveform in the left hemisphere.

This work was also extended to include newborn and infant populations (Molfese & Molfese, 1979). Four CV speech syllables used by Molfese (1978) were presented to 16 infants ages 2–5 months (mean was 3 months, 25 days). AERs to each stimulus were recorded from scalp electrodes placed over the left and right superior temporal regions of the left and right hemispheres. As with children, results showed one component of the cortical AER from the right hemisphere site (which peaked at 144 and 920 msec after stimulus onset) to discriminate between VOT values from different phoneme categories. A second component of the AER which responded similarly was present over both hemispheres and showed peak latencies of 40 and 528 msec.

In a separate study (Molfese & Molfese, 1979), 16 newborn infants were tested to try to determine developmental onset of VOT discrimination as reflected in AERs. The same CV speech stimuli and recording sites described above were used. Results indicated that although both hemispheres were actively involved in processing of VOT stimuli, there was no evidence of any phoneme-categorical VOT effect as seen with older infants, children, and adults. Ability to discriminate VOT stimuli along phoneme boundaries seems to be present in the early months of infancy but not at birth. It may require some period of maturation or experience to develop or become functional.

Three general findings emerged from this series of studies: 1) perception of the VOT cue is controlled by several cortical processes, some restricted to only the right hemisphere site and some common to both hemispheres; 2) there is a developmental pattern to the emergence of mechanisms related to VOT perception; and 3) VOT perception at the cortical level occurs along phoneme boundaries. Our laboratory then addressed the nature of the stimuli that elicited these categorical responses over the right hemisphere. Were such effects elicited only by speech stimuli, or could nonspeech stimuli elicit similar responses? The answer would, of course, have implications for determining the processing units responsible for these responses. To address this question we undertook an experiment to see whether VOT is controlled by mechanisms specific to language, or whether this cue is based on more basic acoustic relationships that are not restricted solely to speech. This study utilized a subset of stimuli tested in a series of behavioral tasks by Pisoni (1977).

Pisoni was one of the first to suggest that discriminating changes in VOT could depend on nonspeech auditory processing units sensitive to temporal changes in the onset of different events. He trained eight subjects with a series of two-tone stimulus sequences. The stimuli for this tone onset time (TOT) training consisted of two tones of 500 Hz (formant 1) and 1500 Hz (formant 2). For one training stimulus (-50 msec), the first formant (F_1) began 50 msec before the second formant (F_2), whereas for the second training stimulus, F_1 began $+50$ msec after F_2. Both tones terminated together. Overall stimulus duration was 230 msec. Subjects were trained to press one button if they heard the -50-msec stimulus and a second button if they heard a $+50$-msec stimulus. Visual feedback was provided after each response. After training, subjects were given identification tests, without feedback, on the original training stimuli plus nine other TOT stimuli which varied in 10-msec steps from -50 to $+50$ msec. Subjects identified the TOT stimuli from -50 to $+20$ msec as one stimulus, whereas stimuli with temporal lags between $+30$ and $+50$ msec were identified as a different stimulus. Subsequent discrimination tests indicated that subjects only discriminated between stimuli from different identification groups; stimuli from the -50- to $+20$-msec category were discriminated from the $+30$- to $+50$-msec category. However, discrimination scores within a temporal category (i.e., from -50 to $+20$ msec or the category from $+20$ to $+50$ msec) were at chance levels.

Because discrimination boundaries for the TOT stimuli closely resembled those for the speech VOT stimuli, Pisoni concluded that VOT perception may depend on properties of the sensory systems that are sensitive to the temporal order between two events. VOT perception, then, would rely on acoustic processing mechanisms that are sensitive to temporal lags between components of particular stimuli. Pisoni suggested that because of the salience of these differences, linguistic systems over time have incorporated this cue as a useful and important one for speech perception.

Given our findings as to the right hemisphere's involvement in the detection of phoneme boundary changes in VOT, we began a series of studies to determine whether similar types of processes might subserve detection of temporal differences for nonspeech stimuli such as those employed by Pisoni (1977). If similar cortical effects were found for both speech and nonspeech, some conclusions could be reached regarding similarities in mechanisms underlying perception of those different stimuli. Specifically, if an acoustic temporal distinction does form the basis for phoneme category distinctions, similar electrocortical responses should be elicited by both the VOT speech and TOT nonspeech materials. Because the 0- and +20-msec VOT stimuli were found to be processed differently in the right hemisphere than the +40- and +60-msec VOT stimuli, similar response patterns should be elicited by TOT stimuli. No differential left hemisphere responses should be noted.

Four TOT stimuli from Pisoni (1977) were used in this series. These stimuli contained temporal relationships comparable to the voicing contrasts of synthesized speech syllables previously used in our laboratory. Use of these four TOT stimuli facilitated comparisons with the earlier electrophysiologic research and controlled stimulus length. Thus, AER differences would not reflect overall differences in stimulus duration (all stimuli were 230 msec in duration). The four two-tone stimuli differed from each other in the onset time of the lower tone in relation to the higher tone. For the 0-msec stimulus, the lower tone began at the same time as the higher tone. The lower tone lagged 20 msec behind the higher tone for the +20-msec stimulus. For the +40-msec stimulus, the lower tone was delayed 40 msec after the onset of the higher tone, whereas for the +60-msec stimulus this delay was increased to 60 msec. Both tones ended simultaneously.

These four stimuli were used by Molfese (1980) in a study of 16 adults with no prior experience with speech perception experiments or electrophysiology procedures. AERs from four scalp sites over each hemisphere were recorded in response to each stimulus and later analyzed by the principal components analysis and analysis of variance procedures noted earlier. Nine factors accounting for approximately 81% of the total variance were isolated and identified. One AER component was common to all four electrode sites over the right hemisphere and discriminated the 0-msec TOT and +20-msec TOT stimuli from the +40-msec TOT and +60-msec TOT stimuli. The right hemisphere lateralized process is evident in the group-averaged AERs shown in Figure 3. This component began 300 msec following stimulus onset and reached its peak 355 msec after onset. The component contributed to the P330 and N405 components of the AERs depicted in the figure. The effect can readily be observed in the relationship between the final two negative components (N260 and N405) of the right hemisphere AERs for the four TOT latencies. These two late negative components reach equal levels of negativity (their lowest points) for the 0- and +20-msec TOT stimuli, whereas the final negative peak appears much larger than the preceding component for the +40- and +60-msec stimuli. No such effect of these two components is seen for the left hemisphere. The left hemisphere could not discriminate between the two TOT categories, although it could make within-category discriminations.

Similarities in findings for VOT and TOT perception measured by scalp-recorded AER techniques suggest that similar processes may underlie perception of these two cues, as hypothesized by Pisoni (1977).

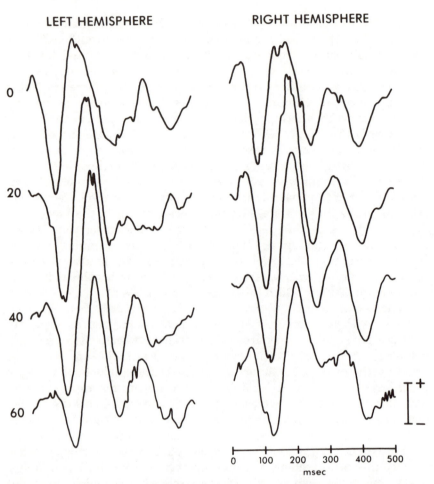

Figure 3. Group-averaged AERs for each hemisphere (but collapsed across electrode sites) elicited in response to each TOT stimulus. The calibration make is $2\mu V$ with positive up. Time course is 500 msec.

VOT perception specifically, and language perception in general, may depend on development and emergence of basic acoustic processes at the cortical level involved in the perceptual activities underlying language comprehension. Because these processes seem to change through development, their role in language development could change over time. Language development, then, would not depend simply on the presence or absence (or degree) of lateralization, but rather on the development of basic acoustic processing mechanisms to detect, identify, and discriminate between certain cues, such as voicing contrasts, critical to speech perception.

Although the mechanisms responsible for processing of voicing contrasts followed a clear developmental pattern in which the right hemisphere seemed to play an important role, independent bilaterally represented processes were also present that appeared to carry on the same functions as the right hemisphere. These findings suggest that there may be some redundancy in the cortical mechanisms employed for this type of perception. Such redundancy could be important in cases of damage to one cortical region in terms of recovery or reemergence of functions.

Although the temporal contrasts described in these series of studies seem important for language perception, our data also suggest that different language-relevant cues are perceived and processed differently. The developmental pattern and the neural substrate for speech-related perceptual mechanisms may differ depending on the specific type of information perceived, as with place of articulation cues.

PLACE OF ARTICULATION CONTRASTS

Several studies were undertaken to identify electrocortical correlates of acoustic and phoneme cues important to perception of place of articulation information for consonants (Molfese, 1978, 1980; Molfese & Molfese, 1979, 1980). In general these studies indicated that multiple processing mechanisms (including left hemisphere and bilateral processes) are involved in perception of such cues as F_2 transition and formant bandwidth. These findings agree with recent behavioral studies which utilized dichotic temporal processing procedures (Cutting, 1974). Cutting found that both bandwidth and transition cues influenced adult discrimination scores. Stimuli with speech formant structure or with an initial transition element were better discriminated by the right ear. Because the majority of the right ear's pathways are thought to project to the left hemisphere, Cutting reasoned that such findings reflected differences in the processing capabilities of the cerebral hemispheres. He concluded that there are different cortical mechanisms involved in processing different cues.

Molfese (1978) attempted to isolate and localize the neuroelectrical correlates of these cues by presenting a series of computer-generated CV syllables in which the stop consonants varied in place of articulation (e.g., /b/ versus /g/), formant structure (nonspeech-like formants composed of sine waves 1 Hz in bandwidth or by speechlike formants with bandwidths of 60, 90, and 120 Hz for F_1, F_2, and F_3, respectively), and phonetic versus nonphonetic transitions (the direction of the frequency changes for F_1 and F_3 were either rising to produce a phonetic transition potentially characterizing human speech patterns, or were falling and therefore occurred in a manner not found in an initial position in human speech patterns). Using principal components analysis to isolate major features of the AERs recorded from the left hemisphere and right hemisphere of 10 adults, Molfese found six major AER components which accounted for 97% of the total variance. Analysis of variance on the gains scores for these factors resulted in identification of these components as sensitive to the various stimulus and subject variables under investigation. One AER component that characterized only the left hemisphere electrode site was found to vary systematically to changes in F_2 transitions.

A replication-extension study (Molfese, 1980) also found that the left hemisphere discriminated consonant place of articulation information. Twenty adults were presented a series of CV syllables which varied in the initial consonant (/b/ or /g/) and the final vowel (/i/, /æ/, /ɔ/). AERs were recorded from three scalp locations over each hemisphere. By means of the analysis outlined above, one component of the brain's AER was found to reflect the ability of only the left hemisphere to differentiate between the consonants /b/ and /g/, independent of the following vowel. Figure 4 presents the group-averaged AERs elicited in response to the /b/ initial syllables (dashed line) and in response to the /g/ initial syllables (solid line). Also shown are the two factors which reflected a left hemisphere-lateralized process (factor 1) and a bilateral process (factor 3). Factor 1 contributed to the AER differences at latencies of 10, 290, and 460 msec, whereas factor 3's contribution between 100 and 230 msec was restricted to the AER component surrounding P200.

These findings are important in terms of their implications for the problem of consonant invariance. Until quite recently (Stevens & Blumstein, 1978; Blumstein & Stevens, 1979), acoustic scientists were unable to isolate a set of acoustic properties that are invariant for a particular consonant place of articulation. Although such invariance exists for vowels, acoustic cues for consonants change as a function of subsequent sounds. Consequently, speech scientists long assumed that consonant and vowel information was processed together as a unit. This electrophysiologic study by Molfese (1980) represents the first direct indication that the brain may in fact respond to consonant sound configurations independent of vowel contexts. Further analysis of these data by Molfese and Schmidt (in press) indicates context-dependent as well as context-independent processing. Factors 5, 6, and 7 of that study (with major peak latencies of 340 msec, 110 msec, and 40 msec, respectively) all reflected consonant sound discriminations when

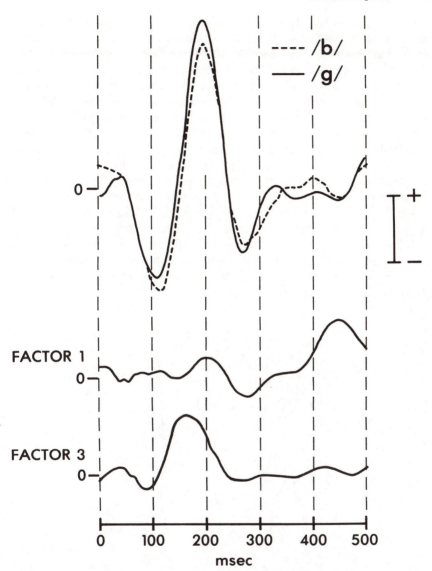

Figure 4.   Group-averaged AERs elicited in response to the /b/ (dashed line) and /g/ (solid line) initial syllables (collapsed across vowels) with factor 1 and factor 3. Calibration marker is 2 μV with positive up. Time course is 500 msec.

those consonants occurred in combination with specific vowel sounds. Cortical processing of speech consonant sounds, then, seems to involve the perception and discrimination of both context-dependent and context-independent cues.

Two studies by Molfese and Molfese (1979, 1980) examined the question of when, developmentally, infants respond differentially to place of articulation contrasts. In the first, AERs were recorded from 16 newborn infants in response to two stop consonants which differed only in F_2 transition and formant bandwidth. As with adults, an AER component found only over the left hemisphere differentiated between consonants. A second, orthogonal AER component which occurred earlier in time and was recorded by electrodes over the left hemisphere and right hemisphere also distinguished between the stop consonants. The contribution of the bilateral (factor 3) and left hemisphere-lateralized processes to the infant AERs (factor 4) can be seen in Figure 5. Here, the left hemisphere component of factor 4 influences the relative size and shape of the initial large negative wave (N230). This portion of the waveform changed in reponse to a rising or falling F_2 transition with speech formant structure over only the left hemisphere recording site. The later AER components between 490 and 704 msec changed over both left hemisphere and right hemisphere regions in response to changes in these same stimulus features.

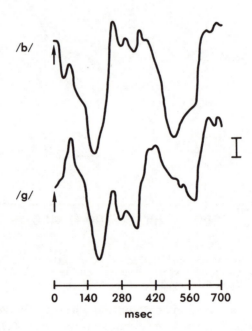

Figure 5.   Reconstructed infant group AERs elicited in response to rising (/b/) and falling (/g/) F_2 transitions.

The later study sought to determine whether left hemisphere processes are present in the responses of preterm infants and whether left hemisphere mechanisms in infants are sensitive to phonetic and non-phonetic transitions. The subjects were 11 preterm infants with conceptional ages ranging from 32 to 37 weeks (mean of 35.9 weeks). They were tested from 1 to 42.5 days (mean of 15 days) after birth. AERs to stimuli identical to those used by Molfese (1978) were recorded again from the T_3 and T_4 electrode sites over the superior temporal regions of left and right hemispheres. As with the full-term newborns, one factor identified in the AERs of preterm infants was a left hemisphere process which distinguished between transition cues in stimuli with speech formant structure, and several factors indicated the presence of general differences in hemisphere activity that were not interactive with other variables. Another factor that also reflected a left hemisphere process differentiated between only the nonphonetic stop consonants (/b/ and /g/). This finding is similar to that reported by Molfese (1978) with adults except that the left hemisphere process for adults was sensitive to both phonetic and nonphonetic stimuli. The difference may be due to maturation and experimental factors. A final factor reflected general hemispheric responsiveness to formant structure (bandwidth) differences. Although Molfese (1978) also found a factor reflecting this process in the AERs with adults, no such effect was found for the full-term infants tested by Molfese and Molfese (1979). This discrepancy may be due to maturation and changes in the processes involved in the discrimination of formant structure such that the mechanisms controlling the discrimination by preterm infants differ from those involved in discrimination by adults.

These studies demonstrate that formant structure, whether it is speechlike or not, is an additional important cue that plays some role in a lateralized response for place of articulation information. In all our studies to date, stimuli with speechlike formant structure have yielded differential effects unique to the left hemisphere for infants (Molfese & Molfese, 1979, 1980) but not for adults (Molfese, 1978, 1980). With infants, the only lateralized effects noted occurred for stimuli with speech formant structure. Stimuli with sine wave formant structure produced no such effect. In the two studies on adults, however, place of articulation contrast effects were noted for stimuli with both speech and nonspeech formant structure. Only bilateral hemisphere effects were noted for formant structure differences. Intriguingly, there are developmental changes in lateralized responses in which the early lateralized process disappears with further development.

There seem to be some basic differences in the organization and localization of brain mechanisms which respond to the temporal information contained in VOT and TOT stimuli and to place of articulation contrasts. Although both contrasts involve both hemispheres (bilateral processes), they differ in important respects. Voicing contracts involve an additional right hemisphere process, whereas place of articulation contrasts involve a left hemisphere process. These mechanisms also appear to develop at different times.

DEVELOPMENTAL ISSUES

Although no evidence for VOT phoneme boundary perception was found for newborn infants, two distinct processing mechanisms sensitive to such differences were present by 2 months of age (Molfese & Molfese, 1979). One mechanism, as reflected by an early AER component common to both hemispheres, responded to the VOT cue along phoneme boundaries. That is, it reflected categorical perception of VOT values. A second mechanism, which was restricted to the right hemisphere and appeared in later portions of the AER waveform, responded in a similar fashion. These different mechanisms persisted into the early childhood years. With 4-year-old subjects, a bilateral process sensitive to phoneme boundaries was reflected in early portions of the AER waveform, whereas a right hemisphere-lateralized process with similar capabilities occurred somewhat later in time (Molfese & Hess, 1978). It was only in the cortical responses of adults that substantially different responses were noted (Molfese, 1978). Here, two distinct, early occurring right hemisphere mechanisms were noted from the anterior temporal recording electrode. No bilateral VOT process was found at these temporal recording sites. Apparently, sometime between 4 years and adulthood the bilateral VOT process either becomes lateralized to the right hemisphere or is replaced by a different mechanism restricted to the right hemisphere. Alternatively, the bilateral process may be displaced (the generators repositioned or their field shrinking) to posterior cortical regions, as suggested by Molfese (1980).

Place of articulation contrasts, however, were detected over the left hemisphere of infants under 30 hr of age (Molfese & Molfese, 1979), 2 months before the right hemisphere mechanisms could make VOT distinctions (Molfese & Molfese, 1979). These place of articulation contrasts do not seem to change to any great extent into adulthood (Molfese, 1978, 1980) except in the manner in which they interact with formant structure characteristics.

In summary:

1.   The different perceptually important cues for speech perception reviewed here seem to be subserved by different regions of the

brain and to develop at different rates. Analyses of the electrophysiologic responses indicate that each cue is processed by a number of distinct mechanisms; some are bilaterally represented and some are lateralized to one cortical region.

2.   How these bilateral and lateral processes interact (excitation,
inhibition, redundancy, process supplement, etc.), or whether they interact, is unknown at the present time. We do know, however, that
these discriminations appear at different points in development. Some
processes change further whereas others do not. Even those processes
that do change may mature at different rates.

3.   Clearly, then, given the findings to date, it seems that language
perception for even relatively simple discriminations must depend on
multidimensional and complex hemispheric processes. Language perception should not be studied solely as a left or right hemisphere task,
but studied for bilateral contributions.

4.   Although the use of electrophysiologic techniques to study language and cognitive development is still very much in its infancy, such
procedures when viewed in the context of other research techniques offer powerful means to increase our knowledge of this area.

REFERENCES

Barnet, A., de Sotillo, M., and Campos, M. 1974. EEG sensory evoked poten-
    tials in early infancy malnutrition. Paper read at the Society for Neuroscien-
    ces, St. Louis.
Blumstein, S. E., and Stevens, K. N. 1979. Acoustic invariance in speech pro-
    duction: Evidence from measurements of the spectral characteristics of stop
    consonants. Journal of the Acoustical Society of America 66:1001–1017.
Cutting, J. E. 1974. Two left hemisphere mechanisms in speech perception.
    Perception and Psychophysics 16:601–612.
Donchin, E., Kutas, M., and McCarthy, G. 1977. Electrocortical indices of
    hemispheric utilization. In: S. Harnad, R. W. Doty, L. Goldstein, J. Jaynes,
    and G. Krauthamer (eds.), Lateralization in the Nervous System. Academic
    Press, New York.
Eimas, P. D., Siqueland, E., Jusczyk, P., and Vigorito, J. 1971. Speech percep-
    tion in infants. Science 171:303–306.
Entus, A. 1977. Hemispheric asymmetry in processing of dichotically pre-
    sented speech and nonspeech stimuli by infants. In: S. Segalowitz and
    F. Gruber (eds.), Language Development and Neurological Theory. Academic
    Press, New York.
Gazzaniga, M. S. 1970. The Bisected Brain. Appleton-Century-Crofts,
    New York.
Geschwind, N. 1965. Disconnection syndromes in animals and man. Brain
    88:585–644.
Geschwind, N., and Levitsky, W. 1968. Human brain: Left-right asymmetries
    in temporal speech regions. Science 161:186–187.

Glanville, B., Best, C., and Levenson, R. 1977. A cardiac measure of cerebral asymmetries in infant auditory perception. Developmental Psychology 13:54–59.

Kimura, D. 1961. Cerebral dominance and the perception of verbal stimuli. Canadian Journal of Psychology 15:166–171.

Kimura, D. 1967. Functional assymmetry of the brain in dichotic listening. Cortex 3:163–178.

Lenneberg, E. 1967. Biological Foundations of Language. John Wiley & Sons, New York.

Liberman, A. M., Cooper, F. S., Shankweiler, D., and Studdert-Kennedy, M. 1967. Perception of the speech code. Psychological Review 74:431–461.

Liberman, A. M., Delattre, P. C., and Cooper, F. S. 1958. Some cues for the distinction between voiced and voiceless stops in initial position. Language and Speech 1:153–167.

Lisker, L., and Abramson, A. S. 1964. A cross language study of voicing in initial stops: Acoustical measurements. Word 20:384–422.

Luria, A. R. 1966. The Higher Cortical Function in Man. Basic Books, New York.

Molfese, D. L. 1972. Cerebral asymmetry in infants, children and adults: Auditory evoked responses to speech and music stimuli. Doctoral dissertation, Pennsylvania State University. Dissertation Abstracts International, 1972, 33. (Available from University Microfilms No. 72-48, 394).

Molfese, D. L. 1978a. Neuroelectrical correlates of categorical speech perception in adults. Brain and Language 5:25–35.

Molfese, D. L. 1978b. Left and right hemisphere involvement in speech perception: Electrophysiological correlates. Perception and Psychophysics 23: 237–242.

Molfese, D. L. 1979. Cortical involvement in the semantic processing of coarticulated speech cues. Brain and Language 7:86–100.

Molfese, D. L. 1980a. Hemispheric specialization for temporal information: Implications for the perception of voicing cues during speech perception. Brain and Language 8:285–299.

Molfese, D. L. 1980b. The phoneme and the engram: Electrophysiological evidence for the acoustic invariant in stop consonants. Brain and Language 9:372–376.

Molfese, D. L., and Hess, T. 1978. Hemispheric specialization for VOT perception in the preschool child. Journal of Experimental Child Psychology 26:71–84.

Molfese, D. L., and Molfese, V. J. 1979a. Hemisphere and stimulus differences as reflected in the cortical responses of newborn infants to speech stimuli. Developmental Psychology 15:505–511.

Molfese, D. L., and Molfese, V. J. 1979b. VOT distinctions in infants: Learned or innate? In: H. A. Whitaker and H. Whitaker (eds.), Studies in Neurolinguistics, Volume 4. Academic Press, New York.

Molfese, D. L., and Molfese, V. J. 1980. Cortical responses of preterm infants to phonetic and nonphonetic speech stimuli. Developmental Psychology 16:574–581.

Molfese, D. L., and Schmidt, A. L. 1983. An auditory evoked potential study of consonant perception. In press.

Morrell, L. K., and Salamy, J. G. 1971. Hemispheric asymmetry of electrocortical responses to speech stimuli. Science 174:164–166.

Pisoni, D. B. 1977. Identification and discrimination of the relative onset time of two component tones: Implications for voicing perception in stops. Journal of the Acoustical Society of America 61:1352–1361.

Regan, D. 1972. Evoked Potentials in Psychology, Sensory Physiological, and Clinical Medicine. John Wiley & Sons, New York.

Shankweiler, D. & Studdert-Kennedy, M. 1967. Identification of consonants and vowels presented to left and right ears. Quarterly Journal of Experimental Psychology 19:59–63.

Stevens, K. N., and Blumstein, S. E. 1978. Invariant cues for place of articulation in stop consonants. Journal of the Acoustical Society of America 64:1358–1368.

Stevens, K. N., and Klatt, D. H. 1974. Role for formant transition in the voiced-voiceless distribution for stops. Journal of the Acoustical Society of America 55:653–659.

Trehub, S., and Rabinovitch, M. 1972. Auditory-linguistic sensitivity in early infancy. Developmental Psychology 6:74–77.

Vargha-Khadem, F., and Corballis M. 1979. Cerebral asymmetry in infants. Brain and Language 8:1–9.

Wood, C. C., Goff, W. R., and Day, R. S. 1971. Auditory evoked potentials during speech perception. Science 173:1248–1251.

Chapter 6

Speech Perception in Infancy and Early Childhood

Rebecca E. Eilers and *D. Kimbrough Oller*

The past decade has witnessed a proliferation of paradigms and data in the study of speech perception in both infants and children. However, the data often seem contradictory and difficult to interpret. In part, this difficulty stems from the newness of the endeavor: from large gaps in existing data and from sketchy theoretical frameworks proposed very early in the data collection process. These scientific gaps include a paucity of knowledge concerning: 1) stages of phonological development and relationships among stages, 2) the perception of relatively complex versus relatively simple stimuli, and 3) processing demands of various speech perception tasks, relationships between different tasks, and the interaction between task demands and development. The goal of this chapter is to reinterpret some of the now classic data and to add a perspective provided by some new findings within a general theoretical framework. To accomplish this task it is first necessary to provide some basic information about current methodologies for assessing speech perception in infants and young children.

This work was supported by the Mailman Foundation and by National Institute of Mental Health Grant MH30634 and National Institute of Neurological Diseases and Stroke Grant NS17604.

METHODS FOR SPEECH PERCEPTION RESEARCH

Infants

Three general methods have been traditionally employed with infants between birth and about 1 year of age: high-amplitude sucking (HAS), heart rate (HR), and visually reinforced infant speech discrimination (VRISD). One laboratory has also successfully employed auditory evoked response (AER) techniques, monitoring brain activity in response to various sound types (Molfese, Freeman, & Palermo, 1975; Molfese & Molfese, Chapter 5, this volume). The AER approach has focused on lateralization of function and is not a major focus in this paper. A brief description of three more familiar and widely used paradigms to study infant speech perception follows with commentary regarding applicability to specific questions and possible modifications.

High-Amplitude Sucking Procedures In the HAS procedure (Eimas et al., 1971) infants sucking on a nonnutritive nipple are presented with a repeating speech stimulus (e.g., /ba,ba,ba . . . /) contingent on the infant's high-amplitude sucking on the nipple. High-amplitude sucks are usually defined for each infant relative to the amplitude of the infant's baseline sucks. The more high-amplitude sucks the infant produces, the more syllables he or she hears, up to a maximum rate of about 1 per second. During the first phase of the experimental run (the acquisition phase), the number of high-amplitude sucks typically increases over baseline until an asymptote is reached and sucking begins to decline. When an arbitrary decrement (e.g., 80% of the prehabituation rate for 2 min) is reached, the infant is assumed to have habituated, that is, to have become less interested in the stimulus, and one of two conditions is applied. Half of the babies are presented with a new speech stimulus (experimental group), and half are maintained on the original stimulus (control group). Discrimination of a new speech stimulus is demonstrated by a significant increase in sucking following habituation for the experimental group relative to the control group.

HAS has undergone several minor variations including redefinitions of high-amplitude sucks and stricter or more lenient criteria for habituation. Spring and Dale (1977) modified the paradigm to increase its sensitivity. In the HAS paradigm infants have only one opportunity to hear the old stimulus (prehabituation) contiguous with the new (posthabituation) stimulus. Should the infant be momentarily inattentive or in a sucking slump, the change might not be apparent. Instead of presenting only one change in stimulus posthabituation, Spring and Dale alternated the two stimuli in question following habituation. They reasoned that if the infant can discriminate stimulus 1 from stimulus 2, then two alternating stimuli presented after habituation would be more interesting and more noticeable to the infant.

Entus (1977) adapted HAS for dichotic listening with one sound presented under headphones to the right ear and a different sound presented to the left. Infants were more likely to detect changes in place of articulation when these changes were presented to the right ear. These results were interpreted to suggest that infants process speech sounds primarily in the left hemisphere.

HAS procedures can be used with infants between about 1 and 4 months of age. In general, data are reported for groups, because single-subject designs are difficult with this procedure. Perhaps the biggest drawback to the procedure is that it tends to yield all-or-nothing effects; that is, it either suggests a stimulus pair is discriminable or does not so suggest. It has not, therefore, been very useful for determining relative ease of discrimination of classes of speech sounds.

Heart Rate Procedure   The HR procedure originally applied to speech perception was first introduced by Moffitt (1971). The procedure differs markedly from HAS in that stimulus presentation is under the experimenter's control rather than under the infants' control. Stimuli are presented in fixed blocks of trials (usually eight blocks with 10 stimulus tokens per block) with a fixed interstimulus interval (1–2 sec) and a longer fixed interblock interval of 40 sec. Heart rate is generally recorded on a polygraph throughout the presentation of stimuli. In the prehabituation phase of the procedure, infant HR decelerates with the onset of each trial block and returns to baseline between blocks. (HR deceleration is thought to be an index of the orienting response in infants.) After several blocks are presented and deceleration no longer occurs, suggesting that the stimulus is no longer interesting to the infant, a new stimulus is introduced. If recovery of the orienting response is found (i.e., renewed deceleration to the stimulus occurs), discrimination is inferred.

The HR procedure, like HAS, has been modified to enhance its sensitivity. Leavitt et al. (1976) noted that the long interblock intervals of the traditional paradigm imposed memory requirements, possibly resulting in failure of infants to show discrimination of contrasts that would be discriminated in other tasks. To reduce the interval over which infants had to remember stimulus 1, Leavitt et al. presented 20 syllables of stimulus 1 (/ba/) followed immediately by 20 syllables of stimulus 2 (/ga/). The interstimulus interval remained constant throughout. Using this 20/20 paradigm, these researchers demonstrated discrimination of place of articulation in 6-week-olds, a discrimination that was not demonstrated with the standard technique. Best and Glanville (1978) and Glanville, Best, and Levenson (1977) have also adapted the HR procedure for a dichotic listening paradigm.

In principle, HR procedures can be used throughout the lifespan, but in practice they are used with infants between about 1 and 6 months of age. With older infants, frequent state changes introduce artifacts into the HR response. The procedure is mainly used in group studies, but it has been successfully adapted for individual subject and within-subject designs (Graham et al., 1978).

Visually Reinforced Infant Speech Discrimination   The visually reinforced head turn paradigm of Eilers, Wilson, and Moore (1976) is the most recent of the widely used infant speech discrimination procedures. The procedure involves presentation of a repeating background stimulus S_B (e.g., /ba/) that is changed to a contrasting stimulus $S\Delta$ (e.g., /pa/) for a fixed time interval, after which the original background is returned. In the change interval (during which $S\Delta$ is being presented) an infant head turn toward the speaker results in the activation of an animated toy (the reinforcer) at the sound source. The toy is housed in an opaque plexiglass box and can only be seen when lighted from within during activation. During testing, infants are entertained at midline with a series of quiet, visually interesting toys. A turn away from these toys toward the reinforcer when an $S\Delta$ is present constitutes a correct experimental trial. Turns toward the reinforcer during fixed intervals when S_B is present (control trials) constitute incorrect control trials. Because trial types are selected randomly, with approximately half of all trials being controls, the probability of success in any sufficiently large number of trials (i.e., 10 through 30) approximates 0.5 and is independent of the infant's probability of head turn. The measure of discrimination depends on the comparison of head turns to $S\Delta$ versus head turns to S_B (during control intervals). Obtained mean correct scores can be compared with theoretically predicted scores (of babies whose behavior is nondiscriminative or of computer-simulated random turning) by using the Z_m statistic (see Eilers, Gavin, & Oller, 1982, for details of the procedure, or Eilers & Gavin, 1981, for details of the simulation and statistics).

The VRISD paradigm has also been modified to accommodate different experimental questions. Kuhl (1976) adapted the procedure for use with multiple-token stimuli rather than single repeating tokens in order to assess perceptual constancy for phonemes. Trehub, Bull, and Schneider (1981b) made more radical changes to adapt the procedure to auditory psychophysics with infants. Their adaptation uses two speakers which alternately emit the background stimulus. $S\Delta$ is presented to one speaker while S_B is maintained in the other. The child's task is to turn toward S∆. Unlike in the standard VRISD paradigm, S∆ is maintained until the infant turns either correctly or incorrectly in this two-forced-choice paradigm. Probabilistic estimation by sequential testing (PEST) procedures are added for threshold and just-noticeable difference evaluation (Trehub, Bull, & Schneider, 1981a).

The VRISD paradigm and its modifications are useful for testing infants between 6 and 18 months of age. The procedure offers a number of advantages over HR and HAS for developmental studies and studies of handicapped populations. First, VRISD can be used to assess infants of broader age range than HAS or HR, although the latter procedures can be used with infants below 6 months whereas VRISD cannot. Second, VRISD can be used repeatedly with the same infant in either the cross-sectional or longitudinal designs to study a wide variety of speech discrimination behaviors. Third, because the reinforcement in VRISD is extrinsic (i.e., not the speech signal itself as in the HAS procedure), no assumptions need be made concerning the relative reinforcing value of different speech signals. Reinforcers may be chosen to maximize individual performance. Finally, VRISD procedures allow comparisons of relative discriminability across stimuli. Such comparisons typically are not possible in HAS or HR.

Discrimination Paradigms for Children 18–30 Months Old

Whereas methodologic attention has been focused on infants between birth and 1 year, the literature is less extensive on speech perception procedures for the 2-year-old. Three basic procedures have been used with varying success and documentation. They all involve the presentation of a stimulus item (syllabic) and a picture or three-dimensional representation of the stimulus item. These are not strictly discrimination tasks but are rather identification tasks; the tasks involve more than judgment of sameness or difference between stimuli. They require an association between a stimulus label and a particular referent. This difference in task content relative to the true discrimination tasks used for infants may help explain some of the discrepancy between the apparent abilities of infants in HR, HAS, and VRISD tasks and the abilities of 2-year-olds in identification tasks. One important future development would be paradigms that can directly compare discriminatory abilities with identification abilities in children 18–30 months old.

Real Word Procedures Each procedure testing identification of words has advantages and disadvantages. The first procedure involves discrimination of real word pairs selected from the child's native language. The child is asked to show, pick up, or look under the named item. The experimenter might say "Show me the bear [or the pear]." To be appropriate, the word pairs must be familiar to the child, differ minimally from a phonological or phonetic perspective, and be representable as objects or pictures the child can recognize. In addition, experimenters must verify that neither member of any pair is highly preferred by the child (who then might tend to select one member of the pair regardless of the instructions). Rigorously conducted studies use random orders of requests for each item and counterbalancing of stimulus position to avoid difficulties of interpretation associated with common response biases of 2-year-olds. Correct identification is inferred from either fixed criteria (e.g., the child achieves eight out of 10 trials correct) or running criteria (i.e., the child reaches a fixed criterion within a specified number of running trials, such as nine out of 10 consecutive correct trials within 30 total trials).

The scarcity of appropriate test pairs restricts this real word procedure. Children of this age usually do not know both members of most easily picturable minimal pairs. Otherwise the paradigm does work well. Locke (1971) used this real word paradigm with children whose mean age was 3 years, 4 months, and found that some 2-year-olds could complete the task. Zlatin and Koeningsknecht (1976) tested 2½- to 3-year-olds on four real word contrasts differing minimally in voice onset time in initial stop consonants. All of the children who passed the inclusion criteria succeeded in the task.

Nonsense Words To remedy the word availability limitation of real word paradigms, procedures may employ made-up words. What is gained in testing flexibility, however, is lost in the extensive training necessary to teach the association of nonsense labels with unfamiliar objects or pictures. In this procedure, two phonotactically acceptable sequences (e.g., for English, /ris/ and /wis/) are presented as the names of two unfamiliar objects, creatures, or drawings. After learning the names, the children are asked to identify the /wis/ or the /ris/. Shvachkin, as reported in Ferguson and Slobin (1973), used this technique with 1- to 2-year-old Russian children, and Garnica (1971) adapted the technique with English-speaking children aged 1 year, 5 months, to 1 year, 10 months. Edwards (1974) used the technique with subjects from 1 year, 8 months, to 3 years, 11 months, to test phonological contrasts for which appropriate real words could not be found.

The made-up word technique is hard to use because extensive teaching sessions are required before the actual discrimination study begins. A third procedure employs both real and made-up words to provide phonetic flexibility not available in the real word procedure while eliminating the teaching time associated with the made-up word procedure.

A Combined Approach—The "Shell Game" Procedure   The shell game is a modification of methodology employed by Vincent-Smith, Bricker, and Bricker (1974) to study receptive vocabulary acquisition. Eilers and Oller (1976) applied the technique successfully with children as young as 1 year, 4 months, and reported data for children aged 1 year, 10 months, to 2 years, 2 months. In the procedure, children are presented with two toys, one real toy familiar to the children (e.g., a ball, /bɔl/), and one unfamiliar nonsense toy, given an unfamiliar but phonotactically English label (e.g., /pɔl/). The children are encourage to play with the toys, name them, perform actions with them, and so on. (More recent versions of the shell game include strict criteria for assessing knowledge of the familiar item as well as of the rules of the game; see Oller & Eilers, 1980, for further details.) After this warm-up period, each object is placed on top of one of two closed containers, one of which houses a tangible reinforcer (usually an edible). The children are taught that the experimenter will tell them where the candy is (e.g., It's under the /bɔl/). If the children respond correctly, they find the edible. If their response is incorrect, they are asked to try again and listen carefully. A fixed number of trials (eight to 10) is presented per contrast; seven out of eight or eight out of 10 trials correct is considered evidence of correct identification.

This task allows investigation of more contrasts than can be studied by means of the real word procedure, because any familiar word can be minimally paired with various made-up words to form suitable testing contrasts. The technique can also be applied in less time than the made-up word procedure, because the child is not required to learn any new words to perform the task. Rather than learn the made-up word, children seem to work by a process of elimination, noticing whether or not the word pronounced by the experimenter is the name of the familiar object. If not, the children can assume the label refers to the unfamiliar object.

The shell game procedure has been modified for use with sign language stimuli instead of orally presented stimuli. Oller, Coleman, and Eilers (1978) found that a group of Down's syndrome children with mental age of about 2 years exhibited superior performance with certain signed stimuli as opposed to oral stimuli in the shell game. The intrinsic high interest in this hide-and-seek game combined with the relatively low memory requirements of the paradigm make this procedure particularly appealing for 2-year-olds and older retarded children.

Speech Perception Paradigms for Children 36 Months to 5 Years

During the age period from 3 to 5 years, methodologies for assessing speech perception are similar to those used with 2-year-olds. The tasks are generally more easily accomplished by the older children due to more advanced cognitive development, longer attention span, larger receptive vocabulary, and the ability to follow more complex directions. Most studies still employ identification paradigms, although some researchers have been successful with same/different discrimination paradigms. Procedures during this period fall into two categories: those using pictures of objects to represent speech items and relying on a pointing response, and those using response boxes or a button-push response. The lines blur between the two procedures when the response box houses pictures of the stimuli. Both procedures often employ tangible rewards, and both often employ pretraining and testing with nonminimal pairs. Sometimes real words are used and sometimes nonsense items. Examples of the use of response box procedures can be found in Krause and Fisher (in press), Abbs and Minifie (1969), and Gilbert (1976). Picture pointing is illustrated in Strange and Broen (1980) and Locke (1971). Locke and Goldstein (1971) provided an example of a true discrimination task for kindergarten-aged children. This study offers, to our knowledge, the youngest successful adaptation of a true discrimination paradigm other than HAS, HR, AER, or VRISD.

RESULTS

Directions

In studying speech perception in infants and children, attention has traditionally been directed toward illustrating a presumed innateness of speech perception capacities. Recently, there have been attempts to show that experience with sound affects speech discrimination skills very early in life and that skills are therefore not entirely innate. The occurrence of a controversy on this matter is surprising because common sense would seem to dictate that both innate and experiential factors are involved in discriminatory skills. It may be best to eschew the controversy and instead seek to characterize the young infant's speech discrimination capability and to describe how that capability changes across time. Future substantial achievements in that characterization will make possible a genuine theory of speech discrimination development and provide an interpretive framework for the role of speech discrimination skills in phonological errors of early childhood and in language disorders.

A useful description of speech perceptual abilities includes determination of the relative ease of speech contrast discrimination at various ages as well as an interpretation as to why some contrasts are easy and some are not. In fulfilling these goals, a clear indication of the underlying organization of the processing system that manages speech reception would be provided. The processing system will undoubtedly be multifaceted, and its description will involve the efforts of many specialists, including anatomists, hearing physiologists, psychologists, and linguists. A broad and comprehensive interdisciplinary approach will be necessary eventually; what can be done now is to provide a psycholinguistically oriented preliminary outline of certain levels of organization of mature speech processing systems, and to speculate about how these levels come to operate in the developing human.

The levels of organization discussed here are familiar to linguists as well as many others. Any novelty in this view is in the suggestions 1) that various theoretical linguistic levels constitute real processing stages of speech signals, and 2) that infants do not begin with all the levels of organization of the mature processor, but rather expand the system of levels with maturation and experience. The level model has been described in some detail by Eilers and Oller (1981) and is presented here in synoptic form only.

An Interpretive Model

The mature perceiver processes speech signals through a number of levels of organization. These levels are not merely features of linguistic competence but represent, in our view, real performance functions. This exposition focuses on a few of the levels and considers only segmental as opposed to suprasegmental perception.

The mature speech perception event begins with reception of an acoustic signal (level 1 in Figure 1). In an early stage of processing (but perhaps not the first stage), this signal is organized by *syllabification;*

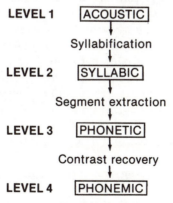

Figure 1.   Certain levels of processing in speech reception.

that is, prominences and low points of intensity in the waveform are located in accordance with the time frames of syllables in natural languages. This process yields syllabic units (level 2). The syllables are in turn analyzed into chunks in a process of *segment extraction,* yielding phonetic units (level 3). The phonetic units are categorized into functional groups in a process of *contrast recovery,* the output of which is a phonemic inventory (level 4).

The processing strategy is not merely an artifact of evolutionary linguistic accidents. Rather, each level serves a concrete function in efficient and accurate recovery of speech information. To comprehend speech, it is to the advantage of the receiver to create or develop these processes and accompanying levels. By syllabification, the perceiver breaks the acoustic waveform into analyzable chunks, and thus determines where in the stream of speech to locate segmental features. By phonetic classification, the perceiver groups together an enormous number of disparate acoustic types into a smaller number of recognizable categories. By contrast recovery, the perceiver unites the still large number of phonetic categories into fewer, more manageable functional phonemic types.

We suggest that infants are not endowed with a full-scale multileveled system, but that they develop it as a strategy for speech processing. The system begins relatively simply, with perhaps only an acoustic level and analysis strategies capable of handling certain distinctions in relatively short, simple signals. Later, infants find it possible to treat a greater variety of acoustic signals if they first seek syllabic prominences and then analyze them. At a still later stage, it is found beneficial to classify into a small number of groups the segmental elements resulting from the analysis of syllables. The classification unites a large inventory of syllable-sized chunks into a more manageable, smaller inventory of segmental phonetic elements. As real words are learned, children come to understand that some contrastive segmental units are relevant to their meaning system whereas others are not. The children then develop a mapping between the segmental phonetic units and functional phonemic ones, ensuring in the process that many phonetic distinctions that are irrelevant can be systemically ignored in real speech events and that the small number of necessary phonemic distinctions can be noticed.

It is possible that children have some innate predisposition to develop a multileveled processing strategy, and they may even have some characteristics of the strategy from the beginning. Our hypothesis is, however, that children do not have the in adult listener's systematic distinction of low-level acoustic categories from high-level linguistic ones. The extent of the difference between low-level and high-level units is much greater in mature listeners, and, we contend, it is developed in response to the needs of the speech processing task.

The Evidence

Normally Developing Infants The present model predicts substantial development of speech reception skills, but does not contend that infants should begin life unable to perceive distinctions among speech sounds. In fact, it is well documented that the human infant has a broad range of discrimination abilities. Infants have been shown to discriminate synthetic speech contrasts involving consonants including: /ba-ga/[1] (Moffitt, 1971, in HR; Morse, 1972, in HAS), /ba-pa/, /da-ta/ (Eimas et al., 1971; Eimas, 1974, in HAS; Eilers et al., 1976, in VRISD), /dæ-gæ/ (Miller & Morse, 1976, in HAS), and /ra-la/ (Eimas, 1975, in HAS). Naturally produced consonantal contrasts shown to be discriminable include: /ba-pa/ (Trehub & Rabinovitch, 1972, in HAS), /sa-va/, /sa-ʃa/ (Eilers & Minifie, 1975, in HAS), and /du-tu/ (Eilers et al., 1981, in VRISD). Further, vowel contrasts have been shown to be discriminable in /i-a/, /i-u/, /pa-pi/, /ta-ti/, /pa-pu/ (Trehub, 1973, in HAS), /i-I/ (Swoboda, Morse, & Leavitt, 1976, in HAS; Eilers & Oller, 1980, in VRISD), and /u-ʊ/ (Eilers, Gavin, & Oller, 1980, in VRISD).

These results have provided a view of infant auditory capabilities that is in stark contrast with earlier assumptions. In the enthusiasm about these abilities, however, recent interpretations were carried too far, and researchers tended to overemphasize the similarities between adult and infant perception. The overemphasis focused on an important pattern, seen in both adult and infant responses to speech; this pattern is referred to as "categorical perception." As an example, consider the continuum of voice onset time (VOT). A syllable phonetically transcribed as [ba] is said to have voicing lead, meaning that vocal cord vibration (voicing) begins before the lips are separated. The amount of voicing lead can be specified by acoustic analysis; for example, in a typical Spanish [ba] the value might be –50 msec VOT. The syllable [pa], on the other hand, usually has a VOT near zero in Spanish as well as in English, and the syllable [pʰa], which occurs in English as phonemic /pa/ but does not occur in Spanish, normally has a VOT of +30 msec or more. The phonemic English contrast of /ba-pa/, transcribed phonetically as [pa-pʰa], has been shown to be perceived categorically, which means that discrimination of VOT within the category of [pa] (for exam-

---

[1]Slashes indicate phonemic (in this paper English phonemic) rather than phonetic transcription. American English elements that are written in slashes as /b,g,d/ and /p,k,t/ here would be rendered as [p,k,t] and [pʰ,kʰ,tʰ], respectively, in phonetic notation.

ple, from − 10 to + 20 VOT) is relatively more difficult for listeners than discrimination of VOT between the categories of [pa] and [pʰa] (as from +10 to +40 VOT). A boundary for the discrimination has been determined at about +30 msec VOT, and that boundary proves to be appropriate for both adults and infants (Eimas et al., 1971, in HAS; Eilers, Wilson, & Moore, 1979, in VRISD). A variety of additional studies have supported the categorical nature of infant speech perception and its similarity with adult patterns (see review in Morse, 1978).

The interpretive error of early studies lies in the assumption that the categoricalness of infant speech perception indicated, in itself, that infants processed speech in a "phonetic" mode (i.e., a special speech mode). That assumption has since been attacked in a number of ways. Detractors of the phonetic processing theory argued that categoricalness by itself could not prove that the mode of processing was special to speech. Other perceptual functions, such as music, might also turn out to be categorical. Indeed, Cutting and Rosner (1974) provided evidence that adults perceived various nonspeech stimuli categorically, and Jusczyk et al. (1977, in HAS) indicated the same to be true of infants. Although some of these results have been questioned with regard to inappropriateness of stimulus preparation (cf. Rosen and Howell, in press), the logical point of their challenge is unimpeached. To show that a particular pattern of perception indicates a "speech mode," it is necessary to show that other modes of perception do not also display the pattern.

Of importance here is a discussion by Eimas (1974, in HAS), who showed continuous (noncategorical) infant discrimination of F_2 transitions cueing /d–g/ when the transitions were presented in a 40-msec isolated chirp. In the same study, infants categorically discriminated /da–ga/ syllables with the very same transitions. Eimas' contention, that the occurrence of categorical perception is dependent upon the contrast being speech, remains uncertain because a variety of differences occur between the isolated F_2 transition stimuli (chirps) and the speech syllable stimuli. One such difference is that the syllables were nearly four times the duration of the chirps. Perhaps categorical perception of such transitions depends on signal duration, in which case the results are not uniquely attributable to a speech mode of processing. Thus, although the results of Eimas' study leave open (and perhaps even weakly support) the involvement of a speech mode of processing, they do not prove its existence in infants.

Beyond the need for additional evidence concerning perception of various kinds of stimuli, detractors of the phonetic processing theory have also argued that support of the theory depends on indications that nonhumans process speech information differently from humans. Yet results of studies on primates and other mammals have noted important similarities between human and nonhuman speech perception. For example, Kuhl and Miller (1975a) gave indications that chinchillas perceive the VOT continuum for labial stop consonants quite the way humans do (i.e., categorically and with near identical boundary values). Morse and Snowdon (1975) showed that rhesus monkeys discriminated a /bæ-dæ/ continuum so that between-category perceptions were better than within-category. Although within-category perception was better than chance in the monkeys, the pattern is still reminiscent of that in humans, who also show within-category discrimination in many cases (cf. Carney, Widin, & Viemeister, 1977; Eilers et al., 1979a). Data on nonhuman speech perception, then, refute the idea that categorical perception is a phenomenon of a special speech mode. Instead the data seem to suggest that categorical perception of certain stimulus types is natural to mammalian audition.

The multileveled speech processing model proposed here offers the possibility of interpreting speech perception of infants as an auditory/acoustic phenomenon in which special speech reception capabilities are not present at the onset. The model allows for the possibility that *some* special speech abilities do obtain in the infant but that these become more elaborate as the child develops.

Even in the early months of life, however, it is reasonable within the model to expect some speech contrasts to be more difficult than others. Although the model makes no claim that any contrasts are absolutely nondiscriminable, it predicts the existence of a hierarchy of difficulty with some speech contrasts easier for infants and some more difficult.

Evidence from a variety of studies supports this view. Eilers and Minifie (1975, in HAS) showed relatively easy discrimination of /sa-ʃa/ but failed to show discrimination of /sa-za/. Eimas et al. (1971, in HAS) found discrimination of English /ba-pa/ (phonetically [pa-pʰa]), but Eimas (1975, in HAS) presented evidence that the homorganic lead contrast (phonetically [ba-pa]) was much more difficult. Similar VOT results have been presented by Eilers et al. (1979) in VRISD and by Aslin et al. (1979) in VRISD. For older infants (6–12 months), Eilers et al. (1980), using the VRISD paradigm, with its greater potential than HAS for comparing contrast difficulty, indicated a wide continuum of difficulty for various minimally paired speech contrasts.

For the present model, one particularly interesting result (Trehub, 1976, in HAS) is that a VOT contrast embedded in a two-syllable nonsense item was discriminable by infants, but the same VOT contrast embedded in a three-syllable context was not. Such results support the idea that infant syllabification strategies are not as advanced as those of older listeners. The model encourages an interpretation of these data in which infants are seen as failing to discriminate sounds in multisyllabic words because they do not have the mature skills needed to chunk acoustic information so that key aspects of contrasting words can be efficiently compared. It seems possible, then, that syllabification strategies do develop in the early months.

The model also predicts that phonetic classification abilities (i.e., abilities to recognize abstract similarities among concretely dissimilar items) develop substantially. Attempts have been made to show such abilities in the first year of life. Fodor, Garrett, and Brill (1975) provided weak indications that infants could recognize the syllables /ba-bi-bu/ as a natural group and the syllables /ga-gi-gu/ as another natural group. The conditioned head turn paradigm (not VRISD) that they employed with these 3- to 4-month-olds has not to our knowledge been successfully used elsewhere (see the description of paradigm difficulties in Kuhl, 1981).

Kuhl and Miller (1975) have demonstrated in a HAS paradigm that infants (4 to 16 weeks old) can discriminate /a/ from /i/ even when pitch contours were varied in a contrast-irrelevant fashion. At the same time, infants failed to demonstrate pitch contours when vowel color ranged from /a/ to /i/ in an irrelevant fashion. Kuhl (1979) pointed out that these results show infant abilities to tolerate phonetic distractions to some extent, but do not demonstate an ability to recognize similarity when critical features of phonetic elements vary. In later work (Kuhl, 1979, 1981; Holmberg, Morgan, & Kuhl, 1977), an elaborated VRISD paradigm was used to illustrate that infants can classify (or at least learn to classify) various exemplars of the vowel /a/ as distinct from exemplars of /u/ or /i/ independent of variations in speaker voice or pitch. Similarly, subjects learned to classify an initial /s/ (in sa–si–su) as distinct from /ʃ/ (in ʃa–ʃi–ʃu), and initial /f/ (in fa–fi–fu) as distinct from /θ/ (in θa–θi–θu). Experiments with /s–ʃ/ and /f–θ/ in syllable final position also showed classificatory abilities.

The results overall show the infant capable to some extent of phonetic classification, at least with some training as provided in the study by Holmberg et al. (1977). In this sense these data represent an important step in verification of infant speech capacities. The results present some difficulties in interpretation due to the use of a running success criterion; infants were judged successful when they reached eight or nine out of 10 consecutive correct trials. Eilers et al. (1981) provided computer simulation data showing that an 8-of-10 criterion is reached by chance in 50% of instances after only 40 trials. Because the subjects studied by Holmberg et al. (1977) reached the generalization criterion on final /f-θ/ after 33–58 trials, it is hard to tell whether they were successful in classification of /f/ and /θ/. Kuhl (1979) used a 9-of-10 criterion (with considerably lower probability of false positives as shown in the computer simulation) in her /a/-/i/ work and presented data showing 19–29 trials to criterion across four subjects who were coping with both talker and pitch variations. In the case of /a–i/, then, classification abilities seem clearly demonstrated. Comparing the various studies, Kuhl (1981) cautiously argued that the larger numbers of trials to criterion in, for example, the case of /f-θ/ indicates a higher discrimination difficulty level for the latter contrast. The higher discrimination difficulty surely would affect classification of /f/s and /θ/s as well.

Classification abilities for speech elements may, then, exist in the first year of life in human infants. The most convincing data are from Kuhl (1979), indicating that /a-i/ contrasts were discriminable in spite of pitch and talker variations even on the first experimental trials in which the variations occurred. The data suggest that infants have substantial natural sorting abilities. With this paradigm, it is possible that the sorting rule used by the infants was formulated during the training trials (an average of 25 training trials occurred before the first experimental trial) but the data show the infant can sort and ignore irrelevant variations as soon as it is necessary to do so in the paradigm. Nevertheless, to say the infant is a natural sorter of /a/ and /i/ is not to say that the capacity for sorting is phonetic as opposed to auditory. Kuhl pointed out that the mammalian auditory system seems to sort vowels such as /a/ and /i/ (cf. Baru, 1975, for the dog; Burdick & Miller, 1975, for the chinchilla). The animal data again offer an important perspective, preventing us from prematurely assuming that infants have established a phonetic level of processing.

One necessary although not sufficient aspect of illustrating the development of a phonetic level is the demonstration of changing infant abilities across time in processing of phonetic segments. Eilers et al. (1977) in a developmental VRISD study showed that discrimination of some speech sound contrasts (e.g., /sa–za/, /θi–fi/) improved from 6 to 12 months of age. Although further studies are needed and the difficulties of comparing across ages given differences in task competency need to be addressed, these results provide an early view of changing speech discrimination abilities. Such changes clearly continue as the child gets older. Zlatin and Koeningsknecht (1976) have provided evidence of boundary sharpening in perception of VOT in children between 2 and 6 years of age.

Not only do children's abilities seem to sharpen, but they also seem to change by contrast facilitation and consequent creation of new categories. Although infants learning English show considerable difficulty in discriminating the Spanish [ba/pa] contrast, children whose languages possess a prevoicing contrast seem to do better with it (Streeter, 1976; Lasky, Syrdal-Lasky, & Klein, 1975). Eilers, Gavin, and Wilson (1979) demonstrated in one study that a group of Spanish-learning babies (6–9 months) were significantly more able to discriminate the Spanish [ba/pa] contrast than were English-learning babies. Both Spanish- and English-learning babies proved readily capable of discrimination of English [pa/p^{h}a]. Such results suggest that babies begin life with a basic auditory tuning which allows relatively free discrimination of VOT in the lag region (English boundary), but that experience is necessary to tune the lead region (Spanish boundary) for discrimination. Because the 6- to 9-month-old Spanish-learning infant has apparently already adopted a new perceptual posture for VOT, it is worth asking whether a phonetic level of processing has been established as well. The answer to that question depends in part on the outcome of studies involving short-term experience in human infants and nonhumans. In any case, additional crosslinguistic studies continue to verify that human infants' speech perception skills adapt to specifics of their language environment (Eilers, Gavin, & Oller, in press; Eilers & Oller, in press) during the first year of life.

The establishment of a phonetic level of processing depends upon the onset of true speech category, not merely auditory category, development. To monitor phonemic processing, it will be necessary to compare performance of young children in real speech identification tasks (e.g., pointing to named objects on command) and strict speech discrimination tasks (e.g., same/different). It is important to determine whether young children ignore nonphonemic contrasts in real speech identification even though the contrasts are discriminable in nonmeaningful contexts. Oller and Eilers (in press) have presented preliminary evidence suggesting that 2-year-olds may ignore certain discriminable contrasts in real speech settings. The study found that children do better in an identification task when they are responding to real phonemic contrasts of their native language (for example, tap versus trill for Spanish-learning children) than when responding to a contrast that is not phonemic in their language (for example, English r versus w for Spanish-learning children). The Spanish-learning children failed to provide evidence of discriminatory identification on the foreign (English) contrast even though the contrast had been shown to be discriminable by Spanish infants in a VRISD paradigm. Thus it seems that, at least in some cases, 2-year-old children may ignore discriminable foreign contrasts in real speech identification. If so, we need to account for the pattern of performance by including a phonemic processing level in the model of speech reception skills.

Handicapped Populations   Although we are just beginning to acquire an adequate data base for theories of normal perceptual development, the same data base is not available for handicapped populations. In fact, only a few isolated studies of handicapped infant speech perception are available in the literature. These studies focus on infants who are expected to show language disorders later in development. The interest in speech perception of handicapped children is twofold. There is both a theoretical interest and a clinical need to determine the speech perception capacities of handicapped infants and children. This section briefly reviews available studies but focuses on results concerning somewhat older children diagnosed as language-disabled.

Research with Infants   Swoboda, Morse, and Leavitt (1976) used the HAS procedure to compare discrimination of isolated vowels by 8-week-old normal and at-risk infants. Stimulus pairs were spaced in logarithmic steps along the /i/ to /ɪ/ continuum such that some pairs were within either the /i/ or the /ɪ/ category and others were between categories. Normal and at-risk infant groups evidenced similar discrimination of both within and between stimuli. Later, Swoboda et al. (1978) investigated the role of memory in infant discrimination of vowels in both normal and at-risk infants. This study used very brief vowels (60 as opposed to 240 msec in the previous study). Results revealed reliable between-category but not within-category discrimination. More importantly, at-risk infants differed in several respects from normals. They differed significantly in initial attention to the stimuli, were significantly poorer at discrimination of short vowels, and were relatively more affected by a long interval between the last presentation of the old stimulus and the first presentation of the new stimulus. The authors suggested that these data may reflect different attentional and memory capabilities. These differences may reflect processes specific to speech perception or, more likely, general neurologic/cognitive constraints imposed by a combination of neonatal stresses or handicaps.

Graham and her colleagues (1978) studied an anencephalic infant's ability to discriminate a /ba–ga/ contrast. In the HR paradigm, the infant evidenced attention to, discrimination of, and memory for the /ba/ and /ga/ stimuli. This startling finding suggests that the HR and HAS paradigm may be reflecting subcortical processing with very young normal infants. Although the results of Graham et al. (1978) and of Swoboda et al. (1978) do not provide unambiguous indications of exactly how speech is processed, they suggest that much of speech (at least with monosyllables) can be handled subcortically and even when there is probable immaturity of or injury to the brain. Our own model of speech perception finds support in this view since it posits possible early discrimination skills for speech in normal infants on the basis of purely auditory function. The work by Graham et al. (1978) is particularly supportive, because the stimulus pair discriminated by the anencephalic babies was one involving a formant transition distinction, precisely the sort of distinction that has traditionally been thought of as quintessentially a speech contrast.

An additional study with children under age 3 on discrimination of vowel and consonant minimal pairs used the VRISD paradigm. Eilers et al. (1980) compared the abilities of normally developing infants (7 months old) to those of severely retarded infants and children (mean IQ was 38.4; mean age was 3 years, 2 months; range was 2 years, 1 month, to 4 years, 2 months). Both groups evidenced discrimination of a /bɪt–bit/ contrast as well as an /awa–ara/ contrast. However, the data suggested that retarded children had relatively more difficulty processing the /awa–ara/ contrast, which was cued by rapid spectral changes (often associated with consonant discrimination) than they did the /bɪt–bit/ contrast, which was cued by steady-state spectral information (often associated with perception of slowly articulated words). The results suggest that retarded children's problems may not be in specific "speech" processing abilities, but rather in handling rapidly presented information. Again the pattern is consistent with a model assuming that basic auditory processing abilities account for the bulk of infant perceptual phenomena related to brief speech stimuli. These results also parallel those of Tallal (1976), who investigated similar phenomena with older dysphasic children.

Research with Older Children   Research of Tallal and colleagues with children who manifest specific language delay (i.e., not global retardation) or dysfunction required overcoming the difficulties of locating homogenous groups. Stark and Tallal (1981) suggested rigorous inclusion and exclusion criteria for specifically language-delayed children.

After eliminating children with sensory, cognitive, or emotional problems, and those with articulation disorders, children still showed marked variation in their language-related disorders. Of the children referred as specifically language-disordered, two-thirds showed evidence of mixed disorders (e.g., cognitive and language delay) or were not sufficiently impaired to differ significantly from normals. The authors noted that younger children were often referred with minimal problems, whereas older children were referred with more substantial problems. Thus, under the best of circumstances, research with such a population must treat a variety of interpretive problems.

Nevertheless, certain points in the literature seem reliable. First, certain perceptual constraints seem to operate with children referred to as developmentally dysphasic or language-delayed. We rely heavily on the work of Tallal and her colleagues, because their populations are precisely and carefully defined, as are their stimulus selection and testing procedures.

Tallal and Piercy (1973b) found that developmentally dysphasic children aged 6–9 years discriminated a 100-Hz tone from a 305-Hz tone at durations of 75–250 msec with large (250 msec) interstimulus intervals (ISI). As the ISI was decreased to less than 150 msec, dysphasics differed from normals in discrimination of tones with durations less than 125 msec. With tone durations of 175 msec and ISI less than 15 msec, dysphasics differed significantly from normals. Thus, dysphasics seemed sensitive to the total duration of the stimulus pattern. Long stimuli were less likely to yield perceptual deficits even when ISIs were short. These authors also reported that tone duration influenced performance on a serial order task. Dysphasics were only successful in ordering sequences when the individual tones exceeded 250 msec. The advantage of longer stimuli for the dysphasic children was not maintained for sequences involving four to five elements. The authors concluded that dysphasics have significant auditory processing deficits that are temporal in nature. They suggested that the deficits adversely affect consonant perception more than vowel perception, because consonants more commonly involve rapidly changing cues.

Tallal and Piercy (1973a) tested the same dysphasic and normal children with synthesized vowel (/ɛ/ and /æ/) and consonant (/ba/ and /da/) patterns. As predicted from the earlier experiment using 250-msec vowels, dysphasic children performed well until as many as five elements were presented. Results with consonants reflected inferior performance by dysphasics when compared to normals or to their own discrimination of vowels. The authors interpreted these results to suggest one of two possibilities. The first is that dysphasics are unable to process the rapidly changing spectral cues that differentiate /ba/ from /da/ because these cues change during a brief 43-msec window; the second possibility is that dysphasics do not process transitional information at all.

To differentiate between these two possibilities, Tallal and Piercy (1975) studied perception of brief vowels and consonants with extended transition durations. They found dysphasic children were relatively poor in discriminating beween two 43-msec vowels as well as between consonants with 43-msec transition durations. Dysphasics did not differ from normals in their ability to discriminate consonant stimuli with 95-msec transition durations. The authors concluded that dysphasics had a specific auditory dysfunction limited to perception of brief components. A lack of ability to process rapidly occurring information in dysphasic children does not suggest a problem that is speech-limited, but rather a problem that may affect speech in especially deleterious ways. Speech includes many rapid spectral changes, and speech comprehension depends on their reception. Dysphasic children, then, may show both problems of speech processing and general deficits in processing of any rapid information. Our model of infant speech perception easily incorporates such thinking, since the data encourage interpretation of speech perception as involving crucial basic auditory or more general sensory capacities without requiring an assumption of speech-specific processing for simple monosyllabic stimuli in discrimination tasks.

Additional data on dysphasic children suggest that their problem of language disability may relate to general auditory detection insufficiencies rather than to speech-specific defects. Springer (1973) and Tobey et al. (1976) suggest higher error rates on dichotic listening tasks for language-delayed children. They note, however, that these children exhibit a right ear advantage comparable to that of normal controls. Rosenthal (1974) used these results and others to suggest that faulty signal detection strategies underlie dysphasic childrens' poor performance on auditory tasks requiring detection of brief segments. He noted that when signals are "detected," the auditory system functions normally.

It is clear that the research reported here represents only a beginning in understanding deviant auditory development. We are just starting to explore basic auditory processes and their relationship with language dysfunction.

CONCLUSION

The study of infant speech perception has come a long way in 10 years. A variety of useful testing paradigms have been developed, and a number of provocative research results have been obtained. We have also come a long way from the original "innateness" model. The multileveled scheme suggested in the present paper offers a quite different view and, it is hoped, a more felicitous interpretive model. The current model may be relatively conservative in requiring specific data from animal studies and studies employing nonspeech stimuli before positing specific speech abilities, but the model is also relatively liberal in assuming a rich linguistic processing system in mature listeners. We look forward to the next 10 years with the hope that in that time we can substantially clarify the nature of speech processing in infants and elucidate the manner of its development.

REFERENCES

Abbs, M., and Minifie, F. 1969. The effects of acoustic cues in fricatives on perceptual confusions in preschool children. Journal of the Acoustical Society of America 45:1535–1542.

Aslin, R. N., Hennessy, B. L., Pisoni, D. B., and Perrey, A. J. 1979. Individual infants' discrimination of VOT: Evidence for three modes of voicing. Paper presented at the Biennial Meeting of the Society for Research in Child Development, San Francisco, March 17, 1979.

Baru, A. V. 1975. Discrimination of synthesized vowels [a] and [i] with varying parameters in dog. In: G. Fant and M. Tathan (eds.), Auditory Analysis and the Perception of Speech. Academic Press, London.

Best, C. T., and Glanville, B. B. 1978. Cerebral asymmetries in speech and timbre discrimination by 2-, 3-, and 4-month-old infants. Paper presented at the International Conference on Infant Studies, Providence, R.I., March 10–12, 1978.

Burdick, C. K., and Miller, J. D. 1975. Speech perception by the chinchillas: Discrimination of sustained /a/ and /i/. Journal of the Acoustical Society of America 58:415–427.

Carney, A. E., Widin, G. P., and Viemeister, N. F. 1977. Non-categorical perception of stop consonants differing in VOT. Journal of the Acoustical Society of America 62(4):961–970.

Cutting, J. E., and Rosner, B. S. 1974. Categories and boundaries in speech and music. Perception and Psychophysics 16:564–570.

Edwards, M. 1974. Perception and production in child phonology: The testing of four hypotheses. Journal of Child Language 1:205–220.

Eilers, R. E., and Gavin, W. J. 1981. The evaluation of infant speech perception skills: Statistical techniques and theory development. In: R. Stark (ed.), Language Behavior in Infancy and Early Childhood. Elsevier North-Holland, New York.

Eilers, R. E. and Minifie, F. D. 1975. Fricative discrimination in early infancy. Journal of Speech and Hearing Research 18(1):158–167.

Eilers, R. E., and Oller, D. K. 1976. The role of speech discrimination in developmental sound substitutions. Journal of Child Language 3:319–329.

Eilers, R. E., and Oller, D. K. 1980. A comparative study of speech perception in young severely retarded children and normally developing infants. Journal of Speech and Hearing Research 23:419–428.

Eilers, R. E., and Oller, D. K. 1981. Cross-linguistic perspective of infant speech perception. Paper presented at the Society for Research in Child Development, Boston, 1981.

Eilers, R. E., and Oller, D. K. 1982. Infant speech perception: Environmental contributions. In: S. Trehub and B. Schneider (eds.), Auditory Development in Infancy. Plenum Press. In press.

Eilers, R. E., Gavin, W. J., and Oller, D. K. 1980. Cross-linguistic studies in infant speech perception. Paper presented at the Boston Child Language Conference, Boston, October 1980.

Eilers, R. E., Gavin, W. J., and Oller, D. K. 1982. Cross-linguistic perception in infancy. The role of linguistic experience. Journal of Child Language. In press.

Eilers, R. E., Gavin, W. J., and Wilson, W. R. 1979a. Linguistic experience and phonemic perception in infancy: A cross-linguistic study. Child Development 50:14–18.

Eilers, R. E., Morse, P. A., Gavin, W. J., and Oller, D. K. 1981. The perception of voice-onset-time in infancy. Journal of the Acoustical Society of America 70:955–965.

Eilers, R. E., Wilson, W. R., and Moore, J. M. 1979. Speech perception in the language innocent and the language wise: The perception of VOT. Journal of Child Language 6:1–18.

Eilers, R. E., Wilson, W. R., and Moore, J. M. 1976. Discrimination of synthetic prevoiced labial stops by infants and adults. Journal of the Acoustical Society of America 60(Suppl. 1):S91(A).

Eilers, R. E., Wilson, W. R., and Moore, J. M. 1977. Developmental changes in speech discrimination by infants. Journal of Speech and Hearing Research 20:766–780.

Eimas, 1974. P. Linguistic processing of speech by young infants. In: R. Schiefelbusch and L. Lloyd (eds.), Language Perspectives: Acquisition, Retardation and Intervention, pp. 55–73. University Park Press, Baltimore.

Eimas, P. D. 1975. Speech perception in early infancy. In: Infant Perception: From Sensation to Cognition, Volume II: Perception of Space, Speech and Sound, pp. 193–231. Academic Press, New York.

Eimas, P. D., Siqueland, E., Jusczyk, P., and Vigorito, J. 1971. Speech perception in infants. Science 171:303–306.

Entus, A. 1977. Hemisphere asymmetry in processing of dichotically presented speech and nonspeech stimuli by infants. In: S. Segalowitz and F. Gruber (eds.), Language Development and Neurological Theory, pp. 63–73. Academic Press, New York.

Fodor, J., Garrett, M., and Brill, S. 1975. Pi ka pu: The perception of speech sounds by prelinguistic infants. Perception and Psychophysics 18:74–78.

Garnica, O. 1971. The development of the perception of phonemic differences in initial consonants by English-speaking children: A pilot study. Stanford University Papers and Reports in Child Language Development 3:1–29.

Gilbert, J. H. V. 1976. Discrimination learning of stops and fricatives in CVC syllables, by five-year-olds. Canadian Journal of Linguistics.

Glanville, B., Best, C., and Levenson, R. 1977. A cardiac measure of cerebral asymmetries in infant auditory perception. Developmental Psychology 13:54–59.

Graham, F., Leavitt, L., Strock, B., and Brown, J. 1978. Precocious cardiac orienting in a human anencephalic infant. Science 199:322–324.

Holmberg, T. L., Morgan, K. A., and Kuhl, P. A. 1977. Speech perception in early infancy: Discrimination of fricative consonants. Journal of the Acoustical Society of America 62(Suppl. 1):S99(A).

Jusczyk, P., Rosner, B., Cutting, J., Foard, C., and Smith, L. 1977. Categorical perception of nonspeech sounds in 2-month-old infants. Perception and Psychophysics 2:50–54.

Kuhl, P. 1976. Speech perception in early infancy: Perceptual constancy for vowel categories. Journal of the Acoustical Society of America 60(Suppl. 1):S90.

Kuhl, P. 1979. Speech perception in early infancy: Perceptual constancy for spectrally dissimilar vowel categories. Journal of the Acoustical Society of America 66(6):1668-1679.

Kuhl, P. 1981. Auditory category formation and developmental speech perception. In: R. Stark (ed.), Language Behavior in Infancy and Early Childhood. Elsevier North-Holland, New York.

Kuhl, P., and Miller, J. 1975a. Speech perception in early infancy: Discrimination of speech-sound categories. Journal of the Acoustical Society of America 58(Suppl. 1):556(A).

Kuhl, P., and Miller, J. 1975b. Speech perception by the chinchilla: Voiced-voiceless distinction in alveolar plosive consonants. Science 190:69-72.

Krause, S. E., and Fisher, H. 1982. Developmental use of vowel duration as a clue to postvocalic voicing: A perception study. Journal of the Acoustical Society of America. In press.

Lasky, R. E., Syrdal-Lasky, A., and Klein, R. E. 1975. VOT discrimination by four to six and a half month old infants from Spanish environments. Journal of Experimental Child Psychology 20:215-225.

Leavitt, L. A., Brown, J. W., Morse, P. A., and Graham, F. K. 1976. Cardiac orienting and auditory discrimination in 6-week-old infants. Developmental Psychology 12:514-523.

Locke, J. L. 1971. Phoneme perception in two- and three-year-old children. Perceptual and Motor Skills 32:215-217.

Locke, J. L., and Golstein, J. I. 1971. Children's identification and discrimination of phonemes. British Journal of Disorders of Communication 6:107-112.

Miller, C., and Morse, P. 1976. The "heart" of categorical speech discrimination in young infants. Journal of Speech and Hearing Research 19:578-589.

Moffitt, A. R. 1971. Consonant cue perception by twenty- to twenty-four-week-old infants. Child Development 42(3):717-731.

Molfese, D. L., Freeman, R. B., and Palermo, D. S. 1975. The ontogeny of brain laterilization for speech and nonspeech stimuli. Brain and Language 2:356-368.

Morse, P. A. 1972. The discrimination of speech and nonspeech stimuli in early childhood. Journal of Experimental Child Psychology 14:477-492.

Morse, P. A. 1978. Infant speech perception origins, processes and alpha centauri. In: F. Minifie and L. Lloyd (eds.), Communicative and Cognitive Abilities—Early Behavioral Assessment, pp. 195-227. University Park Press, Baltimore.

Morse, P., and Snowdon, C. 1975. An investigation of categorical speech discrimination by rhesus monkeys. Perception and Psychophysics 17:9-16.

Oller, D. K., and Eilers, R. E. 1983. Speech identification in Spanish and English-learning two-year-olds. Journal of Speech and Hearing Research. In press.

Oller, D. K., Coleman, D., and Eilers, R. E. 1978. A comparative study of discriminability of signed and spoken vocabulary. Paper presented at the Southeastern Regional Conference on Human Development, Atlanta, April, 1978.

Rosen, S. M., and Howell, P. 1983. Plucks and bows are not categorically perceived. Perception and Psychophysics. In press.

114   Eilers and Oller

Rosenthal, W. S. 1974. The role of perception in child language disorders: A theory based on faulty signal detection strategies. Paper presented at the 50th Annual Convention of the American Speech and Hearing Association, Las Vegas, November, 1974.

Shvachkin, N. 1973. The development of phonemic speech perception in early childhood. In: C. A. Ferguson and D. I. Slobin (eds.), Studies of Child Language Development. Holt, Rinehart and Winston, New York.

Spring, D. R., and Dale, P. S. 1977. Discrimination of linguistic stress in early infancy. Journal of Speech and Hearing Research 20:224–231.

Springer, S. 1973. Hemisphere specialization in linguistically impaired children. Paper presented to the New York State Orton Society Conference, New York, March, 1973.

Stark, R. E., and Tallal, P. 1981. Selection of children with specific language deficits. Journal of Speech and Hearing Research 46(2):114–122.

Strange, W., and Broen, P. 1980. Perception and production of approximant consonants by three-year-olds: A first study. In: G. Yeni-Komshian, J. F. Kavanagh, and C. A. Ferguson (eds.), Child Phonology: Perception, Production and Deviation. Academic Press, New York.

Streeter, L. A. 1976. Language perception of two-month-old infants shows effects of both innate mechanisms and experience. Nature 259:39–41.

Swoboda, P., Kass, J., Morse, P., and Leavitt, L. 1978. Memory factors in infant vowel discrimination of normal and at-risk infants. Child Development 49:332–334.

Swoboda, P., Morse, P., and Leavitt, L. 1976. Continuous vowel discrimination in normal and at-risk infants. Child Development 47:459–465.

Tallal, P. 1976. Rapid auditory processing in normal and disordered language development. Journal of Speech and Hearing Research 19(3):561–571.

Tallal, P., and Piercy, M. 1973a. Developmental aphasia: Impaired rate of nonverbal processing as a function of sensory modality. Neuropsychologia 11:389–398.

Tallal, P., and Piercy, M. 1973b. Defects of non-verbal auditory perception in children with developmental aphasia. Nature 241:468–469.

Tallal, P., and Piercy, M. 1975. Developmental aphasia: The perception of brief and extended stop consonants. Neuropsychologia 13:69–74.

Tobey, E. A., Cullen, J. K., Gallagher, A. F., and Ramp, D. L. 1976. Performance of children with auditory-processing disorders on a dichotic stop-vowel identification task. Paper presented at the 52nd Annual Meeting of the American Speech and Hearing Association, Houston, November, 1976.

Trehub, S. 1973. Infants' sensitivity to vowel and tonal contrasts. Developmental Psychology 9:81–96.

Trehub, S. 1976. Infants' discrimination of two-syllable stimuli: The role of temporal factors. Paper presented at the meeting of the American Speech and Hearing Association, Houston, Texas, November, 1976.

Trehub, S., Bull, D., and Schneider, B. 1981a. Infants' detection of speech in noise. Journal of Speech and Hearing Research 24:202–206.

Trehub, S., Bull, D., and Schneider, B. 1981b. Infant speech and non-speech perception: A review and re-evaluation. In: R. L. Schiefelbusch and D. Bricker (eds.), Early Language: Acquisition and Intervention. University Park Press, Baltimore.

Trehub, S. E., and Rabinovitch, M. S. 1972. Auditory-linguistic sensitivity in early infancy. Developmental Psychology 6:74–77.

Vincent-Smith, L., Bricker, D., and Bricker, W. 1974. Acquisition of receptive vocabulary in the toddler-age child. Child Development 45:189–193.

Zlatin, M. A., and Koeningsknecht, R. A. 1976. Development of the voicing contrast: A comparison of voice-onset-time in stop perception. Journal of Speech and Hearing Research 19(1):93–111.

Chapter **7**

Brainstem Auditory Pathways and Auditory Processing Disorders

Diagnostic Implications of Subjective and Objective Tests

Elizabeth Protti

Functional correlates of brainstem structures suggest that dysfunction might relate to auditory processing disorders in children. Clinical assessment of these disorders in children is based primarily on subjective audiometric tests sensitive to neurologic impairment of the central nervous system in adults. The purpose of this chapter is to stress to clinicians the inappropriateness of utilizing these behavioral tests of CNS function in a site-of-lesion fashion when assessing the central auditory processing skills of children. Implying that a child's CAP disorder relates to CNS involvement at a specific level and site has no support in the literature. Even though authors of these tests indicate that site of dysfunction cannot be inferred, some clinicians continue to assume that test abnormalities are caused by a localized neurologic disorder (e.g., in the brainstem). This overinterpretation is based on the resemblance of the abnormal performance of CAP-disordered children with behaviors associated with central auditory lesions (Cohen, 1980; Keith, 1981a; Richardson, 1977). Test results should be interpreted to describe abnormal auditory behaviors which could interfere with the learning process, and not to diagnose what is believed to be the associated site of neurologic dysfunction.

This chapter discusses brainstem anatomy and functional correlates, followed by a review of CAP tests useful in the evaluation of brainstem disorders in adults. Results of subjective tests sensitive to brainstem disorders in adults are compared to objective electrophysiologic measures of brainstem dysfunction. Binaural Fusion (BF) and Rapidly Alternating Speech (RAS), both from the Willeford Central Auditory Test (CAT) battery, and Katz's Staggered Spondiac Word (SSW) Test are the subject assessment techniques employed. Auditory brainstem response (ABR) is the electrophysiologic measure of brainstem function.

BRAINSTEM ANATOMY

The auditory system is highly redundant and variable. It is that portion of cranial nerve VIII that enters the brainstem in the region of the cerebellopontine angle, and the fibers of the second-, third-, and fourth-order neurons which terminate at the level of the medial geniculate body (Katz, 1978; Willeford & Billger, 1978). Figure 1 presents a schematic of these ascending, or afferent, structures. The eighth nerve, upon entering the brainstem, synapses with cell bodies of second-order

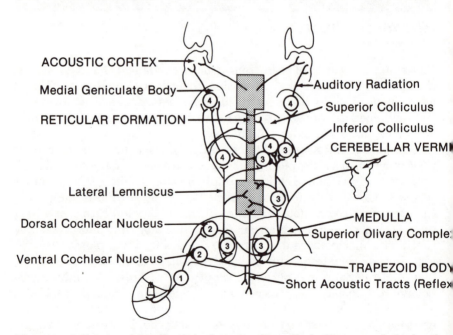

Figure 1.   A diagram of the afferent brainstem auditory fibers. First, second, third, and fourth order neurons and their collateral contact with the reticular formation and cerebellum are indicated. (Reprinted by permission from Gibson, W. 1978. Essentials of Clinical Electric Response Audiometry. Copyright © 1978 Churchill Livingstone, London.)

neurons in the cochlear nuclei (CN). Three subgroupings of cell bodies within the CN relate to auditory functioning: anterior and posterior ventral cochlear nuclei and the dorsal cochlear nuclei, which communicate with each other via interneuronal connections (Durrant & Lovrinic, 1975). The array of the pathways and synapses of nerve fibers exiting the CN is quite diverse, permitting analyses and comparisons of signal parameters processed at various brainstem sites.

Most of the second-order neurons from the CN decussate through the trapezoid body to synapse upon the third-order neurons of the contralateral superior olivary complex (SOC). A significant minority of second-order neurons, however, synapse upon the third-order neurons of the ipsilateral SOC. Other second-order neurons bypass the SOC altogether, ascend through the lateral lemniscus (LL), and, if not synapsing with the nuclei of the LL, synapse at the inferior colliculus (IC).

The third- and fourth-order neurons in a parallel fashion traverse the brainstem with an equal degree of complexity. Most third-order neurons in the audition-specific nuclei of the SOC synapse upon a grouping of cell bodies on a midbrain level (i.e., the IC). At both the level of the LL and more so at the IC, a significant portion of auditory fibers cross over or decussate to the contralateral side. Adding to the intricacy of the system, some third-order neurons bypass the IC, terminating upon a nucleus of the thalamus, the medial geniculate body (MGB). Fourth-order neurons from the IC also terminate in the MGB. All ascending fibers synapse upon the MGB before fifth-order neurons synapse within the auditory cortex of the temporal lobe (Gibson, 1978).

The system is further complicated by the axonal contacts that the afferent auditory fibers have with nonauditory systems on a brainstem level and by the efferent or descending neuronal junctures within the auditory system. The cerebellum, a center for the integration of movement and balance, is in direct contact with the afferent auditory system through collateral contact (Durrant & Lovrinic, 1975). The reticular formation (RF), a generalized neurologic structure receiving multimodal input and forming the central core of the brainstem, also communicates with the ascending auditory fibers (Chusid, 1979). The efferent neurons parallel the afferent system and enable higher brain centers to exercise control upon the neuronal activity of auditory structures.

FUNCTIONAL CORRELATES AND CAP

The auditory cortex and associated cortical structures are the final embellishers of speech perception. Cortical ablation studies performed on cats have shown that they can still respond to the onset of a sound and to changes in intensity and frequency. With only intact subcortical structures, animals display deficits in the ability to discriminate tonal patterns, sound durations, and localization of sounds in space (Durrant & Lovrinic, 1975).

Nonetheless, rudiments of speech perception related to signal onset, frequency, and intensity do occur on a brainstem level. Kiang (1975) reported that individual brainstem neurons may be differentiated from one another on the basis of the uniqueness of their neuronal discharge patterns to various stimuli. He supposed that the activity of certain cells in the CN responsive to stimulus onset may assist in the perception of phonemes, such as sibilants or other vocalic units with periodic glottal pulses. Other cell types of the CN respond only when the signal is on, whereas still others fire at the onset and/or offset of a signal. Some high brainstem neurons at the level of the IC, on the other hand, have been found to be optimally responsive to signals of varying amplitude and/or frequency (Klinke, 1978). Neuronal activity may actually depend upon the direction of these changes (Durrant & Lovrinic, 1975). Pinheiro (1978) stated that some neuronal units of the IC and MGB have periodic responses related to fundamental frequencies and formants. These units are called "vowel detectors." Other neurons of the same nuclei respond asymmetrically; they respond to dynamic signal parameters such as frequency modulation. These neurons are labeled "consonant detectors." Generally, high brainstem auditory structures are more specialized in their response characteristics than low brainstem fibers. "The higher the level of a neuron in the auditory pathway, the more complicated the sound patterns required to excite it" (Klinke, 1978, p. 202).

Intact brainstem structures are necessary for the processing of acoustic signals. Auditory processing, related in part to selective listening skills, is essential for auditory perception or cognition at every CNS level. "Not hearing can be just as essential as hearing" (Cottman & McGaugh, 1980, p. 377). Adequate listening skills are dependent upon the integrity of the afferent and efferent brainstem auditory neurons and RF. Afferent neurons facilitate processing of pertinent auditory input while squelching unwarranted messages by encoding phase and intensity differences between each ear's acoustic input (Durrant & Lovrinic, 1975). Such binaural interaction initially occurs at the level of the SOC, the first decussation site of the auditory CNS (Cottman & McGaugh, 1980). Nerve fibers of the accessory of medial olivary nucleus (AMON), a subdivision of the SOC, appear to be selective regarding sidedness; some specialized neurons are excited by binaural information, others by monaural contralateral input while being inhibited by ipsilateral stimulation. In contrast, neurons from the lateral superior olive (LSO), another part of the SOC, are activated by ipsilateral stimulation but inhibited by contralateral stimulation. AMON neurons are "sensitive to interaural time differences, as small as 10–20 milliseconds," whereas neurons from LSO "have a neural mechanism for frequency spectrum analysis" (Pinheiro, 1978, p. 6). The CN may also play a role in binaural integration due to the effects higher CNS structures have upon lower CNS structures via the descending or inhibitory tracts (Durrant & Lovrinic, 1975).

Proper functioning of these efferent fibers enhances the listening process. Electrical stimulation of the crossed olivocochlear fibers in cats has an inhibitory effect upon the peripheral receptors, depending upon the intensity of the acoustic input (Dewson, 1967; Wiederhold, 1970). Between 40 and 70 dB sound pressure level (SPL), activation of the crossed olivocochlear fibers causes a decreasing sensitivity to as much as 10 dB. Above 70 dB SPL, there is no intensity decrement. Translated into practical terms, this differential inhibitory response triggered by the intensity level of the acoustic input creates a favorable signal-to-noise ratio. Background noise is more apt to be reduced in intensity than the selected auditory message.

Neider and Neider (1970) have shown a release from masking of moderately intense clicks by high-rate, low-intensity clicks upon stimulation of the olivocochlear bundles. Dewson's (1968) research findings have corroborated this. Rhesus monkeys with intact olivocochlear bundles are better able to discriminate moderately intense vowels in a background of noise than those monkeys on whom the bundle has been surgically transected. Activity of efferent fibers apparently facilitates auditory perception in unfavorable acoustic environments.

Activation of the RF also promotes adequate listening. Neuronal communication between the auditory fibers of the CNS and the RF results in a function labeled "cortical tone" by Luria (1973). Excitation of the RF exerts a general activating effect on the cortex, strengthens motoric reactions to stimuli, and sharpens sensitivity. Activation of the RF, which is composed of both inhibitory and activating units, may result in an orienting reflex (attentive behavior), investigative activity, or habituation (Luria, 1973; Sokolov, 1960). Habituation has been described as "the decrement in response to an essentially novel stimulus when it is given repeatedly" (Cottman & McGaugh, 1980, p. 258). Motivational drive has also been attributed by Luria (1973) to RF stimulation.

The question to be addressed at this point is: How do the above processes attributed to functioning of the various brainstem auditory structures relate to CAP and, in turn, to learning disabilities? Integration of binaural cues, activation of RF, and functioning of the efferent fibers facilitate appropriate listening behavior. Approximately 60% of the learning-disabled population has been identified as having deficiencies in selective listening skills (Katz & Illmer, 1972). Auditory figure-ground problems (inability to attend to relevant auditory stimuli in the presence of competing acoustic cues) are characteristic of many learning-disabled children (Clements, 1969; Kasten & Griffin, 1979; Mueller & Kasten, 1978). Some professionals feel that brainstem disorder, associated with CAP functions of arousal, regulation, readiness, and binaural synthesis, may be at the core of learning disabilities (Keith, 1981; Spreen, 1976).

Auditory sensory deprivation associated with conductive hearing loss has been inferred to be related to auditory inefficiencies, including attention, reception, and figure-ground difficulties (Eisen, 1962; Holm & Kunze, 1969; Johnson & Newman, 1979; Lewis, 1976; Mustain, 1979). Webster (Chapter 10, this volume) documents anatomical correlates of sensory deprivation in mice. "Both postnatal auditory deprivation and experimentally produced conductive hearing losses in mice result in incomplete maturation of most brainstem auditory neurons" (Webster & Webster, 1978, p. 2). The authors conclude that adequate sound stimulation must occur during a critical period of brainstem development to realize full growth of these neurons. Similar findings have been observed in guinea pigs subjected to experimental destruction of organ of Corti structures (Webster & Webster, 1977). Effects of sensory deprivation caused by chronic conductive hearing losses, particularly in the first 2–3 years of life, have been associated with linguistic and educational impairments (Johnson & Newman, 1979; Kaplan et al., 1973; Mustain, 1979).

SUBJECTIVE TESTS OF BRAINSTEM FUNCTION

Subjective tests are behavioral measurements which depend upon patient-related variables, such as mental and physical status, intellectual and linguistic capabilities, and patient-environment interaction. These factors may adversely influence the patient's voluntary responses, compromising test specificity. The following tests were employed in the study discussed in this chapter.

Binaural Fusion

The Binaural Fusion (BF) subtest of Willeford's (1976) central auditory battery is a dichotic test sensitive to brainstem dysfunction. This test is based upon the original version developed by Matzker (1959) and subsequent versions (Noffsinger et al., 1972; Smith & Resnick, 1972) in which comparisons were made between a patient's performance on a dichotic and that on a diotic task. Willeford's BF test consists of low-frequency information (500- to 700-Hz bandpass) from 20 spondaic stimulus words presented to one ear, considered the test ear, while high-frequency information (1900- to 2100-Hz bandpass) is presented to the opposite ear in a dichotic mode. The test is then repeated reversing the low-high test stimuli. The presentation level for the low-frequency band is set 30 dB above the pure tone threshold at 500 Hz, while the high frequency component is set 30 dB above the 2000-Hz threshold.

Normal listeners have difficulty with each band presented alone, but when both are played in a dichotic fashion, they easily fuse them (presumably at the level of the brainstem) into an intelligible word. The normative data (Table 1) reveal improved performance and less variability with maturation up to 10 years of age (Willeford, 1977).

Rapidly Alternating Speech

Willeford's (1976) Rapidly Alternating Speech (RAS) subtest is another procedure that is sensitive to brainstem dysfunction in adults. RAS is based on stimulus sentences presented in alternating bursts of 300 msec, first to one ear and then to the other. Ten sentences are presented to each ear. Instructions suggest that the test be administered at 50 dB sensation level (SL) re: pure tone average (PTA) of each ear (Willeford, 1977). However, the presentation level can be modified to 30 dB SL to enhance test specificity (Willeford, 1978). A 5-year-old child should have no difficulty on RAS (Willeford, 1977). Performance should be comparable to that of adults (Table 2).

Lynn and Gilroy (1977) found the RAS procedure to be sensitive to lesions of the lower brainstem at the level of the pons (mean of 38% cor-

Table 1. Normative data of Willeford's BF test, obtained on 40 children at each age level between 6 and 10 years inclusive. The figures represent the percentage of correct responses in the right and left ears. (Modified from Willeford, 1978.)

Age (years)	Mean		Standard deviation		Range	
	Right ear	Left ear	Right ear	Left ear	Right ear	Left ear
6	75.0	74.1	11.4	12.2	55/100	55/95
7	75.5	76.0	11.9	12.5	55/100	55/100
8	76.8	76.8	8.8	10.3	60/100	65/100
9	78.8	79.9	13.2	11.9	55/100	55/100
10	87.6	89.2	5.5	4.8	75/95	80/95

Table 2. Normative data of Willeford's RAS test obtained on 25 children in each age group between 5 and 10 years inclusive. The figures represent the percentages of correct responses in the right and left ears. (Modified from Willeford, 1978.)

Age	Mean		Standard deviation		Range	
	Right ear	Left ear	Right ear	Left ear	Right ear	Left ear
5	99.2	99.2	3.9	2.6	80/100	90/100
6	98.0	98.3	4.6	2.2	80/100	90/100
7	99.5	98.3	2.2	2.2	90/100	90/100
8	99.5	98.8	2.2	1.4	90/100	90/100
9	99.8	98.8	1.4	1.4	90/100	90/100
10	100.0	99.8	0.0	1.4	100/100	90/100

rect). The performance of nine subjects with upper brainstem disorder was close to normal (mean of 83%). Recognition scores of 90–100% were achieved by normal listeners as well as by subjects with unilateral cerebral involvement.

Staggered Spondaic Word Test

The SSW, developed by Katz (1962), utilizes spondaic words as stimuli. The test consists of 40 items, each composed of two partially overlapping spondees. Presentation level is 50 dB re: the three-frequency PTA. All four monosyllabic words are scored for each item: 1) right ear non-competing (R-NC); 2) right ear competing (R-C); 3) left ear competing (L-C); 4) left ear noncompeting (L-NC). From these are derived condition, ear, and total performance scores.

Normative data are available for individuals 11–60 years of age (Katz, 1979). Katz (1978) reported the scoring profile of adults with specific brainstem lesions. Three subjects with lower brainstem involvement demonstrated an overcorrected score for the ear ipsilateral to the lesion and a score within normal limits for the contralateral ear. The profile for four subjects with high brainstem involvement was a severely abnormal score for the ear ipsilateral to the lesion and a score within normal limits for the contralateral ear. The SSW has been used with children down to the age of 5 years. A maturation effect has been noted, however (Table 3), with increasing variability of scores below age 11 years (Johnson et al., 1978; Katz, 1979; Kushner, Johnson & Stevens, 1977; McCroskey & Kasten, 1980; Myrick, 1965).

OBJECTIVE TESTS OF BRAINSTEM FUNCTION

Electrophysiologic measurements are termed objective assessment techniques, because a patient's voluntary responses are not generally

Table 3. Extreme upper limits of normal performance for the four SSW condition scores depending upon age. The figures represent the percentages of error for each condition, approximated to
0.5%. (Modified from Katz, 1979.)

Age	R-NC	R-C	L-C	L-NC
5	7.5	40	60	10
7	7.5	35	42.5	10
8	7.5	17.5	32.5	10
9	7.5	17.5	22.5	10
10	5	10	15	0
11	5	10	10	0

required. Influence of patient-related variables upon test performance
is reduced, enhancing test specificity. The objective test discussed here
is auditory brainstem response (ABR), a technique that relies neither
on the patient's mental state, sleep state, use of sedation, or intelligence. ABR is based upon the recording via scalp electrodes of minute
electrical potentials generated by activity of cranial nerve VIII and
brainstem auditory neurons. When the auditory system is stimulated
by a signal with a fast rise time, such as a click, synchronous neural discharge of brainstem auditory generators occurs. A characteristic waveform (Figure 2) with seven peaks occurs in the averaged trace in the
first 8–12 msec following the click stimuli (Jewett et al., 1970; Jewett &
Williston, 1971). These electrical potentials are extremely small rela-

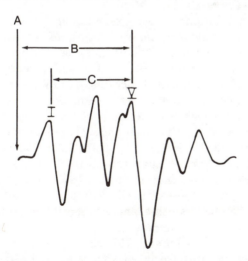

Figure 2.   A characteristic ABR waveform. *A*, stimulus onset; *B*, absolute latency; *C*, interwave latency. (Reprinted by permission from Fira, T. 1980. Monographs in Contemporary Audiology. Copyright © 1980 Maico Hearing Instruments.)

tive to the background EEG activity, so use of an averaging computer is necessary. Onset of the signal is time-locked to the computer, and any neurologic event that occurs at a particular point in time after stimulation will be averaged with previous neurologic responses to an identical stimulus. Random background neuronal and muscle activity, in contrast, would be averaged out. Because the size of an ABR wave component is measured in tenths of a microvolt, it is necessary to enhance the signal-to-noise ratio by relying upon approximately 2000 trials. The interested reader is directed to Berlin and Dobie (1979) regarding instrumentation and procedural requirements.

The integrity and/or functioning of brainstem auditory fibers may be assessed by analyzing the ABR. ABR performance equivalent to that in adults is expected with children approximating 1 year of age (Hecox & Galambos, 1974; Salamy, McKean, & Buda, 1975; Salamy & McKean, 1976). Vital information can be obtained by calculating time delays between stimulus onset and response waveforms (absolute latencies) and by analyzing the time span between waveforms (interpeak latencies), particularly of waves I, III, and V. Differences between the right and left ear responses (interaural latencies) are also considered. Interpeak latencies are reliable within and between normal subjects. The adult standard deviation of these latencies is extremely small, ranging from 0.13 msec (Gilroy & Lynn, 1978) to 0.22 msec (Rowe, 1978), depending upon the test parameters utilized. Abnormal or absent wave configuration can also denote dysfunction in the region of the eighth nerve or the brainstem.

A one-to-one relationship between a particular neuronal generator and a specific ABR waveform cannot be assumed because of redundant neuronal communication along the brainstem. Although "there is no characteristic ABR abnormality for a specific neurologic lesion or disease" (Fria, 1980, p. 30), dysfunctions of cranial nerve VIII and the brainstem can result in atypical ABR recordings. Fria observed that: 1) extrinsic brainstem lesions affecting the cerebellopontine angle may produce an increase in the interwave (II–V) latency (Hashimoto, Ishiyama, & Tozuka, 1979; Starr & Achor, 1975; Stockard & Rossiter, 1977; Stockard, Stockard, & Sharbrough, 1977) or an abnormal wave V interaural latency (House & Brackmann, 1979); 2) an abnormally prolonged III–V interwave latency in the contralateral ear has been seen in cases of large cerebellopontine angle tumors, along with absent or poorly defined waveform components subsequent to wave I in the ipsilateral ear (Selters & Brackmann, 1979; Starr & Achor, 1975); 3) intrinsic brainstem lesions are associated with poorly defined, absent, and/or prolonged latencies of waves III–V (Hashimoto et al., 1979; Starr &

Achor, 1975; Stockard & Rossiter, 1977; Stockard et al., 1977); and
4) the primary effect of midbrain lesions is the prolongation of the
III–V interwave latency (Hashimoto et al., 1979; Starr & Achor, 1975;
Starr & Hamilton, 1976; Stockard & Rossiter, 1977).

Research data related to ABR procedures for assessment of CAP
are minimal and conflicting. Sohmer and Student (1978) have reported
abnormal ABR results with children with minimal brain dysfunction
(MBD). Shimizu and Brown (1981), in contrast, reported that no ABR
differences were seen when MBD children were compared to normals.
Worthington (1981) reported little or no correlation between ABR
results and diagnosed CAP-disordered children. However, Worthington et al. (1981) reported abnormal ABR results with 30% of subjects with moderate to severe language and/or developmental delays.

DIAGNOSTIC IMPLICATIONS OF TESTS

Although CAP disorders on a brainstem level may affect learning, and
subjective tests (e.g., BF, RAS, and SSW) are utilized in the assessment of brainstem dysfunction related to neurologic disease, problems
observed in adults with discrete CNS lesions cannot be directly compared to learning-disabled children who have more vague and generalized problems. Although ABR is specific to brainstem dysfunction, it
cannot be used to rule out a CAP deficiency related to learning problems. A click signal has little in common with speech tasks used in
CAP testing or the language processing required for school activities.
Further, subjective tests may not be specific measures of brainstem
dysfunction, particularly when testing children. Dempsey (1977)
hypothesized that the dichotic presentation mode of the BF test may
require more cortical integration of semantic material than the diotic
mode. Design of initial BF procedures considered brainstem involvement suspect if a significant decrement was observed on dichotic compared to diotic presentations of a stimulus. BF procedures based only
on a dichotic mode do not adequately control for the linguistic variables
mediated on a cortical level.

Auditory memory may also be a variable affecting delineation between cortical and brainstem dysfunction, especially when sentence
material is used (e.g., RAS). Is difficulty exhibited because of a problem
synthesizing dichotic information (brainstem task) or because of deficient auditory memory (cortical variable)? The subject can be asked to
repeat the sentence presented diotically through the audiometer's talk-
over. If he or she is unable to do so, then a memory deficit may be
suspected. Tests of auditory memory, such as are included in the

Detroit Test of Learning Aptitude (Baker & Leland, 1967), can be administered in conjunction with RAS.

Errors on RAS may also relate, at least partially, to a subject's linguistic deficiencies. A review of errors noted on RAS emphasizes a high degree of "syntactical loading" in the task, as is seen in the following:

> *Stimulus:* My dog always does what I ask.
> *Response:* My dog *did* what I *asking.*

Willeford's instructions in scoring RAS are to accept a meaningful approximation as normal. Making the scoring criteria more stringent (as is sometimes done), to sensitize the test battery to subtle linguistic difficulties, seems to make the RAS a test of cortical function. A trend observed in a learning-disabled population is that the "number of syntactic changes made on the RAS task corresponded to the degree to which performance on other (cortical) tests was abnormal" (Dempsey, 1977, p. 303).

Because the cortex is the final embellisher of auditory input, normal performance on the BF, RAS, and SSW necessitates intact linguistic centers on a cortical level. Utilization of such symbolic material makes delineation of brainstem versus cortical dysfunction difficult. Abnormal performance on the BF, RAS, and SSW may reflect cortical instead of, or in addition to, brainstem dysfunction. Indeed, Katz (1979) stated with regard to adults that a moderately to severely depressed score in one or both ears on the SSW may relate to one of three loci of lesion: 1) auditory reception area (Heschl's gyrus) peaking in the opposite ear; 2) high brainstem, usually occurring in the ipsilateral ear; and 3) corpus callosum and/or anterior commissure lesion in the ear opposite the nondominant hemisphere for language. Jerger and Jerger (1975) investigated the clinical utility of various central auditory tests. They report that the SSW is the best procedure for identifying cerebral lesions, but results are variable in brainstem cases. Katz (1978) felt that if the possibility of cortical involvement is eliminated, brainstem dysfunction is plausible, particularly if retrocochlear signs on a conventional audiometric battery are present (e.g., abnormal acoustic reflexes, tone decay, poor speech discrimination). Further, Katz recommended against site-of-dysfunction assumptions and provided no guidelines for evidence of high or low brainstem results on the SSW in children.

Age is another variable that compromises a subjective test's specificity for brainstem dysfunction. The statistical trends of the SSW differ for children under 11 years. The normative data are more variable and are characterized by a maturational effect (Table 3). A child's performance on the SSW cannot be interpreted as if the child were an adult. A statistical review of the BF test results in a similar conclusion. Normal performance at the youngest normed age of 6 years is defined as approximately a ± 20% range of scores around the mean; the range is smaller for older children (Table 1). Such a wide range of performance along with the maturational effect reduces the test's specificity in the determination of brainstem integrity.

ABR was used in a study conducted at the Delaware County Memorial Hospital (DCMH) Hearing, Speech and Learning Center and compared to subjective tests to determine percentage of agreement. ABR is considered to be a more specific measure of brainstem integrity than the subjective tests, yet ABR is not without its limitations regarding its sensitivity toward brainstem dysfunction. As stated earlier, ABR may not be sensitive to diffuse brainstem dysfunction nor to involvement of nonauditory centers, such as the reticular formation. Elicitation of binaural ABR tracings and subsequent comparison of them with predicted binaural tracings (based upon a summing of the monaural ABR results of the right and left ears) may enhance ABR sensitivity to brainstem dysfunction (Dobie & Berlin, 1979). Nonetheless, the ABR procedure utilized in this study is considered to be a more specific, less variable, and less age-dependent procedure in the assessment of brainstem integrity.

Population

Thirteen children ranging in age from 6.0 to 13.5 years, referred to DCMH Hearing, Speech and Learning Center for CAP testing, were chosen for study. The criterion for inclusion was abnormal performance on the BF, RAS, and/or SSW, which was subsequently compared to the child's ABR performance. Abnormal performance was defined as a score falling beyond the limit of normalcy for a specific age on the BF, RAS, or SSW.

Five of the 13 children were undiagnosed as to the basis of their learning difficulties and were attending regular classes. Of six labeled learning-disabled, four were enrolled in self-contained classes, whereas two received assistance in a resource room as an adjunct to the regular classroom. One child was diagnosed as dyslexic and was enrolled in a regular classroom. Another child was classified as emotionally disturbed and was attending a residential classroom for such children. The referring parties reported that the children were of at least average intelligence.

All subjects demonstrated normal hearing sensitivity and normal middle ear function when tested, although seven had a history of recurrent serous otitis media. In 10 out of 13 cases, stapedial reflex studies were negative for retrocochlear involvement as determined by the elicitation of a stapedial reflex at threshold levels of 105 dB hearing level (HL) or less at 500 Hz, 1 kHz, and 2 kHz. In two of the 13 cases, reflex thresholds were elicited at elevated threshold levels. This was considered an ambiguous finding because of abnormal tympanograms (in spite of a negative otologic examination) indicating more than − 150 mm of water pressure within the middle ear cavities. In one case, reflexes were not observed upon stimulating the left ear (ipsilateral and contralateral recording). This child is discussed in the case history section.

Procedure

The test protocols for the BF, RAS, and SSW followed test instructions, with the following modifications: a) an intensity level of 40 dB SL for both the low- and high-pass segment of BF was adopted; b) an error on the RAS test was defined as any change in meaning of a test item. Willeford's (1978) instructions stated that an error exists when a subject cannot perceive the message in any meaningful way.

ABR test design was based on a click signal with the following parameters: rate, 7.9 per second; duration, 100 μsec; intensity, 65 dB SL; polarity, positive and negative clicks utilized in a comfirmatory manner in separate trials. A filter setting of 150–3000 Hz was employed along with a sensitivity setting of 10 μV. Each trace contained the averaged responses of 2000 clicks. In analyzing ABR, interpeak latencies were taken as the critical variables. A response falling above 2 standard deviations from the mean was considered abnormal.

Results

To illustrate the results obtained, three of the 13 cases are discussed below.

Case 1: Positive ABR   T.S., a 9.9-year-old male, was experiencing academic difficulties, particularly in reading comprehension, and was referred to the Center by the school psychologist. Developmental history included a normal 9-month gestation period along with a negative postnatal and childhood history except for a reported speech and language delay. The mother reported that T.S. had started to talk when he was 3 years of age and used two-word sentences when he was 4 years old. He displayed articulation problems at the time of testing and was enrolled in speech-language therapy at school. Language evaluations indicated deficiencies in both expressive and receptive areas. On the expressive and receptive portion of the Northwestern Syntax Screening Test (Lee, 1969), T.S.'s performance was below the 10th percentile. He scored a mental age of 4 years, 9 months, on the Peabody Picture Vocabulary Test (Dunn, 1959) when his chronologic age was 6 years, 7 months. Performance on the Carrow Elicited Language Inventory (Carrow, 1974) was below 1st percentile when he was 7 years, 5 months of age.

At the time of the DCMH study, T.S. was enrolled in a regular third-grade classroom supported by resource room instruction. He was described as highly distractible in school and as having a short attention span. BF and RAS were both positive for brainstem involvement (Table 4). BF scores revealed a depressed right ear score; RAS was severely depressed bilaterally. The SSW R-C and L-C scores were at the extreme limits of normal for a 9-year-old and clearly abnormal for a 10-year-old child.

Results of the ABR were analyzed as being abnormal (Figure 3), with significant wave V interaural latencies of 0.32 msec (positive click) and confirmed by a wave V interaural latency of 0.52 msec (negative click). This suggests an asymmetry between the auditory pathways of both ears, implicating the right ear's responses. In addition, the III–V interpeak latency of the right ear's positive click tracings fell beyond +3 standard deviations of the mean, possibly implicating high brainstem auditory neuronal centers. Stapedial reflex studies were negative for retrocochlear and/or low brainstem involvement.

Referral to a pediatric neurologist was made. T.S. was found to have numerous freckles and at least 13 pale, café-au-lait spots over the trunk of his body. Von Recklinghausen's disease (neurofibromatosis) was suspected and was later confirmed by a dermatologist's examination. In this disease, neurilemmoma (tumors) can occur on both the spinal and the cranial nerves along with meningiomas and gliomas of the CNS (Chusid, 1979). Regular medical follow-up is presently being pursued, along with continued special education considerations. Ac-

Table 4. Subjective CAP scores for three subjects

		BF		RAS		SSW			
Subject	Age (years)	RE	LE	RE	LE	R-NC	R-C	L-C	L-NC
T.S.	9.9	50%	75%	50%	50%	10%	18%	24%	9%
M.K.	8.7	30%	10%	100%	100%	2%	32%	45%	2%
M.A.	6.2	30%	55%	30%	25%	5%	95%	20%	5%

RE, right ear; LE, left ear.

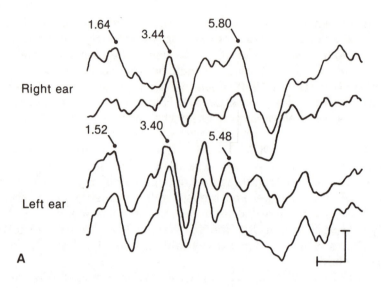

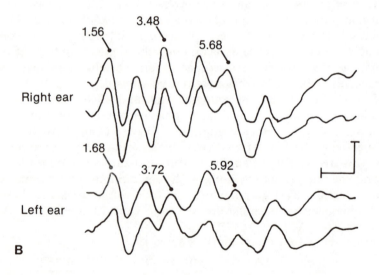

Figure 3.   ABR tracings of T.S. *(A)*, M.K. *(B)*, and M.A. *(C)*. Horizontal scale is 1 msec; absolute latencies are expressed in milliseconds. *A*, Vertical scale is 0.156 mV. Two tracings per ear were elicited. Positive clicks were utilized. *B*, Vertical scale is 0.313 mV. Two tracings per ear were utilized. Positive clicks were utilized. *C*, Vertical scale is 0.156 mV. Right ear and left ear were stimulated with a positive click.

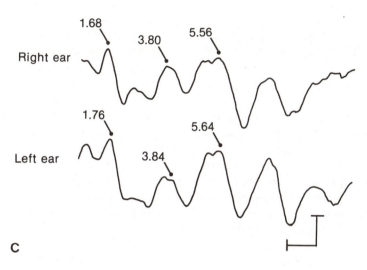

1.68
3.80
5.56

Right ear

1.76
5.64

Left ear
3.84

C

Figure 3, *continued.*

cording to the physician, the ABR and CAT findings were associated with subclinical signs of neurofibromatosis.

Case 2: Positive ABR   M.K., an 8.7-year-old female, was an adopted child who reportedly had a positive birth history. Her biologic mother was on amphetamines during the first four months of pregnancy. Other than a history of ear infections, M.K.'s postnatal and childhood history was essentially insignificant. Speech and language development was considered to be age-appropriate. She was referred to the Center by a psychiatrist, who reported that the child was experiencing reading difficulties. Because M.K. was described as having a short attention span, auditory perceptual skills were suspect. At the time of the study, M.K. was enrolled in a regular third-grade classroom.

CAP testing and ABR were administered. BF revealed depressed scores bilaterally; RAS scores were 100% in both ears. R-C and L-C scores on the SSW fell above the extreme limits of normal for 8-year-olds. The L-C score was depressed more so than the R-C score (Table 4). ABR results confirmed the abnormalities observed on the subjective tests (Figure 3B). The III-V interpeak latency of the right and left ears' responses fell between +2 and +3 standard deviations from the mean (positive click tracings). There seems to be a neurologic substrate to M.K.'s learning problems, partly attributed to brainstem dysfunction and confirmed by impedance reflex studies (absent left ear contralateral and ipsilateral reflexes). A complete psychoeducational evaluation, including a neurologic assessment, was subsequently recommended. The physician attributed positive brainstem signs on ABR tracings to an effect amphetamines had on CNS development during M.K.'s gestation period.

Case 3: Negative ABR   M.A., a 6.2-year-old male, was referred for a complete psychoeducational assessment, including CAP testing by the school physician. M.A. was enrolled in kindergarten, where his behavior in school had been described as very distractible and characterized by a short attention span and discipline problems. Both parents and school personnel reported that M.A. had difficulty paying attention, concentrating, and listening. It is significant to note that the child's responses to pure tones were extremely variable and highly unreliable. Results of a speech-language evaluation indicated an expressive and receptive language delay. The birth process had been stressful for M.A.; the umbilical cord had been wrapped around the child's neck, resulting in physical distress requiring a 3-day stay in an intensive care unit. Except for being a "light eater and restless sleeper," the child's subsequent postnatal and childhood history had advanced without incident.

Both CAP and ABR procedures were administered. A high intertest consistency among BF, RAS, and SSW is noted (Table 4). BF performance is depressed in the right ear, and RAS is bilaterally abnormal. The SSW shows a severely depressed R-C score. Although this profile might strongly implicate brainstem involvement, ABR tracings (Figure 3C) are well within normal limits, with interpeak latencies below 1 standard deviation from the mean. Brainstem involvement is not confirmed by ABR.

All of the children who were chosen for ABR had indications of brainstem involvement on at least one of the subjective tests. Fifty-four percent had what we interpreted as positive brainstem findings on all three subjective tests, 23% on two subtests, and 23% on only one behavioral test. In contrast, only two children (15%) had abnormal ABR tracings; one of these children had absent stapedial reflexes with retrocochlear implications, and both showed positive findings on two out of the three subjective tests. The BF subtest agreed with both positive ABR findings, whereas RAS and SSW were each positive for one child with ABR abnormalities. Of the 54% of cases in which three out of the three subjective tests were positive for brainstem involvement, only one case (14%) had abnormal ABR findings. These findings reinforce our concern that statements of site of brainstem dysfunction in children are tenuous at best when these subjective tests are utilized. One would expect a stronger relationship between BF, RAS, and/or the SSW and ABR if one is to apply labels validly regarding locus of lesion when testing children.

SUMMARY

1. Subjective tests associated with brainstem function are sensitive but not specific to abnormal brainstem functioning. The variability of normal scores and the age effect observed under approximately 11 years of age make the utilization of these tests ambiguous as a site-of-lesion battery with children.
2. Performance on those subjective tests sensitive to brainstem function may be influenced by linguistic variables mediated on a cortical level. However, when substantiated by conventional audiometric site-of-lesion techniques, such as acoustic reflexes and ABR, abnormal performance on subjective tests may have brainstem implications.
3. The clinician must perform a task analysis and statistical review of commercially available tests to utilize the procedures effectively.
4. A strong positive relationship was not observed between abnormal performance on subjective brainstem (BF, RAS, and SSW) and the objective measure of ABR. The authors of the subjective test batteries are correct in cautioning audiologists that one cannot diagnose site of lesion solely on the basis of subjective CAP test findings.
5. Auditory brainstem dysfunction can relate to CAP problems, as indicated by the abnormal ABR findings in two out of the 13 children evaluated. In these cases, the behavioral tests were important in the referral for ABR.
6. Although we used ABR as the criterion for brainstem status, it may not be sensitive to all brainstem involvements. However, positive findings are felt to have site-of-lesion implications and may serve as the basis for medical referral.
7. Negative ABR findings cannot rule out the existence of CAP dysfunction related to a child's abnormal auditory behavior in various acoustic environments. The ABR stimulus is nonspeech in nature and may be classified as a poor identifier of central auditory dysfunction.

ACKNOWLEDGMENTS

Credit is given to Ms. Pamela Mertz and Ms. Joan Evans for their assistance in the compilation of data for this chapter.

REFERENCES

Baker, H. J., and Leland, B. 1967. Detroit Tests of Learning Aptitude. Bobbs-Merrill, Indianapolis.

Berlin, C. I., and Dobie, R. A. 1979. Electrophysiologic measures of auditory function via electrocochleography and brainstem evoked responses. In: W. F. Rintelman (ed.), Hearing Assessment, pp. 425–458. University Park Press, Baltimore.

Carrow, E. 1974. Carrow Elicited Language Inventory. Learning Concepts, Boston.

Chusid, J. 1979. Correlative Neuroanatomy and Functional Neurology, 17th Edition. Lange Medical Publications, Los Altos, Calif.

Clements, S. 1969. A new look at learning disabilities. In: L. Tarnopol (ed.), Learning Disabilities: Introduction to Education and Medical Management, pp. 31–40. Charles C Thomas, Springfield, Ill.

Cohen, R. L. 1980. Auditory skills and the communicative process. Seminars in Speech, Language, and Hearing 1(2):107–115.

Cottman, C., and McGaugh, J. 1980. Behavioral Neuroscience. Academic Press, New York.

Dempsey, C. 1977. Some thoughts concerning alternate explanations of central auditory test results. In: R. Keith (ed.), Central Auditory Dysfunction, pp. 293–317. Grune & Stratton, New York.

Dewson, J. 1967. Efferent olivocochlear bundle: Some relationships to noise masking and to stimulus attenuation. Journal of Neurophysiology 30:817–832.

Dewson, J. 1968. Efferent olivocochlear bundle: Some relationships to stimulus discrimination in noise. Journal of Neurophysiology 31:122–130.

Dobie, R. A., and Berlin, C. I. 1979. Influence of otitis media on hearing and development. Annals of Otology, Rhinology, and Laryngology 88(Suppl. 60):48–53.

Dunn, L. M. 1959. Peabody Picture Vocabulary Test. American Guidance Service, Inc., Circle Pines, Minn.

Durrant, J., and Lovrinic, J. 1975. Bases of Hearing Science. Williams & Wilkins, Baltimore.

Eisen, N. H. 1962. Some effects of early sensory deprivation on later behavior: The quondam hard-of-hearing child. Journal of Abnormal and Social Psychology 65:338–342.

Fria, T. 1980. The auditory brainstem response: Background and clinical applications. Monographs in Contemporary Audiology, Volume 2, Number 2. Educational Publications Division, Maico Hearing Instruments, Minneapolis.

Gibson, W. 1978. Essentials of Clinical Electric Response Audiometry. Churchill Livingstone, New York.

Gilroy, J., and Lynn, G. E. 1978. Computerized tomography and auditory-evoked potentials: Use in the diagnosis of olivopontocerebellar degeneration. Archives of Neurology 35:143–147.

Hashimoto, I., Ishiyama, Y., and Tozuka, G. 1979. Bilaterally recorded brainstem auditory evoked responses: Their asymmetric abnormalities and lesions of the brainstem. Archives of Neurology 36:161–167.

Hecox, K., and Galambos, R. 1974. Brainstem auditory evoked responses in human infants and adults. Archives of Otolaryngology 99:30–33.

Holm, V., and Kunze, L. 1969. Effect of chronic otitis media on language and speech development. Pediatrics 43:833–839.

House, J. W., and Brackmann, D. E. 1979. Brainstem audiometry in neurotologic diagnosis. Archives of Otolaryngology 105:305–309.

Jerger, J., and Jerger, S. 1975. Clinical validity of central auditory tests. Scandinavian Audiology 4:147–163.

Jewett, D. L. 1970. Human auditory evoked responses: Possible brainstem components detected on the scalp. Science 167:1517-1518.

Jewett, D. L., and Williston, J. S. 1971. Auditory evoked far fields averaged from the scalp of humans. Brain 94:681-696.

Johnson, A., and Newman, C. 1979. Central auditory and language disorders associated with conductive hearing loss. Paper presented at the American Speech, Language and Hearing Association Convention, Atlanta, Georgia, November 17, 1979.

Johnson, D. W., Lindgren, J. H., Sherman, R. E., and Enfield, M. L. 1978. Patterns of central auditory function in specific learning disabilities. Paper presented at the American Speech, Language and Hearing Association Convention, San Francisco, 1978.

Kaplan, G., Fleshman, J. K., Bender, T. R., et al. 1973. Long-term effects of otitis media: A ten-year cohort study of Alaskan Eskimo children. Pediatrics 52:557-585.

Kasten, R., and Griffin, B. 1979. Auditory processing of meaningful speech in the presence of competing message in normal children and children exhibiting learning disabilities. Paper presented at the American Speech, Language and Hearing Association Convention, Atlanta, Georgia, 1979.

Katz, J. 1962. The use of staggered spondaic words for assessing the integrity of the central nervous system. Journal of Auditory Research 2:327-337.

Katz, J. 1978. Clinical use of central auditory tests. In: J. Katz (ed.), Handbook of Clinical Audiology, 2nd Edition, pp. 233-243. Williams & Wilkins, Baltimore.

Katz, J. 1979. SSW Workshop Manual. State University of New York at Buffalo, Amherst, N.Y.

Katz, J., and Illmer, R. 1972. Auditory perception in children with learning disabilities. In: J. Katz (ed.), Handbook of Clinical Audiology, pp. 540-563. Williams & Wilkins, Baltimore.

Keith, R. W. 1981a. Tests of central auditory function. In: R. Roeser and M. Downs (eds.), Auditory Disorders in School Children, pp. 159-173. Brian C. Decker, New York.

Keith, R. W. 1981b. Central Auditory and Language Disorders in Children. College-Hill Press, Houston, Texas.

Kiang, N. 1975. Stimulus representation in the discharge patterns of auditory neurons. In: D. Tower (ed.), The Nervous System, Volume 3; Human Communication and Its Disorders, pp. 81-96. Raven Press, New York.

Klinke, R. 1978. Physiology of hearing. In: R. Schmidt (ed.), Fundamentals of Sensory Physiology, p. 202. Springer-Verlag, New York.

Kushner, D., Johnson, D. J., and Stevens, J. 1977. Use of SSW/CES test for identifying children with learning disabilities. Paper presented at the American Speech, Language and Hearing Association Convention, Chicago, 1977.

Lee, L. L. 1969. Northwestern Syntax Screening Test. Northwestern University Press, Evanston, Ill.

Lewis, N. 1976. Otitis media and linguistic incompetence. Archives of Otolaryngology 102:387-390.

Luria, A. R. 1973. The Working Brain: An Introduction to Neuropsychology. Basic Books, New York.

Lynn, G., and Gilroy, J. 1977. Evaluation of central auditory dysfunction in patients with neurological disorders. In: R. Keith (ed.), Central Auditory Dysfunction, pp. 177-217. Grune & Stratton, New York.

McCroskey, R., and Kasten, R. 1980. Assessment of central auditory processing. In: R. Rupp and K. Stockdell (eds.), Speech Protocols in Audiology, pp. 339–389. Grune & Stratton, New York.

Matzker, J. 1959. Two new methods for the assessment of central auditory functions in cases of brain disease. Annals of Otology, Rhinology, and Laryngology 68:1185–1197.

Mueller, K., and Kasten, R. 1978. Auditory processing skills of reading disabled children. Paper presented at the American Speech, Language and Hearing Association Convention, San Francisco, 1978.

Mustain, W. 1979. Linguistic and educational implications of recurrent otitis media. Ear, Nose, and Throat Journal 58:218–222.

Myrick, D. K. 1965. A normative study to assess performance of a group of children aged 7 through 11 on the SSW test. Masters thesis, Tulane University, New Orleans.

Neider, P., and Neider, I. 1970. Crossed olivocochlear bundle: Electric stimulation enhances masked neural responses to loud click. Brain Research 21:135–137.

Noffsinger, D., Olsen, W. O., Carhart, R., et al. 1972. Auditory and vestibular aberrations in multiple sclerosis. Acta Otolaryngologica 303:1–63.

Pinheiro, M. 1978. Examination of central auditory function in adults and children. Paper presented at the Pennsylvania Speech, Language and Hearing Association Annual Convention, Harrisburg, May 6, 1978.

Richardson, S. 1977. Communicating results of central auditory tests with other professionals. In: R. Keith (ed.), Central Auditory Dysfunction, pp. 277–291. Grune & Stratton, New York.

Rowe, J. 1978. Normal variability of the brainstem auditory evoked response in young and old adult subjects. Electroencephalography and Clinical Neurophysiology 44:459–470.

Salamy, A., and McKean, C. M. 1976. Postnatal development of human brainstem potentials during the first year of life. Electroencephalography and Clinical Neurophysiology 40:418–426.

Salamy, A., McKean, C. M., and Buda, F. B. 1975. Maturational changes in auditory transmission as reflected in human brainstem potentials. Brain Research 96:361–366.

Selters, W. A., and Brackmann, D. E. 1979. Brainstem electric response audiometry in acoustic tumor detection. In: W. F. House and C. M. Luetje (eds.), Acoustic Tumors, Volume I: Diagnosis, pp. 225–235. University Park Press, Baltimore.

Shimizu, H., and Brown, F. 1981. ABR in children with MBD. Paper presented at the American Speech Language and Hearing Association Convention, Los Angeles, 1981.

Smith, B. B., and Resnick, D. M. 1972. An auditory test for assessing brainstem integrity: Preliminary report. Laryngoscope 82:414–424.

Sohmer, H., and Student, Q. 1978. Auditory nerve and brainstem evoked responses in normal, autistic, minimally brain damaged and psychomotor retarded children. Electroencephalography and Clinical Neurophysiology 44:380–388.

Sokolov, E. N. 1960. Neuronal models and the orienting reflex. In: M. Brazier (ed.), The Central Nervous System and Behavior, pp. 187–276. Josiah Macy Jr. Foundation, New York.

Spreen, O. 1976. Post-conference review. In: R. Knights and D. Bakker (eds.), The Neuropsychology of Learning Disorders, pp. 445-467. University Park Press, Baltimore.

Starr, A., and Achor, J. 1975. Auditory brainstem responses in neurological disease. Archives of Neurology 32:761-768.

Starr, A., and Achor, J. 1978. Generator of Brainstem Potentials. In: R. Naunton and C. Fernandez (eds.), Evoked Electrical Activity in the Auditory Nervous System, pp. 443-451. Academic Press, New York.

Starr, A., and Hamilton, A. E. 1976. Correlation between confirmed sites of neurological lesions and abnormalities of far-field auditory brainstem responses. Electroencephalography and Clinical Neurophysiology 41: 595-608.

Stockard, J. J., and Rossiter, V. S. 1977. Clinical and pathologic correlates of brainstem auditory response abnormalities. Neurology 27(4):316-325.

Stockard, J. J., Stockard, J. E., and Sharbrough, F. W. 1977. Detection and localization of occult lesions with brainstem auditory responses. Mayo Clinic Proceedings 52:761-769.

Webster, D., and Webster, M. 1977. Cochlear nerve projections following organ of Corti destruction. Paper presented at the 82nd Annual Meeting of the American Academy of Ophthalmology and Otolaryngology, Dallas, Texas, October 2-6, 1977.

Webster, D., and Webster, M. 1978. Auditory brainstem: Sound deprivation and critical period. Paper presented at the 83rd Annual Meeting of the American Academy of Ophthalmology and Otolaryngology, Las Vegas, Nevada, September 9-13, 1978.

Wiederhold, M. L. 1970. Variations in the effects of electrical stimulation of the crossed olivocochlear bundle on cat single auditory-nerve fiber responses to tone bursts. Journal of the Acoustical Society of America 48:966-977.

Willeford, J. 1976. Central auditory function. In: K. Donnelly (ed.), Communicative Disorders: Learning Disabilities. Little, Brown, Boston.

Willeford, J. 1977. Assessing central auditory behavior in children: A test battery approach. In: R. Keith (ed.), Central Auditory Dysfunction, pp. 43-72. Grune & Stratton, New York.

Willeford, J. 1978. Expanded Central Auditory Test Battery Norms. Colorado State University, Fort Collins, Colo.

Willeford, J., and Billger, J. 1978. Auditory perception in children with learning disabilities. In: J. Katz (ed.), Handbook of Clinical Audiology, 2nd Edition, pp. 410-412. Williams & Wilkins, Baltimore.

Worthington, D. 1981. ABR in special populations. Paper presented at ABR workshop, Cleveland, Ohio.

Worthington, D., Beauchaine, K., Peters, J., and Reiland, J. 1981. Abnormal ABR's in children with severe speech/language delays. Paper presented at the American Speech Language and Hearing Association Convention, Los Angeles, 1981.

Chapter **8**

Neuroscience, Pragmatic Competence, and Auditory Processing

Maxine L. Young

This chapter deals with language disorders that may be associated with central auditory processing deficits and the central auditory tests used in their evaluation. Although speech-language pathologists have been the primary investigators in the evaluation of children with language problems, neuroaudiologic test procedures and contributions from the neurosciences can provide a broader understanding of language disorders. Tests of CAP might reveal information regarding the neuromaturational status of the auditory system. Because of the interrelatedness of audition and language, information about a child's developing auditory system may also provide insight regarding the child's language development.

To consider the issue of auditory-perceptually based language disorders, this chapter focuses on several topics. First, neurobiologic evidence is presented to suggest that development of language closely parallels neurologic maturation of the auditory system. Second, selected processing models are reviewed demonstrating the difficulty that language-disordered children have in making auditory perceptual judgments. Third, neuropsychologic research is reviewed that associates language disorders with impairment of lateralized hemispheric functions. Fourth, pragmatic language disorders are related to problems integrating complementary functions of the two hemispheres or to CAP problems involving the right hemisphere.

NEUROBIOLOGIC EVIDENCE

Critical periods of language acquisition (Lenneberg, 1967) seem to parallel certain neuromaturational aspects of the auditory system. Language development occurs along with increased connections in the central nervous system and is dependent upon maturation and interconnectivity of functionally specialized neurons (Milner, 1967; Whitaker, 1976). The diversity and complexity of such interneuronal growth seems to be a prerequisite for both language and cognitive development.

Maturation occurs in the CNS biochemically (McKhann, Levy, & Ho, 1967) and structurally (Scheibel & Scheibel, 1976). Structural aspects correspond closely with progressive development in information processing capacity (Campbell & Coulter, 1976). The structural substrate of the CNS, the neuron, matures in two distinct ways: first, by development of a fatty layer of insulation around the transmitting axon, and second, by multiplication of dendritic synapses. There are two distinct classes of neurons with which we are concerned. Class I neurons (pyramidal cells) are early-developing, long neurons that form an invariant framework of afferent (to the CNS) and efferent (from the CNS) pathways. Class II neurons (stellate cells) develop later, are short and structurally variable, and perform integrative functions between primary afferent and efferent systems. Axons and dendrites of the stellate cells proliferate up and down through all six layers of the cortex, whereas their dendritic branches extend horizontally within each layer. Class II neurons are most susceptible to change as a result of maturation and biochemical stimulation and probably contribute to cognitive and language development (Jacobson, 1975). An infinite number of processing possibilities occur in the developing CNS as a result of this complex network of neurons and their interconnections.

Cortical maturation proceeds upward and from inner to outermost surfaces of the neocortex. Concurrently, maturation proceeds anteriorly from the occipital to the frontal lobes, as shown in Figure 1. Functionally specialized cortical centers develop with a specific rate of interneuronal maturation and in an orderly sequence. This results first in connections between peripheral and primary zones of sensorimotor, visual, and auditory cortices followed by connections between primary and association areas. Last to develop are the interneuronal connections between the association areas themselves, including the arcuate

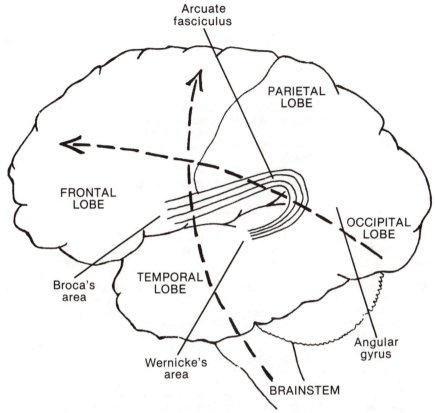

Figure 1.   Maturational development of the CNS. Arrows show direction of brainstem-to-brain and anterior-to-posterior maturation.

fasciculus and the corpus callosum (Figure 2, 9) the major pathway connecting the hemispheres (Whitaker, 1976).

Of primary concern to language development is maturation of the association areas of the cortex, which occupy 80% of the cortex. Higher-order skills such as cognition, language, and learning are mediated by functionally specialized centers and association areas of the cerebral cortex. Centers that subserve language are among the later developing components of the CNS (Lecours, 1975).

Neuroanatomical Asymmetries

Functional and anatomical asymmetries exist between the two hemispheres. The left may be distinguished from the right by such dichotomies as linguistic/nonlinguistic, analytic/gestalt, and sequential/

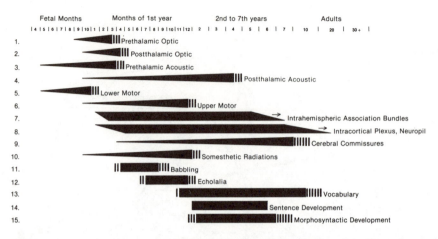

Figure 2.   Myelogenetic cycles of CNS systems that subserve speech-language and approximate schedules of development. *1*, Prethalamic optic pathways begin myelination during the 9th fetal month and are completed during the 4th postnatal month. *2*, By the 5th postnatal month the postthalamic optic pathway is fully myelinated. *3*, Prethalamic acoustic fibers start their myelogenetic cycle during the 20th fetal week and are completed up to the collicular level 1 month before birth; the inferior colliculus is fully myelinated by the 3rd or 4th postnatal month. *4*, Some myelination of the acoustic radiation is evident at birth; however, it is not fully mature until 4 years of age. *5*, Myelinated fibers of the lower motor components of the spinal and cranial nerves are evident by the 16th fetal week and are fully developed during the 1st trimester of postnatal life. *6*, Corticobulbar and corticospinal tracts progressively myelinate cephalocaudally. The pyramidal pathways are completely mature by 12 or 15 months after birth. *7*, Between 4 and 8 months postnatally, some fibers between primary and adjacent secondary cortices are myelinated. Fibers linking specific association areas begin myelination before fibers to and from nonspecific association areas, including afferents to and efferents from the angular region. Heschl's gyrus is myelinated before the posterior half of the first temporal convolution. *8*, The intracortical neuropil of primary projection areas (including Heschl's gyrus) begins myelination before the neuropil of specific association cortices such as Wernicke's area; neuropil myelination in the angular regions proceeds into 5th year of life, with some fibers still maturing into the 4th decade of life. *9*, Myelination of long association and commissural fiber systems continues into the 3rd decade of life, with corpus callosum still maturing beyond the first decade in some cases. *10*, Somesthetic (kinesthetic) radiations begin myelination at 9 months gestation and are completed during the first half of the 2nd year. *11–15*, See text. (Modified from Lecours, 1975.)

simultaneous. Investigators such as Witelson and Pallie (1973) have estimated that the left temporal planum is one-third longer than the right planum, and that a secondary division of the auditory cortex (the posterior portion of the superior temporal gyrus) is seven times larger in the left. The inferior frontal gyrus, comprising part of Broca's area, was also determined to be larger in the left hemisphere (Galaburda, 1980). Auditory-oral cortical areas predominantly involved in processing language thus seem to have greater left hemisphere representation in most individuals. Recent neuroanatomical research reveals structural asymmetries, suggesting that the right hemisphere is larger in volume and has more white matter than gray compared to the left (Galaburda et al., 1978; Gur et al., 1980; LeMay, 1976). Goldberg and Costa (1981) concluded that the left hemisphere has greater sensory and motor representation and is characterized by "intraregional" neuronal connectivity, whereas the right hemisphere has more associative cortex and neuronal growth is predominantly "interregional." The right hemisphere may better deal with informational complexity, whereas the left may be superior in tasks involving fixation upon a single mode of representation.

Auditory Neuromaturation and Language Development

The basic premise of tests employed to assess CAP is the interrelatedness of structural and functional maturation of the auditory system. Maturation of the CNS can also be related to the progressive differentiation of behavioral patterns, including the development of speech and language (Yakovlev, 1962). Figure 2 provides a timetable of myelogenetic cycles of the CNS, modified from Yakovlev and Lecours (1967), and the corresponding milestones of speech and language development.

A striking aspect of the developing brain is seen in comparing pre- and postthalamic maturational components of the auditory and visual pathways, the two primary learning modalities. As seen in Figure 2, pre- and postthalamic visual systems are fully myelinated by the 4th and 5th postnatal months (Figure 2, 1 and 2); however, development of the acoustic pathways differs markedly. Myelinated fibers are detected up to the collicular level (high brainstem) between the 8th and 9th fetal months, and are observed in the thalamic area by the 3rd or 4th postnatal months (Figure 2, 3). The geniculotemporal or cortical radiations, however, are only first being myelinated at birth and will not be completed until approximately 3½ to 4 years of age (Figure 2, 4).

A relationship between these neuromaturational features and the development of speech and language may be inferred. Babbling occurs during the first 6 months of life and continues into the 2nd year (Figure 2, 11). Fibers related to babbling that are fully myelinated during this period are the motor roots of the cranial nerves, the lower motor neurons (Figure 2, 5), and the facial area of the motor strip. The lower motor neurons (Figure 2, 6) and association fibers between Broca's and Wernicke's areas (Figure 2, 7) are beginning to myelinate and remain immature until 12 months of age. Prosodic components, imitated in the early repertoire of infant vocalizations, include melodic and suprasegmental patterns similar to those heard in adult speech. Intonation and rhythm provide the basic patterns upon which the child builds sound sequences and syntactic structures and which may serve as the basis for connotative or paralinguistic features of language (Liberman, 1977). Echolalic responses of infants develop from 6 to 12 months of age and may continue into the 2nd year of life (Figure 2, *12*). Both echolalia and prosodic imitation depend upon proprioceptive feedback (Lecours, 1975), presumably related to the increase of the arcuate fasciculus (Figure 2, *7*) and to the well (but not fully) developed maturation of the sensorimotor substrate. Imitation improves as maturation of the arcuate fasciculus continues to develop and facilitate transmission of auditory stimuli to motor speech areas (Lecours, 1975).

Vocabulary growth beyond 12 months of age is probably dependent upon progressive maturation of the auditory-visual-somesthetic association areas (Figure 2, *7* and *10*), which according to Yakovlev and Lecours (1967) continue to mature into the 3rd and 4th decades of life. Lecours (1975) related increase in language production and comprehension to neuromaturational development of association areas and to developing interneuronal connections and connections to and from angular regions.

Between 24 and 36 months of age, children begin to produce more complex syntactical structures (Figure 2, *14* and *15*) and attain the relatively complex sounds and forms of adult language by age 4 or 5. This coincides with the age at which postthalamic acoustic fibers are fully myelinated (Figure 2, *4*). Lecours (1975) paralleled the acquisition of syntax and semantics with a) protracted myelogenesis of the postthalamic acoustic radiations, b) maturation of intra- and interhemispheric association cortices, and c) developing intercortical neuropil (interwoven dendrites and axons; Figure 2, *8*). Language development, then, seems in part dependent upon neuromaturational auditory processes. Speech and language disorders may result from delays or idiosyncrasies in that system.

PROCESSING MODELS

The route from auditory reception to perception involves numerous neural transformations so that acoustic stimuli are eventually perceived as meaningful language. Disorder of the auditory periphery may ultimately affect the final perception. Adequate reception of the acoustic aspects of the speech signal is an important prerequisite of language acquisition. The global language disorder of deaf children demonstrates that inadequate reception so completely disrupts speech perception that a severe deficit in communication results. Serous otitis media, which causes a temporary reduction in hearing, has been correlated with speech and language disorders (Holm & Kunze, 1969; Lewis, 1976; Needleman, 1977). Webster (Chapter 10, this volume) suggests that, in animals, temporary sensory deprivation can cause irreversible structural abnormalities in brainstem structures involved in auditory perception.

Theories of speech perception focusing primarily on early stages of auditory processing suggest deficits in feature detection as possible causes of language disorder (Abbs & Sussman, 1971; Cole, 1977; Liberman et al., 1967). Tallal and colleagues (1976, a and b; 1980) theorized that the speech and language disorders of some children may be associated with difficulty in processing rapid auditory signals occurring during formant transitions. The difficulty was observed for both speech and nonspeech stimuli, suggesting that the problems in sound identification and discrimination are associated with transmission of very rapid acoustic rather than linguistic information. Language disorders may result from a primary auditory perceptual deficit in temporal analysis in the language-dominant hemisphere (Cutting, 1974; Efron, 1963b; Halperin, Nachshon, & Carmon, 1973).

LANGUAGE AND HEMISPHERIC SPECIALIZATIONS

Functionally, the cerebral hemispheres are cognitively and perceptually asymmetric, with the left hemisphere having superiority in sequential, logical, and verbal-linguistic abilities and the right specialized in nonverbal, visuospatial, and holistic processes (Dimond & Beaumont, 1974; Kinsbourne, 1978). Some theories of specialization suggest that left hemispheric processing of language is due to a simultaneous suppression of the minor hemisphere (Kinsbourne, 1976). Others propose that language requires global involvement with contributions and complementary integration of both hemispheres (Milner, 1974). There seems to be an equivalence of both hemispheres for language capacity, with language functions not fully lateralized until puberty (Penfield & Roberts, 1959; Lenneberg, 1967). Kimura's (1963) data, however, suggest a left hemispheric predominance for language in children as young as 3 years. Recent evidence also indicates a left hemisphere specialization for language in infants (Eimas et al., 1971; Entus, 1975; Molfese, Freeman, & Palmero, 1975; Molfese and Molfese, Chapter 5, this volume).

Although the left hemisphere has been traditionally viewed as language-dominant, increasing evidence supports the notion that the right hemisphere plays a role in linguistic processing. Zangwill (1967) associates language deficits with right hemisphere damage more frequently in children than in adults. According to Witelson (1977), the right hemisphere has a greater role in language processing in children than in adults; the left hemisphere has relative rather than complete dominance in mediating language functions. Further, Witelson concluded, the neural substrate of language changes with age, becoming more focused in one hemisphere rather than exclusive to one hemisphere.

The complementary contributions to language and the specialized functions of each hemisphere involve a right ear (left hemisphere) advantage (REA) in the identification of the stop consonants p, b, t, d, k, and g (Cutting, 1973) and a REA in the perception of rapid acoustic cues found in formant transitions (Tallal and Newcombe, 1976; Tallal, Stark, & Curtiss, 1976; Tallal, 1980). Left hemisphere specializations include verbal memory, conceptualization, grammar, syntax, and temporal ordering (Dennis & Kohn, 1975; Dennis & Whitaker, 1976; Efron, 1963a; Milner, 1974; Nebes & Briggs, 1974).

Evidence from neurologically involved and commissurotomy patients has provided knowledge of right hemisphere specializations. Memory for faces and visual forms, perception of human emotion, visuospatial orientation, gestalt-syntactic perception, simultaneous processing, and concrete perceptual insight are functions of the right hemisphere (Carmon & Nachshon, 1973; DeRenzi, 1968; Geffen, Bradshaw, & Wallace, 1971; Levi-Agresti & Sperry, 1968; Milner, 1974). Sentence stress cues that aid comprehension are processed in the right hemisphere (Blumenstrin & Cooper, 1974; Zurif, 1974). A left ear advantage (LEA) has been shown for processing melodies and speech intonation patterns (Darwin, 1969). The right hemisphere has connotative, associative, and imaginable language characteristics and may function in a language-supportive role in processing visual or auditory gestalts and in attending to extralinguistic context (Zaidel, 1977).

The complementary role of the hemispheres in processing language can be demonstrated by the sentence, "Well, what do you know?" First, say the sentence with the primary stress on the words "Well" and "you," as if angrily asking a question of someone who has offered advice on a topic about which they know little. Then say the sentence with the primary stress on the words "what" and "do," making an exclamation, as if finding that your cat named Tom gave birth to kittens. The syntax, temporal ordering, grammar, and articulation are identical in each utterance and are functions of left hemisphere processing. The meaning of each, however, is entirely different due to the melodic line, intonation, and stress. These aspects are mediated by the right hemisphere and contribute to the comprehension of each utterance. As Broadbent (1974) stated, speech perception requires processes of both hemispheres involving integrated performance.

PRAGMATICS AND THE RIGHT HEMISPHERE

Language is described through the dimensions of phonology, syntax, semantics, and pragmatics. Pragmatics can be defined as rules of communicative interaction between two or more persons and uses extralinguistic cues to convey intentions. Pragmatics utilizes the context of the physical, verbal, social, and psychologic environments.

Emerging evidence suggests that pragmatic aspects of language may be mediated in the right hemisphere. Language deficits in right-handed adults with unilateral right cerebral damage included diminished responses to contextual cues, literal rather than conceptual interpretation, and overall communicative ineffectiveness significantly different from normals (Myers & Linebaugh, 1980). Pragmatic deficits in patients with right hemisphere damage included poor vocal intonation, limited eye contact, and a lack of facial expression (Burns, 1979). These patients were unable to take a listener's perspective or to clarify communication inadequacies, and assumed they knew more than they really did.

Cicone, Wapner, and Gardner (1980) studied aphasics who in spite of formal language test deficits showed use of "pragmatic devices" such as the ability to take turns in conversation, use appropriate intonation and body language, maintain eye contact, and make inferences that gave the impression that they comprehended language discourse. The investigators felt these were attributes of the right hemisphere and contributed to the aphasics' communicative competence.

Although the speech of right hemisphere-damaged individuals is literally acceptable, they often fail to comprehend utterances in context or the tone of conversational exchange, and they experience difficulty in the comprehension of abstract sentences and logical reasoning (Caramazza et al., 1976; Lezak, 1979). The work of Gardner et al. (1975) shows they have difficulty understanding humor. They use a limited range of intonation and have difficulty interpreting figures of speech (Ross & Mesulam, 1979; Winner & Gardner, 1977). Right hemisphere-damaged patients were often unable to appreciate fictive, imaginary, and humorous material and had even greater difficulty processing contextually bound information (Wapner, Hamby, & Gardner, 1981). This pragmatic aspect of language communication may, then, involve the right hemisphere.

Although most of these studies dealt with neurologically impaired adults, some language-disordered children seem to have similar deficits of pragmatic communication (Lucas, 1980; Rees & Wollner, 1981; Simon, 1979). The youngsters' disorders in communication are subtle, appear to be similar to right brain-damaged adults' language, and may go undetected in a speech and language evaluation using language tests designed to evaluate other aspects of communication. Bryan, Donahue, and Pearl (1981) determined that learning-disabled children have pragmatic deficits that affect social relationships and academic achievement.

LANGUAGE DISORDERS AND CENTRAL AUDITORY TESTS

This relationship between auditory perception and language development has caused increased interest in tests of CAP (Brandes & Ehinger, 1981; Johnson, Enfield, & Sherman, 1981; Tallal, 1980). A study was conducted at the Hearing, Speech and Learning Center of Delaware County Memorial Hospital to determine any differences in patterns of performance among children with normal speech and language, those with speech and language disorders (articulation, syntactic, and semantic disorders), and those whose primary communication disorder involved pragmatic functions of language. Katz's Staggered Spondaic Word (SSW) Test and Willeford's Central Auditory Processing Battery (WCAP) were administered to subjects because of the diversity of these tests, their normative data for children, and their value in diagnosing deficient and language-disordered children (Johnson et al., 1981; Katz & Illmer, 1972; Protti, Young, & Byrne, 1980; Stubblefield & Young, 1975; Willeford & Billger, 1978).

Method

The sample included 75 normal hearing youngsters, 53 males and 22 females, between the ages of 5 and 19, who were referred because of suspected auditory perceptual problems. The data were obtained retrospectively from a review of clinical records. All of the children had normal intelligence. All experienced reading difficulty. Forty subjects (53.3%) were classified as learning-disabled by educational personnel using a battery of psychoeducational tests. All other subjects were in regular classrooms, but some received speech and language therapy or academic help through services such as resource rooms. None were included who had visual or physical handicaps or had known neurologic involvement. Subjects demonstrated normal hearing for pure tones and had excellent speech discrimination. First-generation reel-to-reel or cassette tape versions of the SSW and WCAP were administered according to test instructions. The Auditory Attention Span for Unrelated Words and Related Syllables subtests of the Detroit Test of Learning Aptitude (Baker & Leland, 1967) were also administered to determine whether auditory memory deficit contributed to test performance.

Each child was placed into one of three categories: 1) normal speech and language (NSL), including those with delayed onset and acquisition but whose language was normal at the time of the central auditory evaluation ($N=24$); 2) speech and/or language delayed (SLD; $N=33$) determined by a speech-language pathologist; 3) pragmatically disordered (PD; $N=18$). Ten (56%) in the PD group had immediate family members who also experienced learning problems (Table 1). The PD subjects were divided into two subgroups of 6- to 9-year-olds ($N=8$) and 11- to 19-year-olds ($N=10$) corresponding to data provided by Katz (1978), Lecours (1975), and Willeford (1978) suggesting that the auditory CNS is functionally mature by 10–11 years of age. Subjects in the PD group had full-scale IQs between 100 and 125 as assessed by the Wechsler Intelligence Scale for Children—Revised (WISC-R; Wechsler, 1974).

Pragmatic disorder was determined in part by parent and teacher ratings of communicative competence. Spontaneous conversation was assessed with Loban's Oral Language Scale (Loban, 1961) as cited in Simon (1979). This scale rates seven characteristics of oral language. The items that most characterized the oral skills of the PD group were poor prosody and vocal inflection, difficulty getting to the point and verbal irrelevancy (conversational postulates), inability to express ideas adequately (presupposition), difficulty attending to others (presupposition), and passivity in group discussion (performative). Vocabulary and structural aspects of language were rated within normal limits by teachers for all but two subjects. Some youngsters were rated as very verbal in the classroom; however, the quality of their language

Table 1.   Percentage of subjects by group who experienced serous otitis media (SOM), who were left-handed for writing skills, and whose immediate family members experienced learning difficulties.

Group	SOM	Left-handed	Familial
NSL (24)[a]	42% (10)	29% (7)	13% (3)
SLD (33)	67% (22)	15% (5)	21% (7)
PD (18)	28% (5)	0% (0)	56% (10)
Total (75)	49% (37)	16% (12)	27% (20)

[a]Number of subjects (N) is given in parentheses.

was judged inadequate and ineffective within the communicative context. Parents usually gave higher ratings to their children than the teachers did.

A history of serous otitis media (SOM) was reported for more SLD subjects (67%) than for any other group (Table 1). Subjects were included if they had thresholds of 15 dB hearing threshold level (HTL) or better, had tympanometric results with no more than −150 mm of water pressure, and had negative otoscopic findings at the time of the evaluation. Articulation disorders in SLD youngsters 8 years and older usually occurred for sibilants and glides (particularly the /r/ phoneme). These subjects were frequently reported as having difficulty learning the phonics approach to reading and had vowel discrimination difficulties and auditory memory and sequencing deficits.

Modified versions of Fisher's Auditory Checklist, one for educators and one for parents, provided an assessment of listening skills (Protti et al., 1980). Attributes most characteristic were: easily distracted, short auditory attention span, inability to relate what was seen with what was heard, and poor learning through the auditory channel. The teacher's assessment was particularly relevant, because the child was observed in the context of social communication within a peer group. Observations checked by the teachers were: poor eye contact, social and communicative "rudeness," lack of facial expression and intonation while talking, literal interpretations, and failure to get the punchline of jokes. These characteristics are often associated with the learning- and language-disordered child (Wiig & Semel, 1976).

SSW Test Results   Forty-one of the 75 children in this study had abnormal SSW results, quantitative and/or significant response biases (Katz, 1978). Twenty-three (70%) of the SLD group, 13 (54%) of the NSL group, and five (28%) of the PD group had abnormal results (Figure 3). Those subjects judged more severely learning-disabled by educational personnel had more errors in competing conditions (more so in the left competing stimulus mode), had more reversals, and exhibited greater ear and order effects, which White (1977) considered significant in children. Subjects typically showed ear low-high (fewer errors on the right-ear-first items) and order high-low (more errors on the first spondee) patterns. SSW reversals occurred in 21 subjects, many of whom were determined as having auditory sequencing and memory problems.

WCAP Test Results   Results showed 88% had abnormal Competing Sentences (CS) test performance, with 90% of the subjects showing a REA. On the Filtered Speech (FS) test, 66% had difficulty; most showed symmetrical (less than 16% difference between ears) but low scores.

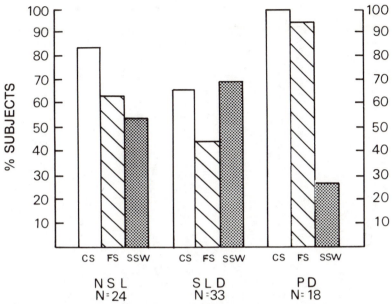

Figure 3.   Percentage of subjects exhibiting a significant number of errors on the CS, FS, and SSW tests, for the NSL, SLD, and PD groups.

A comparison of the NSL, SLD, and PD subjects' performances is summarized in Figure 3. Of the 24 children in the NSL group, the largest proportion had difficulty on the CS test. The proportions showing difficulty on the FS and SSW tests were nearly equal but smaller than that seen on the CS test. The NSL group had more difficulty on the dichotic tests (CS and SSW) than on the FS test.

All 18 PD subjects had difficulty on the CS test; 13 (73%) had better right ear scores. Seventeen (94%) exhibited abnormal performance on the FS test, with 16 showing significant differences in symmetry. Thirteen (81%) had ear differences of between 20% and 60%. Significant asymmetry between ear scores on the FS test occurred for eight subjects in the 11- to 19-year-old group but for only five of the younger subjects (Table 2). The CS and the SSW consistently agreed as to affected ear. The range of performance for the 6- to 9-year-olds on the CS test showed generally poorer results than the normal range reported by Willeford (1978). The range, however, on the FS test for the 11- to 19-year-olds suggests they had even greater difficulty when compared to Willeford's norms.

Discussion

Quantitative scores on the SSW were often developmentally normal (Katz, 1978), but response biases were significant. Response bias in

Table 2. Means and standard deviations for pragmatically disordered subjects on the CS and FS tests and the range of performance compared to Willeford's normative data (Willeford, 1978).

| | Right ear | | Left ear | | Percentage range | | | |
| | | | | | Subjects | | Normals | |
	Mean	SD	Mean	SD	Right	Left	Right	Left
6- to 9-year-olds (N=8)								
Competing Sentences	48.0	24.49	33.0	24.74	20–100	0–80	90–100	0–100
Filtered Speech	55.6	10.46	53.2	13.84	56–84	52–84	42–92	44–92
11- to 19-year-olds (N=10)								
Competing Sentences	96.0	5.16	85.0	4.9	90–100	70–100	90–100	90–100
Filtered Speech	75.6	8.31	59.2	17.7	56–84	24–84	74–100	74–100

children may indicate developmental delay or idiosyncrasy in areas that contribute to language perception (White, 1977). None of the subjects who exhibited SSW reversals had reported episodes of SOM; however, fine motor difficulties, clumsiness, and incomplete cerebral dominance seemed to be related to this phenomenon. When little or no improvement is seen on SSW test scores and the individual continues to experience auditory language and auditory learning problems, a deficit rather than a developmental delay may be implied. The abnormal CAP test results of the 6- to 9-year-old PD group may represent developmental delay that may resolve with time. Performance of the 11- to 19-year-old PD group could reflect auditory CNS idiosyncrasy or deficit, which is less likely to resolve.

Willeford (1978), Katz (1978), and others have reported developmental trends and a REA on dichotic test performance. This was first reported by Kimura (1963) as due to greater contralateral auditory representation of the left hemisphere, which is dominant for language processing. Right ear scores were consistently better than left ear scores on the CS test, and symmetrical results were observed in subjects who had no difficulty on this test by age 10. It would seem that the normative data, showing 90–100% scores symmetrically at age 10, coincide with the age at which the corpus callosum has nearly completed its myelogenetic cycle. It is suggested that youngsters 10 years of age and older whose CS scores are abnormal may have immature development or idiosyncratic function of the corpus callosum. Another explanation involves transmission time across the corpus callosum, which has been determined to be 6 msec for auditory information (Pirozzolo & Rayner, 1977) but can range to several hundred milliseconds. Central transmission time between the two hemispheres must be synchronous so that specialized but different functions of each are adequately processed.

The PD group was distinguished from the other groups by consistently abnormal performance on the CS and FS tests. Even when quantitative scores were borderline normal, difficulty reported by these subjects (for example, something wrong with the earphones or their hearing) revealed qualitative difficulties on dichotically competing tests. This suggests an auditory perceptual deficit. Difficulty on these tests may be related to CNS transmission time involving the corpus callosum or the right hemisphere, which can be seen by examining the test profile of a subject who typified the PD group in this study.

A male age 14 years, 9 months (B.J.) was referred for testing because of his inability to follow oral directions, poor attentional skills in the classroom, and the discrepancy between academic performance and intellectual potential (WISC-R Verbal IQ=137, Performance

IQ=105). His parents were middle socioeconomic class professionals; both held master's degrees. Birth history was negative, postnatal development was normal, and speech and language milestones were normal. B.J. seemed to be a passive but polite adolescent.

Teachers judged B.J.'s class participation as poor, stating that he rarely offered answers or participated in group discussions. He was quite popular with classmates but was generally considered to be quiet and a "bookworm." In English literature, his interpretation of *Animal Farm* was a literal one. After several weeks of class discussion, he described the book as a "strange story about talking animals." His voice quality was monotone and eye contact was poor during conversation. He was reportedly more serious than peers and siblings and was described by teachers as having poor written and oral expressive skills in spite of having a good vocabulary. A psychoeducational evaluation revealed that B.J. had incomplete cerebral dominance and a mild deficit in visual-motor integration, with his major academic handicap in reading. Although he had superior intelligence and performed at an eighth-grade level in other subjects, his independent reading (without teacher assistance) was at the fourth-grade level. Results of a speech and language evaluation showed that B.J. had the necessary linguistic skills (articulation, syntax, and semantics) to function effectively, but difficulty was observed on the auditory closure subtest of the Illinois Test of Psycholinguistic Abilities (Kirk, McCarthy, & Kirk, 1968). This is frequently observed at Delaware County Memorial Hospital in children whose FS tests are significantly asymmetrical.

Several suggestions were offered as to why this subject had reading difficulty. One interpretation is that meanings of sentences may be affected by intonation, melody, and stress patterns. If an individual fails to interpret how a passage is to be read according to the intended suprasegmental stress, pauses, and inflection, then reading comprehension could suffer.

Let us examine the CAP test results. Scores on the CS test should be 100% for both ears in subjects 14 years of age. Quantitatively the scores are in the normal range, but responses for all left ear presentations were qualitatively poor (hesitations and numerous self-corrected errors). Difficulty on the CS test may reflect idiosyncratic corpus callosum function or a right hemisphere processing deficit. Scores for FS were markedly asymmetrical (right=84%, left=56%); this is not, however, a dichotic test, so no ear advantage should occur. Stimuli presented to the right ear (left-hemisphere-direct route) were adequately processed, so processing of the left ear signals in the right temporal lobe or transmission via the corpus callosum to the left hemisphere may be implicated.

The monotonous voice quality may be related to an inability of both hemispheres to integrate melodic intonation simultaneously with linguistic processing during speech production, or a right hemisphere processing deficit that would inhibit B.J. from perceiving the prosody of others' speech. A deficit that affects prosody is known to occur in adults with right brain damage (Sidtis, 1980). Asymmetrically significant FS test results are frequently found in subjects who lack normal prosodic and inflectional voice qualities.

With normal linguistic abilities suggesting adequate left hemisphere function, with voice quality and auditory closure difficulties suggestive of limitations of more right hemisphere functions, it is not surprising that the central auditory tests suggested a deficit in the auditory processing of the right hemisphere.

This chapter suggests that pragmatic communication disorders and CAP deficits may be related; these deficits may involve interhemispheric transmission or right hemisphere auditory processes. The right hemisphere may mediate pragmatic aspects of communication. Diagnostic and therapeutic strategies employed with children should assure that pragmatic difficulties do not go undetected during a speech and language evaluation (Scott & Taylor, 1978). Ways need to be explored to facilitate communication skills in learning-disabled youngsters with pragmatic disorders. A broader approach would include assessment of language in context as well as peripheral and central auditory function.

REFERENCES

Abbs, J. H., and Sussman, H. M. 1971. Neurophysiological feature detectors and speech perception. A discussion of theoretical implications. Journal of Speech and Hearing Research 14:23–36.

Baker, J., and Leland, B. 1967. Detroit Test of Learning Aptitudes. Test Division of Bobbs-Merrill, Indianapolis.

Blumenstein, S. E., and Cooper, W. E. 1974. Hemispheric processing of intonation contours. Cortex 10:146–158.

Brandes, P. J., and Ehinger, D. M. 1981. The effects of early middle ear pathology on auditory perception and academic achievement. Journal of Speech and Hearing Disorders 46(3):301–306.

Broadbent, D. E. 1974. Division of function and integration of behavior. In: F. O. Schmitt and F. G. Worden (eds.), The Neurosciences, Third Study Program, pp. 31–41. MIT Press, Cambridge, Mass.

Bryan, T., Donahue, M., and Pearl, R. 1981. Studies of learning disabled children's pragmatic competence. Topics in Learning and Learning Disabilities 1(2):29–40.

Burns, M. S. 1979. Communication deficits associated with right cerebral brain damage. Paper presented at American Speech and Hearing Association Annual Convention, Atlanta, 1979.

Campbell, B. A., and Coulter, X. 1976. The ontogenesis of learning and memory. In: M. R. Rosenzweig and E. L. Bennet (eds.), Neural Mechanisms of Learning and Memory, pp. 209–235. MIT Press, Cambridge, Mass.

Caramazza, A., Gordon, J., Zurif, E. B., and Deluca, D. 1976. Right-hemispheric damage and verbal problem solving behavior. Brain and Language 3:41–46.

Carmon, A., and Nachson, I. 1973. Ear asymmetry in the perception of emotional non-verbal stimuli. Acta Psychologica 37:351–357.

Cicone, M., Wapner, W., and Gardner, H. 1980. Sensitivity to emotional expressions and situation in organic patients. Cortex 16:145–158.

Cole, R. A. 1977. Invariant features and feature detectors. Some developmental implications. In: S. J. Segalowitz and F. H. Gruber (eds.), Language Development and Neurological Theory. Academic Press, New York.

Cutting, J. E. 1973. Parallel between degree of encodedness and the ear advantage: Evidence from an ear monitoring task. Journal of the Acoustical Society of America 53:368.

Cutting, J. 1974. Different speech processing mechanisms can be reflected in the results of discrimination and dichotic listening tasks. Brain and Language 1:363–373.

Darwin, C. J. 1969. Auditory perception and cerebral dominance. Unpublished Ph.D. thesis, University of Cambridge, England.

Dennis, M. D., and Kohn, B. 1975. Comprehension of syntax in infantile hemiplegia after cerebral hemidecortication. Left hemisphere superiority. Brain and Language 2:472–482.

Dennis, M. D., and Whitaker, H. A. 1976. Language acquisition following hemidecortication. Linguistic superiority of the left over the right hemisphere. Brain and Language 3:404–433.

DeRenzi, E. 1968. Non-verbal memory and hemispheric side of lesion. Neuropsychologia 6:181–189.

Dimond, S. J., and Beaumont, J. G. 1974. Hemispheric function in the human brain. Halstead Press, New York.

Efron, R. 1963a. Temporal perception, aphasia and deja vu. Brain 86:403–424.

Efron, R. 1963b. Effect of handedness on the perception of simultaneity and temporal order. Brain 86:261–284.

Eimas, P. D., Siqueland, E., Jusczyk, P., and Vigorito, J. 1971. Speech perception in infants. Science 171:303–306.

Entus, A. K. 1975. Hemispheric asymmetry in processing of dichotically presented speech and non-speech sounds by infants. Paper presented at the meetings of the Society for Research in Child Development, Denver, Colo., 1975.

Galaburda, A. M. 1980. Paper presented at the 13th Annual Winter Conference on Brain Research, Keystone, Colo., January 19–26, 1980.

Galaburda, A. M., LeMay, M., Kemper, T. L., and Geschwind, N. 1978. Right-left asymmetries in the brain. Science 199:852–856.

Gardner, H., Ling, K., Flamini, L., and Silverman, J. 1975. Comprehension and appreciation of humor in brain-damaged patients. Brain 98:399–412.

Geffen, G., Bradshaw, J. L., and Wallace, G. 1971. Interhemispheric effects on reaction time to verbal and non-verbal visual stimuli. Journal of Experimental Psychology 85:415–422.

Goldberg, E., and Costa, L. D. 1981. Hemisphere differences in the acquisition and use of descriptive systems. Brain and Language 14:144–173.

Gur, R. C., Packer, I. K., Hungerbuhler, J. P., Reivick, M., Obrist, W. D., Amarnek, W. S., and Sackeim, H. A. 1980. Differences in the distinction of grey and white matter in human cerebral hemisphere. Science 207:1226–1228.

Halperin, Y., Nachshon, I., and Carmon, A. 1973. Shift of ear superiority in dichotic listening of temporally patterned nonverbal stimuli. Journal of the Acoustical Society of America 53:46–50.

Holm, V. A., and Kunze, L.H. 1969. Effect of chronic otitis media on language and speech development. Pediatrics 43:833–839.

Jacobson, M. 1975. Brain development in relation to language. In: E. H. Lenneberg and E. Lenneberg (eds.), Foundations of Language Development— A Multidisciplinary Approach, Volume I, pp. 105–119. Academic Press, New York.

Johnson, D. W., Enfield, M., and Sherman, R. E. 1981. The use of the Staggered Spondaic Words and the Competing Environmental Sounds tests in the evaluation of central auditory function of learning disabled children. Ear and Hearing 2(2):70–77.

Katz, J. 1978. SSW Workshop Manual. Allentown Industries, Buffalo, N.Y.

Katz, J., and Illmer, R. 1972. Auditory perception in children with learning disabilities. In: J. Katz (ed.), Handbook of Clinical Audiology, pp. 540–563. Williams & Wilkins, Baltimore.

Kimura, D. 1963. Speech lateralization in young children as determined by an auditory test. Journal of Comparative and Physiological Psychology 56:899–902.

Kinsbourne, M. 1976. The ontogeny of cerebral dominance. In: D. R. Aaronson and R. W. Reiber (eds.), Developmental Psycholinguistics and Communication Disorders. New York Academy of Sciences, New York.

Kinsbourne, M. 1978. Asymmetrical Function of the Brain. Cambridge University Press, Cambridge, England.

Kirk, S. A., McCarthy, J. J., and Kirk, W. D. 1968. Illinois Test of Psycholinguistic Abilities (Revised Edition). University of Illinois Press, Urbana, Ill.

Lecours, A. R. 1975. Myelogenetic correlates of the development of speech and language. In: E. H. Lenneberg and E. Lenneberg (eds.), Foundations of Language Development—A Multidisciplinary Approach, Volume I, pp. 121–135. Academic Press, New York.

LeMay, M. 1976. Morphological cerebral asymmetries of modern man, fossil man and non-human primate. In: S. R. Harnad, H. D. Steklis, and J. Lancaster (eds.), Origins and evolution of language and speech. Annals of the New York Academy of Sciences 280:349–366.

Lenneberg, E. H. 1964. Speech as a motor skill with special reference to nonaphasic disorders. Monographs of the Society for Research in Child Development 29:115–127.

Lenneberg, E. H. 1966. The natural history of language. In: F. Smith and G. Miller (eds.), The Genesis of Language. MIT Press, Cambridge, Mass.

Lenneberg, E. H. 1967. Biological Foundations of Language. John Wiley & Sons, New York.

Levi-Agresti, J., and Sperry, R. W. 1968. Differential perceptual capacities in major and minor hemispheres. Proceedings of the U.S. National Academy of Sciences 61:1151.

Lewis, N. 1976. Otitis media and linguistic incompetence. Archives of Otolaryngology 102:387–390.

Lezak, M. D. 1979. Behavioral concomitants of configurational disorganization in the hemisphere damaged patients. Unpublished paper, Portland, Ore.

Liberman, P. 1977. Speech Physiology and Acoustic Phonetics. Macmillan, New York.

Liberman, A. M., Cooper, F. S., Shankweiler, D., and Studdert-Kennedy, M. 1967. Perception of the speech code. Psychological Review 74:431–461.

Loban, W. 1961. Language Ability in the Middle Grades of Elementary Schools. U.S. Office of Education, Washington.

Lucas, E. V. 1980. Semantic and Pragmatic Language Disorders. Aspen Systems Corporation, Bethesda, Md.

McKhann, G. M., Levy, R., and Ho, W. 1967. Biochemical studies of myelinization. In: A. Minkowski (ed.), Regional Development of the Brain in Early Life, pp. 189–197. Blackwell, Oxford, England.

Milner, E. 1967. Human Neural and Behavioral Development. Charles C Thomas, Springfield, Ill.

Milner, E. 1974. Hemispheric specializations: Scope and limits. In: F. O. Schmitt and F. G. Worden (eds.), The Neurosciences, Third Study Program, pp. 75–92. MIT Press, Cambridge, Mass.

Molfese, D. L., Freeman, R. B., and Palmero, D. S. 1975. The ontogeny of brain lateralization for speech and non-speech stimuli. Brain and Language 2:356–368.

Myers, P. S., and Linebaugh, C. W. 1980. The perception of contextually conveyed relationships by right brain damaged patients. Paper presented at ASHA Annual Convention, Detroit.

Nebes, R. D., and Briggs, G. C. 1974. Handedness and the retention of visual materials. Cortex 10:209–214.

Needleman, H. 1977. Effects of hearing loss from early recurrent otitis media on speech and language development. In: B. F. Jaffe (ed.), Hearing Loss in Children, pp. 640–649. University Park Press, Baltimore.

Penfield, W., and Roberts, L. 1959. Speech and Brain Mechanisms. Princeton University Press, Princeton, N.J.

Pirozzolo, F. J., and Rayner, K. 1977. Hemispheric specialization in reading and word recognition. Brain and Language 4:248–261.

Protti, E., Young, M., and Byrne, P. 1980. The evaluation of a child with auditory perceptual deficiencies: An interdisciplinary approach. In: R. W. Keith and J. L. Northern, Seminars in Speech, Language and Hearing 1(2):167–180.

Rees, N., and Wollner, S. G. 1981. A taxonomy of pragmatic abilities. The use of language in conversation. Paper presented at the American Speech and Hearing Association Eastern Regional Convention, Philadelphia, 1981.

Ross, E. D., and Mesulam, M. M. 1979. Dominant language functions of the right hemisphere. Prosody and emotional gesturing. Archives of Neurology 36:144–148.

Scheibel, M. E., and Scheibel, A. B. 1976. Some thoughts on the ontogeny of memory and learning. In: M. Rosenzweig and E. L. Bennett (eds.), Neural Mechanisms of Learning and Memory, pp. 241–310. MIT Press, Cambridge, Mass.

Scott, C., and Taylor, A. 1978. A comparison of home and clinic gathered language samples. Journal of Speech and Hearing Disorders 43:482–495.

Sidtis, J. 1980. On the nature or cortical function underlying right hemisphere auditory perception. Neuropsychologia 18:321–333.

Simon, C. S. 1979. Communicative Competence: Functional Pragmatic Approach to Language Therapy. Communication Skill Builders, Tucson, Ariz.

Stubblefield, J., and Young, E. 1975. Central auditory dysfunction in learning disabled children. Journal of Learning Disabilities 8:89–94.

Tallal, P., and Newcombe, F. 1976. Impairment of auditory perception and language comprehension in residual dysphasia. Journal of the Acoustical Society of America 59:585.

Tallal, P., Stark, R., and Curtiss, B. 1976. The relation between speech perception impairment and speech production impairment in children with developmental dysphasia. Brain and Language 3:305–317.

Tallal, P. 1980. Auditory processing disorders in children. In: P. J. Levinson and C. Sloan (eds.), Auditory Processing and Language—Clinical and Research Perspectives. Grune & Stratton, New York.

Wapner, W., Hamby, S., and Gardner, H. 1981. The role of the right hemisphere in the apprehension of complex linguistic materials. Brain and Language 14:15–33.

Wechsler, D. 1974. Wechsler Intelligence Scale for Chilren—Revised. The Psychological Corporation, New York.

White, E. 1977. Children's performance on the SSW test and Willeford's Battery: Interim clinical data. In: R. Keith (ed.), Central Auditory Dysfunction. Grune & Stratton, New York.

Whitaker, H. 1976. Neurobiology of language. In: E. C. Carterette and M. P. Friedman (eds.), Handbook of Perception, Volume 7, pp. 121–144. Academic Press, New York.

Wiig, E. H., and Semel, E. M. 1976. Language Disabilities in Children and Adolescents. Charles E. Merrill, Columbus, Ohio.

Willeford, J. 1978. Procedures for Tests of Central Auditory Function. Colorado State University, Fort Collins, Colo.

Willeford, J., and Billger, J. 1978. Auditory perception in children with learning disabilities. In: J. Katz (ed.), Handbook of Clinical Audiology, pp. 410–426. Williams & Wilkins, Baltimore.

Winner, E., and Gardner, H. 1977. Comprehension of metaphor in brain-damaged patients. Brain 100:719–727.

Witelson, S. F. 1977. Early hemispheric specialization and interhemispheric plasticity. An empirical and theoretical review. In: S. J. Segaliwitz and F. A. Gruber (eds.), Language Development and Neurological Theory, pp. 213–275. Academic Press, New York.

Witelson, S. F., and Pallie, W. 1973. Left hemisphere specialization for language in the newborn. Neuroanatomical evidence of asymmetry. Brain 96:641–646.

Yakovlev, P. I. 1962. Morphological criteria of growth and maturation of the nervous system in man. Research Publications, Association for Research in Nervous and Mental Disease 39:3–46.

Yakovlev, P. I., and Lecours, A. R. 1967. The myelogenetic cycles of regional maturation of the brain. In: A. Minkowski (ed.), Regional Development of the Brain in Early Life, pp. 3–70. Blackwell, Oxford, England.

Zaidel, E. 1977. Auditory vocabulary of the right hemisphere following brain bisection or hemidecortication. Cortex 12(3):191–211.

Zangwill, O. L. 1967. Speech and the minor hemisphere. Acta Neurologica et Psychiatrica Belgica 67:1013–1020.

Zurif, E. B. 1974. Auditory lateralization: Prosody and syntactic factors. Brain and Language 1:391–404.

Chapter 9

Auditory Processing Skills of Hyperactive, Language-Impaired, and Reading-Disabled Boys

Christy L. Ludlow, Edward A. Cudahy,
Celia Bassich, and *Gerald L. Brown*

The assessment of central auditory processing has received a great deal of attention in recent years as a potentially useful diagnostic tool. This chapter is concerned with the diagnostic significance of CAP testing of children. The first section discusses information derived from testing CAP in adults with acquired brain lesions. Next, recent studies of CAP in normal children and those with central pathologies are reviewed. The final section discusses implications of these data for interpretation of central pathologies underlying auditory processing deficits.

Many tests of CAP have been developed since Bocca and Calearo (1963) reported that brain-lesioned adults had impaired speech recognition skills for filtered stimuli. Their findings suggested that performance on speech recognition tests is sensitive to central auditory pathway pathology. Most tests that are sensitive to neuropathologies of the central auditory system use monaural speech stimuli that have been degraded through masking, distortion, or binaural speech stimuli which complement or compete with each other at the two ears. Validation of these measures of central auditory pathology came from studies of adults with brain tumors, following cerebrovascular lesions, or following surgery for intractable epilepsy. Before the advent of computerized tomography (CT), verification of site of lesion was poor. Because a subject's speech perception can be severely compromised by a central language disorder such as aphasia, the diagnostic implications of CAP test results can be severely compromised when only speech materials are employed with such patients. Language disorders impair speech perception skills regardless of whether there are independent lesions in the auditory association cortex, the primary auditory cortex, or the medial geniculate and/or geniculocortical tracts. Lesions in the central language regions of the cortex can now be determined with the improved resolution of new CT scanners.

Many tests of CAP assess speech perception rather than nonverbal auditory perception (the perception of frequency, intensity, and temporal order characteristics of auditory signals). In most CAP tests the speech signals have been degraded by noise, or redundancy has been reduced. Thus, linguistic deficits could account for poor performance on these tests rather than disturbances in the central auditory system. Function at various levels of the central auditory system can be assessed with nonverbal test stimuli. Comparing performance for nonverbal stimuli with performance for speech stimuli will determine both whether deficits are confined to speech stimuli and the relation between specific deficits with given stimuli and the site of lesion. This work has just begun in adults, and early data suggest that nonverbal auditory processing and speech perception can be independently impaired depending upon the location of acquired brain lesions (Auerbach, Naeser, & Mazurski, 1981).

Interpretation of CAP tests in children is more difficult. Speech recognition skills in children are shaped through speech exposure and linguistic development (Aslin & Pisoni, 1980). Therefore, speech recognition skills of language-impaired children may be impaired, reflecting the central language disorder. To assess higher-level auditory perceptual skills of language-impaired children independent of their language functioning, it is crucial to test with nonspeech signals and nonverbal operant conditioning procedures. Tallal and Piercy (1973) synthesized complex tones of 100 and 305 Hz and used operant conditioning tasks to determine the ability of language-impaired children to discriminate the two stimuli when presented at different rates. They found the language-impaired subjects had greater difficulty processing nonverbal stimuli than did normal subjects when the stimuli were reduced in length, the interval between stimuli was reduced, or an increasing number of stimuli had to be remembered.

Tallal and Piercy (1974) repeated the experiments with speechlike stimuli to test discrimination between the isolated vowels /ɛ/ and /æ/ and between the consonant-vowel (CV) syllables /ba/ and /da/. The language-impaired group discriminated between the vowels as well as they had the complex tones. They had only perceptual difficulties in comparison with normals when stimuli were reduced in length or presented in rapid succession. However, on the /ba/ and /da/ syllables, which normal children recognize as speech syllables, the language-impaired subjects had much more difficulty; they could not accurately discriminate between the two stimuli. Many of the children who had easily discriminated the complex tones and vowel sounds were unable, even with training, to discriminate between the syllables. Only when the rate of formant change was reduced did the language-impaired subjects discriminate between speech stimuli.

Tallal and Piercy (1978) interpreted their results to indicate that perceptual deficits of language-impaired children were specific to rapidly occurring acoustic events, because the expansion of the formant transition from 40 msec to 80 msec improved the subjects' performance. Thus, they concluded that "...some cases of developmental dysphasia are the direct consequence of defective processing of rapidly changing acoustic information and an associated, possibly consequential reduced memory span for auditory sequence" (Tallal & Piercy, 1978, p. 82).

In a subsequent study using similar CV syllables, however, Stark and Tallal (1980) failed to replicate the finding of a significant improvement in syllable discrimination skills in language-impaired children when the formant transitions were expanded to 80 msec. Another view of Tallal and Piercy's results could be that although children with language disorders had impaired perception of temporal order for rapid nonverbal stimuli, they were significantly more impaired in their perception of speech stimuli. The finding that their speech perception deficits were not commensurate with their nonverbal auditory processing difficulties could suggest that language impairment interfered with speech perception.

Independence of specific speech processing deficits from deficits in auditory nonverbal processing could be supported if similar nonverbal auditory and visual perceptual difficulties were found in groups of learning-disordered children with and without language disorders. Strauss and Lehtinen (1947) first described the frequency of nonverbal perceptual deficits in learning-disabled children. Several investigators have reported auditory and visual perceptual deficits in children with impaired language, impaired reading, minimal brain dysfunction, or learning disability (Aten & Davis, 1968; Lowe & Campbell, 1965; Poppen et al., 1969; Birch & Belmont, 1964; Bakker, 1971; Corkin, 1974; Stark, 1966, 1967). Tallal et al. (1981) reported both visual and auditory nonverbal deficits in language-impaired children between 5 and 7 years, although only auditory deficits reached statistical significance in older children. Tallal (1980) and Stark and Tallal (1980) demonstrated the same difficulties in reading-impaired children when discriminating between shortened complex tones of 100 and 305 Hz and sequencing such tones presented at a rapid rate. Further, the reading-impaired children's phonic reading skills were correlated with their degree of nonverbal auditory perceptual dysfunctions (Tallal, 1980). None of the reading-impaired children had impaired language or a history of language impairment, although they had nonverbal auditory processing deficits very similar to those found in language-impaired subjects by Tallal and Piercy (1973).

Similar perceptual deficits in different subtypes of learning-disordered children may indicate that these deficits are symptoms often associated with various forms of learning disability but not generic to a particular primary learning disability, such as reading or language impairment. Thus, the nonverbal auditory processing deficits of the language-impaired may be independent of their speech perception deficits if nonverbal auditory processing deficits are also found in other groups of children without specific language disorders. Nonverbal deficits may be closely related to difficulties with attention and distractibility frequently found in learning-disabled children and most notable in "hyperactive" children with specific attention deficits but without specific impairments in language or reading (Douglas, 1976). To determine the possible independence of nonverbal auditory processing from speech recognition and reading and language comprehension, highly selective subtypes of normal, learning-impaired, hyperactive, and language-impaired children were selected for study of their nonverbal auditory processing skills.

GENERAL EVALUATION PROCEDURE

These studies are part of an ongoing program of the National Institute of Mental Health to investigate hyperactive and learning-disabled boys aged 6–12 years at the National Institutes of Health Clinical Center. On admission, all subjects were evaluated by a multidisciplinary team including a psychiatrist, a psychologist, a school teacher, a speech-language pathologist, and a social worker. All subjects were comprehensively evaluated by each team member to determine classification according to the Third Edition of the Diagnostic and Statistical Manual of the American Psychiatric Association (DSM-III). All subjects were free of medications for 2 weeks prior to speech and language testing, which included standardized speech and language tests in one session and experimental tests of nonverbal auditory processing on a second testing session in the same week. The standardized speech and language tests included the Auditory Association, Grammatic Closure, and Auditory Perception subtests of the Illinois Test of Psycholinguistic Abilities (ITPA; Kirk, McCarthy, & Kirk, 1968); the Peabody Picture Vocabulary Test (PPVT; Dunn, 1965); the Goldman-Fristoe-Woodcock Selective Attention Test (GFW; Goldman, Fristoe, & Woodcock, 1976); and the Children's Token Test (DiSimoni, 1978). Psychologic testing included the Wechsler Intelligence Scale for Children—Revised (WISC-R; Wechsler, 1974) and the Reading Recognition, Reading Comprehension, and Spelling subtests of the Peabody Individual Achievement Test (PIAT; Dunn & Markwardt, 1970). Conners' Teachers Rating Scale (CTRS) Factor IV (Conners, 1973) ratings were obtained from school teachers for each subject before admission as well as during the multidisciplinary evaluation period.

SUBJECT SELECTION CRITERIA

Subject selection criteria for boys with hyperactivity without language or learning disabilities (H) included: 1) age-inappropriate excess motor activity, poor attention span, and impulsive behavior as defined in the DSM-III; 2) no other psychiatric diagnoses or neuropsychologic abnormalities; 3) a CTRS Factor IV rating of 3.0 or greater (2.86 is equal to 2 standard deviations over the norm) (Werry, Sprague, & Cohen, 1975); 4) a Verbal and Performance IQ of 90 or greater on the WISC-R; 5) performance within 1 standard deviation of age norm on all tests of expressive and receptive language; 6) performance within 1 grade of age-expected grade level on tests of reading and spelling achievement; and 7) hearing within normal limits as determined by audiometric screening at 30-dB hearing level (HL) in both ears at 500, 1000, 2000, and 4000 Hz (American National Standards Institute, 1969).

The subject selection criteria for hyperactive boys with a reading disability (HRD) were identical to those for hyperactive boys without a reading disability except for reading achievement. Those in the HRD group performed at least one grade below age-expected grade level on tests of reading achievement.

Subject selection criteria for language-impaired boys without hyperactivity (LI) included: 1) absence of emotional, behavioral, or cognitive disturbance other than a language impairment as determined by the multidisciplinary team; 2) a Performance IQ of 80 or greater on the WISC-R; 3) a Performance minus Verbal IQ score difference of

15 points or greater, to indicate cognitive deficits only in language; 4) a score 2 standard deviations or more below age norm on tests of expressive and receptive language; 5) reading achievement scores 1 grade level or more below expected for chronologic age-equivalent grade level; 6) hearing within normal limits as determined by audiometric screening at 30 dB HL in both ears at 500, 1000, 2000, and 4000 Hz; and 7) a score of 2 or below on the CTRS Factor IV.

Subject selection criteria for language-impaired boys with hyperactivity (LIH) included those criteria for language-impaired boys plus: age-inappropriate excess motor activity, poor attention span, and impulsive behavior as defined by DSM-III and determined by the multidisciplinary team.

Four groups of normal control boys were selected so that one normal control was the same age as one subject in the impaired groups. Selection criteria for each normal control included: 1) no signs by history or current physical examination of behavioral, emotional or cognitive disorders; 2) performance within 1 standard deviation of age-expected level on tests of language and intelligence; 3) a CTRS Factor IV rating of 2 or less; 4) hearing within normal limits as determined by audiometric screening at 30 dB HL in both ears at 500, 1000, 2000, and 4000 Hz; and 5) performance at age-expected levels in all subjects in school.

EXPERIMENTAL AUDITORY PROCESSING TESTING

The experimental auditory processing testing was conducted in a sound-treated room with two examiners. One examiner was seated next to the child to ensure correct sitting position and earphone placement, and the other examiner scored the subject's responses. All stimuli were presented monaurally through TDH 49 headphones to the preferred ear at 80 dB re 0.0002 dynes/cm^2. Modular programming equipment in an adjoining room was used to administer all tasks and automatically score responses from a two-button response box. All testing except the vigilance task was subject-paced; a subsequent trial was not presented until the subject responded to the previous one.

Threshold for a 1000-Hz tone in 80-dB sound pressure level (SPL) of white noise was determined for each subject by means of a two-interval forced-choice adaptive procedure. Subjects pressed one of two panels on the response box to indicate whether the tone was contained in the first or second noise burst. If the subject's response was correct, a small light was automatically activated on the response box. This demonstrated the subject's ability to respond to the test stimuli, provided training for the two experimental tasks to follow, and established a subject's threshold for use in the vigilance task. Throughout the auditory testing, the reinforcement light provided feedback to subjects on all tasks except the vigilance task.

The vigilance test (a continuous performance test) measured the subject's ability to attend to stimuli and consisted of 180 trials over 15 min. A 1000-Hz, 50-msec tone was randomly presented on 50% of the trials at 10 dB above the subject's previously determined threshold in 1 sec of white noise presented for each trial at 80 dB SPL. Subjects were instructed to press a response button only when they detected a tone in noise. Total percent correct was computed by summing the number of hits and correct rejections, dividing by the number of trials, and multiplying by 100. On each signal trial, signal onset triggered a clock which counted milliseconds until a response occurred or 2.4 sec had elapsed, whichever came first. Reaction time was then recorded by the experimenter. Only reaction times for correct responses were used to compute mean response time for a subject.

Two experimental tests of auditory perception of nonverbal acoustic stimuli were administered. A gap detection task was used to assess temporal resolution. For each trial of the task, two 80-dB SPL, 750-msec noise bursts were separated by 300 msec of silence. A short gap of silence was inserted into the middle of either the first or second noise burst. Subjects responded by pressing one of two buttons corresponding to whether the first or second noise burst contained the gap. Gap duration was held constant for each block of 40 trials. The first block had a 20-msec gap. If necessary, gap duration was adjusted until a subject identified placement of the gap with greater than 90% accuracy. Gap duration was then systematically reduced on each subsequent block of 40 trials until a subject responded no better than 60% correct.

The perception of temporal order of acoustic stimuli was assessed utilizing Hirsh and Sherrick's (1961) procedure. Two 50-msec, 80-dB SPL pure tones of 1000 and 2500 Hz were presented on each trial and separated initially in their onset times by an interstimulus interval (ISI) of 500 msec. The order of the two tones was varied randomly, and the subjects responded by pressing one of two buttons, depending upon which tone came first. The duration of the ISI was constant for each block of 40 trials. If necessary, ISI was adjusted until a subject achieved greater than 90% accuracy. Then ISI duration was decreased for subsequent blocks of 40 trials until a subject responded no better than 60% correct.

Percent correct was computed for each block of 40 trials in the gap detection and temporal order tasks. Least-squares curves (psychometric functions) were derived for each subject between 60% and 90% correct relating percent correct to the temporal dimension varied (i.e., gap duration or ISI). The 75% correct point was determined from these curves and termed the threshold for gap detection or temporal order.

RESULTS

Twenty-six of the children admitted to the National Institutes of Health Clinical Center over a period of 4 years met the subject selection criteria for one of four subject groups: six subjects were language-impaired without hyperactivity (LI), with a mean age of 9.3 years and a range of 6–12 years; six were language impaired with hyperactivity (LIH), with a mean age of 10.1 years and a range of 8–12 years; eight were hyperactive without language or reading disability (H), with a mean age of 8.0 and a range of 7.9–10 years; six were hyperactive with reading disability (HRD), with a mean of 9.4 years and a range of 8.4–11 years.

The results of the standardized language and reading testing (Table 1) confirmed that the four groups had distinctive characteristics. The LI and LIH groups had marked language impairments and differed from each other only in their behavioral characteristics. The H and HRD subjects had similar behavioral and language characteristics but differed in their reading achievement.

Twenty-six boys met the normal criteria on speech, language, reading, and intelligence testing. They were matched for age with each patient and assigned to one of four normal control groups. They underwent the same experimental auditory processing testing as the patient groups.

Five scores were derived for each subject from the three experimental CAP testing conditions: 1) mean percent correct on the vigilance task; 2) mean reaction time for correct detections (vigilance task); 3) standard deviation for reaction time; 4) mean gap duration at 75% correct (gap threshold); and 5) mean ISI at 75% correct for temporal order (temporal order threshold). Performance for the subject groups was analyzed with two-way ANOVAs, blocking on age, using log transform data.

The results for signal detection performance on the vigilance task are presented in Table 2. Only the H group performed significantly poorer than the respective normal controls, although poorer performance was also noted for the HRD group. Also note the larger, although not significant ($p \leq 0.05$) standard deviations for each impaired group relative to its control. These results are in agreement with

Table 1. Language and reading achievement test results of LI, LIH, H, and HRD groups

Language and reading measures	Subject groups							
	LI (N=6)		LIH (N=6)		H (N=8)		HRD (N=6)	
	Mean	SD	Mean	SD	Mean	SD	Mean	SD
WISC-R Verbal IQ	79.0	6.6	77.5	9.1	106.8	12.5	96.0	8.6
ITPA quotient scores[a]								
Auditory Reception	83	12	70	16	97	22	105	10
Auditory Association	65	6	74	10	96	16	105	18
Grammatic Closure	72	13	75	19	100	10	95	6
PIAT Z scores[b]								
Reading Recognition					0.8	1.1	−1.6	0.5
Reading Comprehension					1.41	1.2	−1.4	0.6
Spelling					0.0	1.5	−1.9	0.6

SD, standard deviation.

[a]Quotient score=100×mental age equivalent of obtained test score/chronologic age.

[b]Z scores=(mean score for grade level−obtained score)/standard deviation of grade level scores.

Table 2. Comparisons of mean percent correct on the vigilance task of each patient group with respective age-matched normal control group

Group	Percent correct		F ratio	p of F	df
	Mean	SD			
Language-impaired	97.20	4.00	1.2	0.32	1,5
Normal control	98.80	0.75			
Language-impaired hyperactive	98.50	8.09	1.2	0.32	1,5
Normal control	99.20	0.41			
Hyperactive	95.80	3.40	5.66	0.05	1,7
Normal control	98.80	0.46			
Hyperactive reading-disabled	95.67	3.93	4.74	0.08	1,5
Normal control	99.17	0.41			

SD, standard deviation.

previous findings of poor performance on continuous performance tasks by hyperactive children (Sykes, 1969; Sykes, Douglas, & Morgenstern, 1973). Examination of the types of errors of the group indicated 28 false alarms and only 11 misses. Thus, the majority of the H subjects' errors were due to impulsivity rather than poor attention to the stimuli.

The mean reaction times of the four patient groups in comparison with their respective controls are presented in Table 3. Only one group, the LIH group, was significantly impaired compared to the normals on this measure. Previous studies using an alerting signal prior to the target on continuous performance tasks found hyperactive children had slower reaction times than normal (Cohen, 1970; Parry, 1973; Firestone, 1974). The presence of a noise burst on each trial of our vigilance task may have served as an alerting stimulus for subjects. The H group had significantly more commission errors than the normals, whereas the LIH children were slow to respond but responded correctly. Thus, both the H and the LIH children were impaired on the vigilance task, but in different ways.

The standard deviation in a subject's reaction times, a measure of response variability, may reflect the attention disorders of hyperactive children (Cohen, Douglas, & Morgenstern, 1971). The results in Table 4 demonstrate that all four patient groups had significantly greater variability in their reaction time than the normals on the vigilance task. Thus, even though an alerting stimulus was provided to warn subjects when a target could be presented, the impaired subjects were still more variable than the normals in their responses. This occurred in all three hyperactive groups (LIH, H, and HRD) and in the LI group. Therefore, although these latter subjects responded correctly to the stimuli, all of the impaired subjects were more variable than the normals in their reaction speed.

The mean gap duration required to achieve 75% correct for each subject group is presented in Table 5. Only the LI subjects were significantly impaired relative to the normals on this task; they required a longer interval of silence for detection of the gap than the normal subjects. The H group had the longest mean gap duration, but it was also the youngest group. Tallal et al. (1981) has shown developmental aspects to temporal order perception, and perhaps this also occurs with gap detection. Note that the highest mean found in a normal group is for the youngest, those whose ages were matched to the H groups.

Examination of the data reveals some interesting individual differences within and across the groups. In particular, three of the H group had longer gap thresholds than their age-matched normal controls, and

Table 3. Comparison of mean reaction time on the vigilance task of each patient group with respective age-matched normal control group

Group	Reaction time (msec)		F ratio	p of F	df
	Mean	SD			
Language-impaired	424	105	0.10	0.75	1,5
Normal control	415	133			
Language-impaired hyperactive	716	281	17.90	0.008	1,5
Normal control	303	89			
Hyperactive	495	191	1.49	0.26	1,7
Normal control	384	133			
Hyperactive reading-disabled	501	255	0.26	0.63	1,5
Normal control	423	134			

SD, standard deviation.

Table 4.   Comparison of variance in reaction time on the vigilance task of each patient group with respective age-matched normal control group

Group	SD in reaction time (msec) Mean	SD in reaction time (msec) SD	F ratio	p of F	df
Language-impaired	222	121	10.5	0.02	1,5
Normal control	133	46			
Language-impaired hyperactive	377	83	66.3	0.0004	1,5
Normal control	126	33			
Hyperactive	256	118	11.79	0.01	1,7
Normal control	122	49			
Hyperactive reading-disabled	250	138	6.76	0.05	1,5
Normal control	138	35			

SD, standard deviation.

Table 5.   Comparisons of mean gap size thresholds on the gap detection task of each patient group with respective age-matched normal control group

| Group | Threshold gap size (msec) | | F ratio | p of F | df |
	Mean	SD			
Language-impaired	5.79	2.76	8.95	0.03	1,5
Normal control	3.25	0.56			
Language-impaired hyperactive	4.86	2.95	0.4	0.57	1,4
Normal control	3.57	0.40			
Hyperactive	7.60	7.20	2.19	0.18	1,7
Normal control	4.16	1.09			
Hyperactive reading-disabled	3.63	0.79	0.95	0.37	1,5
Normal control	3.26	0.57			

SD, standard deviation.

two of these had gap thresholds longer than any of the LI subjects. Furthermore, the LIH group did not differ from their normal controls, and only one LIH subject had a gap threshold longer than any of the normals. Thus, temporal resolution deficits were not restricted to those with language impairment, and not all subjects with language deficits were impaired in gap detection.

On the temporal order task, presented in Table 6, all four patient groups were significantly impaired relative to normal controls. All of the impaired groups required longer than normal ISIs to identify the temporal order of the stimuli. These data replicate, and go beyond, the data of Tallal and Piercy (1973) and Tallal (1980) with regard to language-impaired and reading-impaired children. In addition to these groups, hyperactive children without these disorders showed the same deficit in temporal order perception. This suggests that deficits in temporal processing are not restricted to individuals with impairments in language and/or reading and may be independent of these impairments. Examination of the individual data supports this point. Six of the eight H subjects had longer ISIs at threshold than any LI subject. Furthermore, of nine subjects with thresholds of 100 msec or longer, five were from the H group, three from the HRD group, and one from the LIH group. Thus, subjects with the greatest deficits on this task were all hyperactive, whereas only one had a significant language impairment.

There were large differences among subjects on each of the five CAP measures, particularly among the hyperactive subjects. To determine whether CAP skills of gap detection and temporal order were related to subjects' attention deficits on the vigilance task, Pearson correlation coefficients were calculated. The relationships examined in each group were between subjects' mean reaction times and their gap detection thresholds, between subjects' mean reaction times and their threshold ISIs, between subjects' variation in reaction time and their gap detection thresholds, and between subjects' variation in reaction time and threshold ISIs. No significant ($p \leq 0.05$) relationships were found between either mean reaction time or variance in reaction time and performance on the gap detection task for any group. Only the HRD group showed a statistically significant relationship between the temporal order task and performance on the vigilance task ($r=0.75$, $p=0.04$ for mean reaction time; $r=0.80$, $p=0.03$ for variation in reaction time). Subjects with the slower reaction times and those with more variable responses to acoustic stimuli in the reading-disabled group required longer ISIs to determine temporal order between stimuli. No significant relationships between auditory attention and temporal resolution or temporal order perception were found in any of the other groups.

Table 6. Comparisons of mean ISI thresholds (msec) on the temporal order task of each patient group with respective age-matched normal control group

Group	Threshold ISI (msec) Mean	SD	F ratio	p of F	df
Language-impaired	72.1	37.4	48.6	0.002	1,4
Normal control	14.3	3.2			
Language-impaired hyperactive	61.8	17.3	15.7	0.01	1,4
Normal control	17.8	10.9			
Hyperactive	269.4	229.9	6.90	0.03	1,7
Normal control	36.1	23.21			
Hyperactive reading-disabled	167.2	162.3	10.57	0.02	1,5
Normal control	17.2	9.9			

SD, standard deviation.

DISCUSSION

Our studies of nonverbal auditory processing in language-impaired subjects replicated and extended those of Tallal and Piercy (1973) and Tallal et al. (1981). These subjects learned to discriminate accurately temporal changes in signals on the gap detection task but required longer than normal gap durations to do so. Furthermore, on the temporal order task, the LI subjects could accurately perceive the order of the two tones, but again required longer ISIs than normal subjects.

An exclusive relationship between language impairments and auditory temporal processing deficits, suggested by previous authors, was not found in our research. Temporal order perceptual capabilities were poorest for the hyperactive subjects with normal language and reading skills. This suggests that auditory temporal processing performance may be related to some central auditory processing function independent of language function. Further, we found that temporal order deficits occurred independently of gap detection deficits. Our findings suggest that nonverbal temporal processing deficits may be present in a child with intact language. Conversely, when language is impaired, nonverbal temporal processing deficits may be only one of many contributing factors.

Difficulties in maintaining attention were seen in all groups of learning-disabled children regardless of the specific disability. All groups were more variable than normal in their performance, although (with one exception on the vigilance task) they were able to do all tasks and achieve a high performance level. All impaired groups, regardless of type of impairment, completed all tasks and achieved greater than 90% correct. The tasks were all self-paced; a trial was presented only after the subject responded to the previous stimulus. Reinforcement followed each response. Thus, the influence of attention deficits was kept to a minimum. With one exception there was no relation between variability of response and performance. Thus, differences in performance between the impaired groups and their normal peers were most likely the result of processing deficits and not attention deficits.

Findings of nonverbal processing deficits in the presence of language impairment and a difficulty in discriminating speech stimuli have led some authors to speculate on the basis for the poor performance. Tallal and Stark (1981) suggested abnormalities in auditory masking. Performance on a gap detection task can be viewed in the context of auditory masking (Smiarowski & Carhart, 1975). The detection of the offset of the noise at the beginning of the gap would be dependent on the rate of decay of the masker in the auditory system (forward masking), whereas the detection of onset of the noise at the end of the gap would be dependent on the rise time of excitation in the auditory system (backward masking). Abnormalities in temporal masking should, therefore, produce longer than normal gap thresholds. Impairments in hearing sensitivity result in longer than normal gap thresholds (Church & Cudahy, 1978; Fitzgibbons, 1979) and abnormal temporal masking (Cudahy, 1982). Both of these deficits can occur in regions of normal hearing, suggesting that central factors may play a role in both of these deficits. However, Ludlow et al. (1981) found that patients with normal hearing who were in the early stages of Huntington's disease had abnormal gap thresholds. Presumably in such cases the neuropathology was primarily in the basal ganglia and cortical functioning was not yet affected, because language functioning was still within normal limits. These adult patients, therefore, had an auditory masking deficit but did not evidence language impairment. Thus, in adults, the presence of auditory masking deficits does not alter language functioning, contrary to Tallal and Stark's (1981) hypothesis.

An alternative hypothesis is that CAP performance deficits reflect differences in central neural transmission in some hyperactive and language-impaired subjects. It has been suggested that beneficial effects of stimulants in hyperactive children are due to an increase in neural conduction speed. One possible test of this hypothesis is to examine the effects of stimulants on nonverbal auditory processing performance in other groups with deficits in gap detection.

Whereas only one group of listeners had longer than normal gap thresholds, all disorder groups had longer than normal temporal order thresholds. This lack of a strict relationship between temporal resolution and temporal order perception challenges the view that temporal order deficits are the result of poor temporal resolution. Rather, it suggests that these two types of temporal processing are performed by two different mechanisms.

Our findings do have some import in the light of recent work on phonetic (linguistic) and psychoacoustic (nonverbal) modes of auditory information processing. Investigators have reported on the discrepancies between the discrimination functions associated with verbal and nonverbal stimuli (Warren et al., 1969). Other investigators have reported on similarities in discrimination functions for verbal and nonverbal stimuli (Pisoni, 1979; Kuhl & Miller, 1975). Recently, Best, Morrongiello, and Robson (1981) have attempted to distinguish between "phonetic" (linguistic processing) of speechlike stimuli and "psychoacoustic" (nonverbal auditory processing) of speechlike stimuli. Their data suggest that adult perception of sine wave analogues of speech stimuli depends upon the listener's impression of whether or not the stimuli are speech. In particular, the locations along the time domain where listeners indicate their categorical perception of two different signals depend on the "mode" of processing. In addition, the acoustic cues employed for categorical perception seem to differ depending on the "mode" of processing. The authors admit their results are preliminary and that more work is needed before the "processing mode" notion is fully supported. The present data provide some interesting insights into the relation between psychoacoustic performance and speech perception. Because all the disordered groups had longer than normal temporal order thresholds, we may hypothesize that their "psychoacoustic" discrimination functions may be displaced relative to normal. However, the hyperactive children had developed normal language and reading skills, implying independence between phonetic and psychoacoustic modes of processing. Aslin and Pisoni (1980) argued that certain perceptual skills, such as categories discrimination, although present in infants and specific to a particular language, are maintained and modified during language development. Considered in this light, our study suggests that the processes necessary for verbal and nonverbal discrimination may develop independently, although both may be affected by central pathologies.

Nonverbal auditory perception and linguistic capabilities develop with age, but not necessarily in parallel. The limits of nonverbal psychoacoustic functioning as assessed in studies such as this one may reflect impaired neural transmission, whereas speech perception tasks, which require less temporal resolution, may not reflect psychoacoustic deficits. Hence speech perception tests may be insensitive to changes in neural transmission with maturation. Thus, even though the neural transmission of hyperactive children may not show normal maturational changes with age, these children may develop speech perception skills normally, because the latter depend upon both psychoacoustic skills and linguistic maturation. Their linguistic maturation may compensate for their psychoacoustic deficits. Language-impaired subjects, however, may have exhibited the co-occurrence of two unrelated deficits: slow neural transmission time and impaired linguistic development.

This investigation studied nonverbal auditory processing in hyperactive and nonhyperactive children with and without language impairment. The major findings were: 1) the presence of CAP deficits in hyperactive children who had developed normal language and reading skills; and 2) a lack of a relationship between temporal resolution and temporal order perception. These findings lead us to conclude that: a) there is not an exclusive relationship between language impairment and auditory temporal processing as measured in this study; b) temporal resolution deficits as evidenced on gap detection tasks are not the basis for language impairment, because children with temporal resolution deficits can develop normal language; and c) auditory processing for nonverbal stimuli is sensitive to central pathologies. Furthermore, the deficits in psychoacoustic and phonetic discrimination of the language-impaired children may have different bases. The disturbed auditory comprehension of language-impaired children is probably due to linguistic development difficulties rather than impaired nonverbal acoustic processing.

REFERENCES

American National Standards Institute. 1969. Specifications for audiometers (ANSI 3.6). American National Standards Institute, New York, 1969.

Aslin, R. N., and Pisoni, D. 1980. Some development processes in speech perception. In: G. Yeni-Komshian, J. Kavanagh, and C. Ferguson (eds.), Child Phonology, Volume 2: Perception, pp. 67–95. Academic Press, New York.

Aten, J., and Davis, J. 1968. Disturbances in the perception of sequence in children with minimal cerebral dysfunction. Journal of Speech and Hearing Research 11:236–245.

Auerbach, S., Naeser, M., and Mazurski, P. 1981. Primary auditory cortical function and auditory comprehension in aphasia: A functional approach. Paper presented at the Academy of Aphasia, London, Ontario, October 11–13, 1981.

Best, C. T., Morrongiello, B., and Robson, R. 1981. Perceptual equivalence of acoustic cues in speech and nonspeech perception. Perception and Psychophysics 3:191–211.

Bakker, D. J. 1971. Temporal Order in Disturbed Reading: Developmental and Neuropsychological Aspects in Normal and Reading Retarded Children. Rotterdam University Press, Rotterdam.

Birch, H. G., and Belmont, L. 1964. Auditory-visual integration in normal and retarded readers. American Journal of Orthopsychiatry 34:852–861.

Bocca, E., and Calearo, C. 1963. Central hearing processes. In: J. Jerger (ed.), Modern Developments in Audiology, pp. 337–368. Academic Press, New York.

Church, G., and Cudahy, E. 1978. Gap detection as a function of age. Paper presented at the Annual Meeting of the American Speech-Language-Hearing Association, San Francisco, California, November 17–24, 1978.

Cohen, J. 1970. Psychophysiological concomitants of attention in hyperactive children. Unpublished doctoral dissertation, McGill University, Montreal.

Cohen, N. J., Douglas, V. I., and Morgenstern, G. 1971. The effect of methylphenidate on attentive behavior and autonomic activity in hyperactive children. Psychopharmacologia 22:282–294.

Conners, C. K. 1973. Rating scales for use in drug studies with children. Psychopharmacology Bulletin (special issue on pharmacotherapy with children): 24–84.

Corkin, S. 1974. Serial-ordering deficits in inferior readers. Neuropsychologia 12:347–354.

Cudahy, E. 1982. Changes in the temporal processing of acoustic signals in hearing-impaired listeners. In: R. P. Hamernik, D. Henderson, and R. Salvi (eds.), New Perspectives on Noise-Induced Hearing Loss. Raven Press, New York.

DiSimoni, F. 1978. The Token Test for Children. Teaching Resources, Boston.

Douglas, V. I. 1976. Effects of medication on learning efficiency. Research findings review and synthesis. In: R. P. Anderson and C. G. Halcomb (eds.), Learning Disability/Minimal Brain Dysfunction Syndrome: Research Perspectives and Applications. Charles C Thomas, Springfield, Ill.

Dunn, L. M. 1965. Peabody Picture Vocabulary Test. American Guidance Service, Circle Pines, Minn.

Dunn, L. M., and Markwardt, F. C. 1970. Peabody Individual Achievement Test. American Guidance Service, Circle Pines, Minn.

Eimas, P. O., Siqueland, E. R., Jusczyk, P., and Vigorito, J. 1971. Speech perception in infants. Science 171:303–306.

Firestone, P. 1974. The effects of reinforcement contingencies and caffeine on hyperactive children. Unpublished doctoral dissertation, McGill University, Montreal.

Fitzgibbons, P. J. 1979. Temporal resolution in normal and hearing impaired listeners. Unpublished doctoral dissertation, Northwestern University, Evanston, Ill.

Goldman, R., Fristoe, M., and Woodcock, R. W. 1976. Goldman-Fristoe-Woodcock Auditory Selective Attention Test. American Guidance Service, Circle Pines, Minn.

Hirsh, I. J., and Sherrick, E. C. 1961. Perceived order in different sense modalities. Journal of Experimental Psychology 62:423–432.

Kirk, S. A., McCarthy, J. J ., and Kirk, W. D. 1968. The Illinois Test of Psycholinguistic Abilities, Revised Edition. University of Illinois Press, Urbana, Ill.

Kuhl, P. K., and Miller, J. D. 1975. Speech perception by the chinchilla: Voiced-voiceless distinction in alveolar plosives. Science 190:69–72.

Lowe, A. D., and Campbell, R. A. 1965. Temporal discrimination in aphasoid and normal children. Journal of Speech and Hearing Research 8:313–314.

Ludlow, C., Caine, E., Cudahy, E., Nutt, J. G., and Bassich, C. 1981. Auditory processing deficits in Huntington's disease. Submitted for publication.

Lynn, G. E., and Gilroy, J. 1977. Evaluation of central auditory dysfunction in neurological disorders. In: R. Keith (ed.), Central Auditory Dysfunction, pp. 177–222. Grune & Stratton, New York.

Mills, L., and Rollman, G. B. 1980. Hemispheric asymmetry for auditory perception of temporal order. Neuropsychologia 18:41–47.

Parry, P. 1973. The effect of reward on the performance of hyperactive children. Unpublished doctoral dissertation, McGill University, Montreal.

Pisoni, D. B. 1979. On the perception of speech sounds as biologically significant signals. Brain Behav. Evol. 16:330–350.

Poppen, R., Stark, J., Eisenson, J., et al. 1969. Visual sequencing performance of aphasic children. Journal of Speech and Hearing Research 12:288–300.

Remez, R. E., Rubin, P. E., Pisoni, D. B., and Carrell, T. D. 1981. Speech perception without traditional speech cues. Science 212:947-950.

Smiarowski, R. A., and Carhart, L. 1975. Relations among temporal resolution, forward masking and simultaneous masking. Journal of the Acoustical Society of America 57:1169-1174.

Stark, J. 1966. Performance of aphasic children on the ITPA. 1966. Exceptional Children 33:153-158.

Stark, J. 1967. A comparison of the performance of aphasic children on three sequencing tests. Journal of Communication Disorders 1:31-34.

Stark, R. E., and Tallal, P. 1980. Sensory and perceptual functioning of young children with and without delayed language development. Final Report for DHHS-NIH Contract NO1-NS-5-2322.

Strauss, A. S., and Lehtinen, L. E. 1947. Psychopathology and Education in the Brain-Injured Child. Grune & Stratton, New York.

Swisher, L., and Hirsch, I. J. 1972. Brain damage and the ordering of two temporarily successive stimuli. Neuropsychologia 10:137-151.

Sykes, D. H. 1969. Sustained attention in hyperactive children. Unpublished doctoral dissertation, McGill University, Montreal.

Sykes, D., Douglas, V. I., and Morgenstern, G. 1973. Sustained attention in hyperactive children. Journal of Child Psychology and Psychiatry 14: 213-220.

Tallal, P. 1980. Auditory temporal perception, phonics, and reading disabilities in children. Brain and Language 9:182-198.

Tallal, P., and Piercy, M. 1973. Defects of nonverbal auditory perception in children with developmental aphasia. Nature 241:468-469.

Tallal, P., and Piercy, M. 1974. Developmental aphasia: Rate of auditory processing and selective impairment of consonant perception. Neuropsychologia 12:83-93.

Tallal, P., and Piercy, M. 1978. Deficits of auditory perception in children with developmental dysphasia. In: M. A. Wyke (ed.), Developmental Dysphasia, pp. 63-84. Academic Press, London.

Tallal, P., and Stark, R. E. 1981. Speech acoustic-cue discrimination abilities of normally developing and language impaired children. Journal of the Acoustical Society of America 69:568-574.

Tallal, P., Stark, R. E., Kallman, C., and Mellits, D. 1981. A re-examination of some nonverbal perceptual abilities of language impaired and normal children as a function of age and sensory modality. Journal of Speech and Hearing Research 24:351-357.

Warren, R. M. 1974. Auditory temporal discrimination by trained listeners. Cognitive Psychology 6:237-256.

Warren, R. M., Obusek, C. J., Farmer, R. M., and Warren, R. P. 1969. Auditory sequence: Confusion of patterns other than music or speech. Science 164:586-587.

Wechsler, D. 1974. Wechsler Intelligence Scale for Children—Revised. Psychological Corporation, New York.

Werry, J., Sprague, R. L., and Cohen, M. N. 1975. Conners' Teacher Rating Scale for use in drug studies in children: An empirical study. Journal of Abnormal Child Psychology 3:217-229.

Chapter 10

Effects of Peripheral Hearing Losses on the Auditory Brainstem

Douglas B. Webster

Peripheral hearing losses occur as a result of malfunction in some part of the peripheral organ (external, middle, and/or inner ear). It has been tacitly assumed that if this malfunction can be corrected and the ear restored to normal, hearing will also be normal. Contrary to expectation, however, experience has shown that completely normal hearing is seldom, if ever, regained after long-term hearing losses, regardless of the means used to correct the peripheral malfunction. A possible explanation could be the existence of a functional-structural interdependence between the peripheral ear and the central auditory pathway. This chapter explores the possibility of such an interdependence.

EFFECTS OF CONDUCTIVE LOSSES

By far the most common cause of conductive hearing loss is otitis media, which is particularly prevalent in infants and preschool children. A recent study of Boston-area children revealed that 71% had experienced at least one bout of otitis media, and 33% had suffered three occurrences or more by 3 years of age (Teele, Klein, & Rosner,

Original research reported here was supported by National Institutes of Health grants NS-12510, NS-11647, and BRSG SO7-RR-5376.

1980). When otitis media is accompanied by effusions, whether they be serous, purulent, or mucoid, there is a concomitant conductive hearing loss. Children who have recurrent or chronic otitis media with effusions (OME), therefore, not only suffer from the disease itself but also endure a continual or recurring hearing loss, which averages between 20 and 30 dB (Bluestone, Beery, & Paradise, 1973; Kokko, 1975).

Dobie and Berlin (1979) indicated that many significant speech sounds cannot be heard by such children under normal listening conditions. A failure to hear speech sounds is particularly devastating for young children in the process of learning language. Therefore, at the very least, children with chronic OME are at risk for delayed speech and language development.

In addition to problems involving language skills, it is possible that a conductive hearing deficit during the first few years of life, when the brain is still maturing, may affect an individual's eventual auditory ability. In the case of the visual system, it has been amply shown that normal peripheral stimulation during postnatal development is required for the eventual integrity of the system. If the auditory system is similarly dependent upon environmental input, a chronic conductive loss in early life could result in a permanent central auditory disorder. The remainder of this section on the effects of conductive losses examines data pertinent to this proposition from nonhuman behavioral, neurophysiologic, and anatomical experiments, as well as human correlative studies.

Nonhuman Studies of Conductive Losses and Auditory Deprivation

The effects of neonatal conductive hearing loss have been commonly studied either by raising animals with occluding earplugs, or by assuming that sound deprivation will have the same effect as conductive loss and raising them instead in a very quiet environment. Both these approaches have some inherent technical problems.

Because neonatal animals grow rapidly, earplugs must be frequently replaced. Each time this is done, the cerumen and proliferating epithelium they trap within the external auditory meatus must be removed with great care not to damage the tympanic membrane. Acoustically, earplugs have the effect of mass loading the auditory periphery, which enhances low-frequency conduction and decreases high-frequency conduction.

Problems are also encountered in rearing animals in a quiet environment, and rearing in total silence is impossible because animals themselves produce noises by their vocalizations, movements, and metabolic processes. Because we are interested in conductive loss rather than total deafness, however, this is not a serious problem; if environmental noise can be eliminated, a model of human conductive loss will have been approximated.

The earliest report suggesting long-term effects from early conductive loss was from an unusual behavioral experiment by Wolf (1943), using two groups of rats. One group was raised with bilateral ear plugs from 11 to 26 days of age; a second group was raised with visual deprivation from 16 to 26 days. At 40 days both groups were put on a food deprivation schedule and trained to avoid a shock and obtain a morsel of food by attending to either an auditory or a visual stimulus. At 52 days of age, a visually deprived animal was paired with an auditorily deprived animal, and the pair was presented with either an auditory or a visual stimulus for the single morsel of food. Under this stressful situation, the visually deprived animals most frequently obtained the food when the stimulus was sound, and the auditorily deprived animals most frequently obtained the food when the stimulus was light. Wolf (1943) also described the stressed rats' behavior as neurotic and interpreted these data to mean that failure to take appropriate action when stressed is often the result of experimental deprivation in early life.

Several years later, Gauron and Becker (1959) replicated this complicated experiment as closely as they could and found the same result, with one exception: as the number of competitive tests became quite large, the advantage of the nondeprived animals (e.g., the visually deprived animals when the stimulus was sound) became "hardly noticeable." Because their rats showed no neurotic behavior, Gauron and Becker interpreted the results to mean that sensory deprivation weakens sensory ability, and discounted the importance of stress.

Tees (1967, a and b) raised rats with earplugs (changed every other day) in a sound-reduced environment from the 5th day of life. They were behaviorally tested starting at 60 days of age, with the earplugs removed only during testing. Tees found that the rats learned both intensity and frequency discriminations as well as did normal control rats, but were deficient in learning both temporal sound patterns and durations, which suggested that the deprivation affected higher-order auditory processing.

In another behavioral study, Clements and Kelly (1978) demonstrated that unilateral earplugging of newborn guinea pigs resulted in impaired auditory localization even after removal of the earplug. This also suggests an effect on higher-order processing.

Rajecki (1974) found that after prehatch exposure to specific sounds, chicks after hatching were more responsive to those same sounds. Kerr, Ostapoff, and Rubel (1979) found that chicks that had

had earplugs were less able to make sharp frequency generalizations after earplug removal, again suggesting an effect on higher-order auditory processing.

There have also been neurophysiologic studies of animals with early conductive loss or auditory deprivation. One group of studies concerns audiogenic seizures in mice. There are several strains of mice that are susceptible to audiogenic seizures if they are first "primed" by a 120-dB noise when about 17 days old. Mice from some other, non-seizure-prone strains can be made seizure-prone in two ways: by destroying their tympanic membranes at 20 days of age (Gates, Chen, & Bock, 1973), or by plugging their ears at 17 days of age (McGinn, Willott, & Henry, 1973). Destruction of the tympanic membrane causes a 40-dB reduction in the cochlear microphonic (Gates, Chen, & Bock, 1973). The earplugs cause a 40-dB attenuation in evoked responses recorded from the inferior colliculi; a 12-dB attenuation remains after the earplugs are removed (McGinn et al., 1973). Saunders et al. (1972, a and b) were the first to suggest that audiogenic seizures are the result of disuse supersensitivity. Their reasoning was as follows: in non-seizure-prone strains of mice that have been acoustically primed, both the cochlear potential and the eighth nerve action potential have reduced sensitivity at all intensities, whereas both the cochlear nuclei and inferior colliculus have reduced sensitivity at low intensities but increased sensitivity at high intensities.

Henry and Haythorn (1975) extended this line of thought and suggested that genetic defects, earplugging, tympanic membrane destruction, and overstimulation all cause loss of peripheral auditory sensitivity. When this loss occurs during a critical period of auditory system maturation, it causes abnormalities in the physiology of the auditory brainstem. The net result of stimulation deprivation during the critical period is disuse supersensitivity in brainstem neurons, which induces the audiogenic seizure. All these data on audiogenic seizures are consistent with the broader hypothesis that normal auditory brainstem maturation is partially dependent upon proper stimulation from the peripheral organs.

Batkin et al. (1970) studied the effects of auditory deprivation on auditory evoked cortical potentials. They raised rats in a sound-attenuated chamber placed in the crater of an extinct volcano. To reduce the noise produced within the chamber, the toes of the newborn rats were amputated and the mothers were made avocal by laryngeal cauterization. After 8 months of this deprivation, the cortical evoked potentials of the deprived animals were about 30 dB less sensitive than those of littermate controls. Three weeks after the deprived rats were placed in a normal ambient noise environment, there was partial, but not complete, recovery of sensitivity.

Silverman and Clopton (1977; Clopton and Silverman, 1977) produced a conductive loss by ligating the external auditory meatus of neonatal rats. Recording from individual neurons of the inferior colliculus, they found partial to complete loss of binaural interaction even after the ligation was reversed, provided: 1) that the ligation was unilateral, and 2) it was done between 10 and 30 days of age.

Inferior collicular neurons are affected not only by early sound deprivation, but also to some degree by early sound exposure, depending upon the type of exposure. If neonatal rats are exposed to specific sound patterns, for instance, individual inferior collicular neurons, when tested later, will be more sensitive to those patterns than to patterns not previously experienced (Clopton & Winfield, 1976). However, Moore and Aitken (1975) found no effect on inferior collicular tonotopic organization or single unit tuning curves in kittens exposed neonatally to a 1000-Hz pure tone for 5–8 hr per day.

These behavioral and physiologic data are consistent with the concept that, in young animals, both conductive loss and auditory deprivation cause central auditory disorder(s) affecting primarily durational, binaural, and sensitivity perception. To determine possible structural correlates of these disorders, we have been doing anatomical studies on the brainstems of mice that have undergone neonatal conductive loss or auditory deprivation (Webster & Webster, 1977, 1979b, 1980).

Mice were chosen for these experiments because: 1) they are deaf at birth and do not start hearing until about 10 days of age (Mikaelian & Ruben, 1965; Ehret, 1976); 2) hearing is mature by 18–20 days of age (Ehret, 1976); and 3) hearing is very poor below 1000 Hz, which facilitates adequate auditory deprivation. CBA/J mice, a standard normal hearing mouse strain, were used in each experiment.

One group of mice was given a conductive loss at 3–4 days of age by bilateral removal of the developing connective tissue and epithelium that would normally form the external auditory meatus. When these animals were killed at 45 days of age, their middle and inner ears were normal but they lacked an external auditory meatus. Thus they were similar to humans with atresias of the external auditory meatus, except that they lacked the ossicular and other osseous malformations commonly found in human congenital atresias. A second group of mice was raised from 3 or 4 days of age by an avocal mother in a deprivation chamber consisting of a small-animal IAC chamber lined with indoor-outdoor carpeting and supported by acoustic springs in a walk-in, double-walled IAC chamber. Ambient noise within this chamber is at least 10 dB below normal mouse auditory thresholds at all frequencies. A third group of control mice was raised by normal mothers in our animal colony.

All three groups were killed at 45 days of age. Tracings were made at a magnification of $1400\times$ of identified neurons of the cochlear nucleus, superior olivary complex, and inferior colliculi. These tracings were then digitized on a microprocessor-based image analysis system, which calculated the cross-sectional area of each neuron. After all measurements were made, the code was broken and the measurements were assigned to the proper experimental or control group for analysis.

Analysis of the data demonstrated that, for all 11 neuronal groups measured, there was no significant difference ($p > 0.05$) in the neuronal cross-sectional areas of mice with conductive loss and auditorily deprived mice. However, neuronal cross-sectional areas of normal mice were significantly larger ($p < 0.05$) than those of the two experimental groups of mice in the following neuronal areas: in the cochlear nuclei, the octopus, globular, small spherical, and large spherical neurons; in the superior olivary complex, neurons of both the lateral superior olivary nucleus and medial nucleus of the trapezoid body. The only analyzed neuronal groups that showed no significant differences ($p > 0.05$) between normal and experimental groups were: in the cochlear nuclei, the multipolar neurons and neurons of the central region of the dorsal cochlear nuclei; and the central nucleus of the inferior colliculus. In both the multipolar neurons and the central nucleus of the inferior colliculus there was a tendency for neurons to be smaller in experimental animals than in normal animals, but the difference was not statistically significant ($p > 0.05$). These data demonstrate that after greatly reduced auditory input during postnatal development, the neurons of many brainstem auditory neuronal groups are smaller than normal. Although the functional significance of this finding is not known, it is possible that they would be less capable of complex information processing than would normal neurons.

To test whether or not this phenomenon is reversible, a group of mice was raised from 3 to 45 days by an avocal mother in the auditory deprivation chamber and then transferred to the normal animal colony for an additional 45 days. Their brains were then compared to those of normal 90-day-old mice. In this experiment, neurons were significantly smaller ($p < 0.05$) in the deprived-reversal mice than in the normal mice in the following areas: in the cochlear nuclei, the multipolar, globular, small spherical, and large spherical neurons; in the superior olivary complex, neurons of both the lateral superior olivary nucleus and the medial nucleus of the trapezoid body; and in the inferior colliculus, its central nucleus. Only the octopus neurons of the ventral cochlear nucleus and the neurons of the central region of the dorsal cochlear nucleus showed no differences ($p > 0.05$) between groups. It therefore appears that, at least in mice, the adverse effects of postnatal auditory deprivation are for the most part not reversible by later normal acoustic stimulation. Because multipolar neurons and inferior collicular neurons were not different than normal in the 45-day deprived animals, but were smaller than normal in the 90-day deprived-reversal animals, it is possible that the effects of early postnatal deprivation may become more severe as the animals grow older.

A postnatal developmental study of normal CBA/J mice showed that neurons in the auditory brainstem double in cross-sectional area between days 3 and 12 and then do not change through day 90 (Webster & Webster, 1980); the size attained by day 12 is therefore considered to be adult. It is logical that this rapid growth to adult size must be under genetic control only, rather than dependent upon environmental stimulation, because mice do not hear at all until 10 days of age and do not achieve mature hearing until 18–20 days. The data cited above, however, argue that there must be some minimal auditory activity for adult neuronal size to be maintained once it has been reached, and that this level of activity is not achieved in animals that have external auditory meatus atresias or have been raised in auditory deprivation.

Both Coleman and O'Connor (1979) and Feng and Rogowski (1980) have also demonstrated anatomical brainstem effects from postnatal conductive losses. Coleman and O'Connor (1979) showed that removing the left auditory ossicles in 10-day-old rats resulted in smaller than normal large spherical neurons in the left ventral cochlear nucleus when the rats were 50 days old. Feng and Rogowski (1980) reported that monaural earplugging of 12-day-old rats resulted in significantly more medial superior olivary neurons, with dendrites extending only toward the nonplugged side.

All of these experimental anatomical data are consistent with the behavioral and physiologic data from nonhuman experiments, and indicate that in experimental rodents auditory processing is jeopardized by neonatal conductive loss or auditory deprivation.

Human Studies of Conductive Losses and Auditory Deprivation

Whereas human studies on the effects of conductive loss and auditory deprivation cannot have the control and rigor of nonhuman studies, they can directly study the important question of whether the acquisition of speech and language is affected by early sound deprivation. Several human studies have examined children with histories of chronic or recurring OME and looked for later effects. Eisen (1962) reported on a 7-year-old child with normal hearing but a history of repeated bouts of OME during his first 3 years. The child was reported to be inattentive in school and to have learning difficulties and poor social adjustments. Although this child was audiologically normal, psychophysical testing showed poor auditory localization, difficulty in word finding, and poor word discrimination; these deficits became more severe under stressful conditions. A case history report must be regarded as merely anecdotal, but this child's poor auditory localization, learning difficulties, and difficulty under stress are impressively similar to the experimental animal findings (Wolf, 1943).

A few years later, Holm and Kunze (1969) reported a pilot study of 16 children with chronic OME who were compared to 16 children with no history of otitis media. The two groups were matched for age, socioeconomic background, and schools attended. Standardized tests showed that the children in the otitis media group were inferior in both receptive and expressive language.

In an extensive 10-year study of Alaskan Eskimo children, Kaplan et al. (1973) concluded that early onset of OME impairs verbal development and that this impairment increases as the children grow older. Similar conclusions were drawn by Hamilton and Owrid (1974) and by Lewis (1976), following retrospective studies of normal children compared with chronic otitis media children. These studies lacked rigorous control.

In the best controlled retrospective study to date, Sak and Ruben (1981) compared 18 normal hearing children with documented histories of OME before the age of 5 to their normal hearing siblings. All 36 children were in the bright-to-normal range of verbal ability as tested by the WISC-R test, and none had been diagnosed as learning-disabled. Nevertheless, the children with a history of OME performed more poorly in verbal ability, auditory decoding, and spelling than their sibling controls.

Whereas these studies examined children with histories of otitis media and looked for effects, another group of studies has started with known learning, auditory, speech, and/or language disorders and correlated them with present and past otitis media. Katz and Illmer (1972) found that 33% of a population of children with learning disabilities also had hearing problems, usually conductive losses. Freeman and Parkins (1979) found that 48% of their population of learning-disabled children failed an airborne hearing test at 15 dB hearing threshold level (HTL) and 25% at 25 dB HTL; 38% failed tympanometric testing (-100 mm H_2O criterion), and 20% had active middle ear disease at the time of testing. Gottlieb, Zinkus, and Thompson (1979) reported on a group of 213 learning-impaired children, none of whom had active otitis media when examined. Of these children, 177 had a significant auditory processing handicap; 46% of those had a history of recurrent otitis media during the first 3 years of life, whereas only 22% of the 36 children without an auditory processing handicap had such a history. A study of 53 learning-disabled children was done by Bennett, Ruuska, and Sherman (1980): 23% had a history of recurrent otitis media, whereas only 9% of a control group of 56 children had such a history. There have also been several other studies noting similar relationships (Brookhouser, Hixon, & Matkin, 1979; Cook & Teel, 1979; Downs, 1977; Howie, Plousard, & Sloyer, 1975; Ling, 1959; Naremore, 1979; Omer, 1972; Paradise, 1976; Zinkus & Gottlieb, 1978; Zinkus, Gottlieb, & Shapiro, 1978).

Thus, there is presently an extensive literature that can be interpreted as supporting a causative link between recurrent or chronic OME and a variety of language-related or central disorders. Reviews have been published by Katz (1978), Ruben and Rapin (1980), Ventry (1980), and Webster (1980); the proceedings of a special workshop sponsored by the Communicative Disorders Program of the National Institute of Neurological and Communicative Disorders and Stroke (NINCDS) have also been published (Hanson & Ulvestad, 1979). The NINCDS publication is the most exhaustive review, whereas Ventry's (1980) is the most severely critical but also presents some suggestions for improving the quality of future studies.

To varying degrees, all these reviews point out shortcomings of most or all published reports which suggest that early auditory deprivation causes permanent central disorders. Indeed, these reports are inconclusive; the reasons include problems inherent in retrospective studies, the uncertainty that attends both definitions and diagnoses of otitis media, and poor control of confounding variables such as possible neurologic problems unrelated to hearing, as well as that familiar gremlin, socioeconomic factors.

No "perfect" study has yet been published demonstrating a causative link between early auditory deprivation and later auditory processing disorders. Nevertheless, the bulk of the evidence to date makes it almost certain that any early childhood hearing disorder puts the child at risk for poor speech and language development. In addition, a broad range of data from nonhuman studies supports the hypothesis that there is some critical postnatal period during which adequate sound stimulation is necessary for full development and maintenance of the auditory brainstem to occur.

Nonhuman experiments demonstrate that animals without adequate stimulation during this critical period have abnormal neuronal physiology in their central auditory systems, which also causes poor performance on such higher-order processing tasks as sound localization, sound pattern discriminations, durational discriminations, and loudness recruitment. This is as far as nonhuman experimentation can go toward showing a link between early deprivation and language deficits. It would therefore be most informative to discover how persons with known postnatal conductive losses perform on the types of tasks on which the experimental rodents performed poorly.

EFFECTS OF SENSORY LOSSES

If conductive losses cause auditory brainstem dystrophies, as seems most certainly to be the case, one would expect sensory losses to be even more harmful. The pertinent literature is far too extensive to discuss here; instead I review the nonhuman experimental data from my own laboratory. For the past few years we have been studying the effects of total organ of Corti loss in mice and guinea pigs. With the increased interest in cochlear prostheses for the totally deaf, this subject has become of practical as well as academic significance.

In our laboratory, Trune (1979) ablated the right cochlea in 6-day-old mice, killed the mice at 45 days, and quantitatively examined their cochlear nuclei to determine volume, number of neurons, size of neuronal somas, extent of dendritic fields, and axonal projections to the contralateral inferior colliculi. The cochlear nuclei on the ablated side were reduced to 54% of normal size and contained only 34% of the normal number of neurons. Most of the remaining neurons were significantly smaller than normal in both soma size and extent of dendritic fields. However, their axons projected to the contralateral inferior colliculi in an apparently normal manner.

In separate experiments, we have been studying the long-term effects of organ of Corti loss in juvenile (not newborn) guinea pigs. The organ of Corti was destroyed at 1 month of age, either by surgical removal of the cochlear capsule and stria vascularis or by the combined drug treatment of kanamycin followed 2 hours later by ethacrynic acid. A third experimental group was the genetic waltzing strain, which has normal hearing at birth but undergoes gradual loss of organ of Corti and ensuing deafness during the first months of life.

In all three groups, organ of Corti loss is followed by a slow but insidious loss of spiral ganglion neurons until, between 8 months (drug and surgically deafened) and 2 years (waltzing guinea pigs), only

10-15% of the spiral ganglion neurons remain (Webster & Webster, 1978a, 1981b). As the majority disappear, their degenerating axons can be traced into the cochlear nuclei, where there is a massive loss of presynaptic structures (Webster & Webster, 1978a). Most of the remaining 10-15% gradually sprout new processes, thereby becoming multipolar (Webster & Webster, 1981a); their axons, however, continue to project to the cochlear nuclei in a normal cochleotopic pattern (Webster & Webster, 1978b). There is no loss of cochlear nuclear neurons, but the ventral cochlear nucleus is reduced to 64% of normal volume, and its neurons are reduced to 79% of their normal soma size; the dorsal cochlear nucleus retains normal size and its neurons are unaffected (Webster & Webster, 1979a).

These morphologic data demonstrate that organ of Corti loss results in drastic dystrophies of the cochlear nuclei which are more damaging to neonatal than to juvenile animals, assuming that the biologic systems of mice and guinea pigs are similar.

This finding is relevant to the subject of cochlear prostheses for totally deaf patients if one makes two further assumptions: 1) that candidates for cochlear prostheses have long-term organ of Corti loss, and 2) that the biologic system in humans is similar in certain respects to that in mice and guinea pigs. In that case, one must conclude that although prostheses may be implanted, and may function properly, the long-deprived cochlear nuclei of such patients may be severely limited in their ability to process the auditory information brought in by the prosthesis. Additionally, these problems may be expected to be even more pronounced for patients who were either born deaf or became deaf at a very early age.

CONCLUSIONS

1. Either sound deprivation or conductive loss during a critical postnatal period in experimental animals leads to anatomical and physiologic alterations of the auditory brainstem as well as complex auditory processing disorders.
2. Chronic or recurring otitis media with effusion in children between ages 0 and 5 years places them in jeopardy for language-related disorders.
3. Sensory hearing losses have a more drastic effect on auditory brainstem structures than do conductive losses and therefore must more severely limit auditory processing ability.

ACKNOWLEDGMENTS

Molly Webster has been of invaluable aid in editing this chapter. Judy Knight typed the entire manuscript. Equipment important to this research was provided by Zenetron, Inc.

REFERENCES

Batkin, S., Groth, H., Watson, J. R., and Ansberry, M. 1970. Effects of auditory deprivation on the development of auditory sensitivity in albino rats. Electroencephalography and Clinical Neurophysiology 28:351-359.

Bennett, F. C., Ruuska, S. H., and Sherman, R. 1980. Middle ear function in learning-disabled children. Pediatrics 66:254-260.

Bluestone, C. D., Beery, Q. C., and Paradise, J. L. 1973. Audiometry and tympanometry in relation to middle ear effusion in children. Laryngoscope 83:594-604.

Brookhouser, P. E., Hixon, P. K., and Matkin, N. D. 1979. Early childhood language delay: The otolaryngologist's perspective. Laryngoscope 89: 1898-1913.

Clements, M., and Kelly, J. B. 1978. Auditory spatial responses of young guinea pigs *(Cavia porcellus)* during and after ear blocking. Journal of Comparative and Physiological Psychology 92:34-44.

Clopton, B. M., and Silverman, M. S. 1977. Plasticity of binaural interaction. II. Critical period and changes in midline response. Journal of Neurophysiology 40:1275-1280.

Clopton, B. M., and Winfield, J. A. 1976. Effect of early exposure to patterned sound on unit activity in rat inferior colliculus. Journal of Neurophysiology 39:1081-1089.

Coleman, J. R., and O'Connor, P. 1979. Effects of monaural and binaural sound deprivation on cell development in the anteroventral cochlear nucleus of rats. Experimental Neurology 64:553-566.

Cook, R. A., and Teel, R. W., Jr. 1979. Negative middle ear pressure and language development. Clinical Pediatrics 18:296-297.

Dobie, R. A., and Berlin, C. I. 1979. Influence of otitis media on hearing and development. Annals of Otology, Rhinology, and Laryngology 88 (Suppl. 60): 48-53.

Downs, M. P. 1977. Expanding imperatives of early identification. In: F. Bess (ed.), Childhood Deafness: Causation, Assessment, and Management. pp. 95-107. Grune & Stratton, New York.

Ehret, G. 1976. Development of absolute auditory thresholds in the house mouse *(Mus musculus)*. Journal of the American Auditory Society 1:179-184.

Eisen, N. H. 1962. Some effects of early sensory deprivation on later behavior: The quondam hard-of-hearing child. Journal of Abnormal and Social Psychology 65:338-342.

Feng, A. S., and Rogowski, B. A. 1980. Effects of monaural and binaural occlusion on the morphology of neurons in the medial superior olivary nucleus of the rat. Brain Research 189:530-534.

Freeman, B. A., and Parkins, C. 1979. The prevalence of middle ear disease among learning impaired children. Does a higher prevalence indicate an association? Clinical Pediatrics 18:205-212.

Gates, G. R., Chen, C. S., and Bock, G. R. 1973. Effects of monaural and binaural auditory deprivation on audiogenic seizure susceptibility in BALB/c
mice. Experimental Neurology 38:488–493.

Gauron, E. F., and Becker, W. C. 1959. The effects of early sensory deprivation
on adult rat behavior under competition stress: An attempt at replication of a
study by Alexander Wolf. Journal of Comparative and Physiological Psychology 52:689–693.

Gottlieb, M. I., Zinkus, P. W., and Thompson, A. 1979. Chronic middle ear
disease and auditory perceptual deficits. Is there a link? Clinical Pediatrics
18:725–732.

Hamilton, P., and Owrid, H. L. 1974. Comparisons of hearing impairment and
sociocultural disadvantage in relation to verbal retardation. British Journal
of Audiology 8:27–32.

Hanson, D. G., and Ulvestad, R. F. 1979. Otitis media and child development:
Speech, language and education. Annals of Otology, Rhinology, and Laryngology 88 (Suppl. 60):1–111.

Henry, K. R., and Haythorn, M. M. 1975. Auditory similarities associated with
genetic and experimental acoustic deprivation. Journal of Comparative and
Physiological Psychology 89:213–218.

Holm, V. A., and Kunze, L. H. 1969. Effect of chronic otitis media on language
and speech development. Pediatrics 43:833–839.

Howie, V. M., Plousard, J. H., and Sloyer, J. L. 1975. The "otitis-prone" condition. American Journal of Diseases of Children 129:676–678.

Kaplan, G. J., Fleshman, J. K., Bender, T. R., Baum, C., and Clark, P. S. 1973.
Long term effects of otitis media: A 10-year cohort study of Alaskan Eskimo
children. Pediatrics 52:577–585.

Katz, J. 1978. The effects of conductive hearing loss on auditory function.
Asha 20:879–886.

Katz, J., and Illmer, R. 1972. Auditory perception in children with learning
disabilities. In: J. Katz (ed.), Handbook of Clinical Audiology, pp. 540–563.
Williams & Wilkins, Baltimore.

Kerr, L. M., Ostapoff, E. M., and Rubel, E. W. 1979. Influence of acoustic experience on the ontogeny of frequency generalization gradients in the chicken.
Journal of Experimental Psychology: Animal Behavior Processes 5:97–115.

Kokko, E. 1975. Chronic secretory otitis media in children: A clinical study.
Acta Otolaryngologica (Suppl.) 327.

Lewis, N. 1976. Otitis media and linguistic incompetence. Archives of Otolaryngology 102:387–390.

Ling, D. 1959. The education and general background of children with defective
hearing. Unpublished doctoral dissertation, Cambridge University, Cambridge, England.

McGinn, M. D., Willott, J. K., and Henry, K. R. 1973. Effects of conductive
hearing loss on auditory evoked potentials and audiogenic seizures in mice.
Nature: New Biology 244:255–256.

Mikaelian, D., and Ruben, R. J. 1965. Development of hearing in the normal
CBA/J mouse. Acta Otolaryngologica 59:451–461.

Moore, D. R., and Aitkin, L. M. 1975. Rearing in an acoustically unusual environment—Effects of neural auditory responses. Neuroscience Letters
1:29–34.

Naremore, R. C. 1979. Influences of hearing impairment on early language development. Annals of Otology, Rhinology, and Laryngology 88 (Suppl. 60):54–63.

Omer, J. L. 1972. The incidence of hearing impairment in students identified as learning-disabled. Language, Speech, and Hearing Services in the Schools 3:34–43.

Paradise, J. L. 1976. Management of middle ear effusions in infants with cleft palate. Annals of Otology, Rhinology, and Laryngology 85 (Suppl. 25): 285–288.

Rajecki, D. W. 1974. Effects of prenatal exposure to auditory or visual stimulation on postnatal distress vocalizations in chicks. Behavioral Biology 11: 525–536.

Ruben, R. J., and Rapin, I. 1980. Plasticity of the developing auditory system. Annals of Otology, Rhinology, and Laryngology 89:303–311.

Sak, R. J., and Ruben, R. J. 1981. Recurrent middle ear effusion in childhood: Implications of temporary auditory deprivation for language and learning. Annals of Otology, Rhinology, and Laryngology 90:546–551.

Saunders, J. C., Bock, G. R., Chen, C-S., and Gates, G. R. 1972a. The effects of priming for audiogenic seizures on cochlear and behavioral responses in BALB/c mice. Experimental Neurology 36:426–436.

Saunders, J. C., Bock, G. R., James, R., and Chen, C-S. 1972b. Effects of priming for audiogenic seizure on auditory evoked responses in the cochlear nucleus and inferior colliculus of BALB/c mice. Experimental Neurology 37:388–394.

Silverman, M. S., and Clopton, B. M. 1977. Plasticity of binaural interaction. I. Effect of early auditory deprivation. Journal of Neurophysiology 40: 1266–1274.

Teele, D. W., Klein, J. O., and Rosner, B. A. 1980. Epidemiology of otitis media in children. Annals of Otology, Rhinology, and Laryngology 89 (Suppl. 68): 5–6.

Tees, R. C. 1967a. The effects of early auditory restriction in the rat on adult duration discrimination. Journal of Auditory Research 7:195–207.

Tees, R. C. 1967b. Effects of early auditory restriction in the rat on adult pattern discrimination. Journal of Comparative and Physiological Psychology 63:389–393.

Trune, D. R. 1979. Influence of neonatal cochlear removal on cochlear nuclear development. Unpublished doctoral dissertation. Louisiana State University Medical Center, New Orleans.

Ventry, I. M. 1980. Effects of conductive hearing loss: Fact or fiction. Journal of Speech and Hearing Disorders 45:143–156.

Webster, D. B. 1980. Do conductive losses compromise the central auditory system? In: C. I. Berlin (ed.), Studies in the Use of Amplification for the Hearing Impaired, pp. 56–65. Excerpta Medica, Princeton, N.J.

Webster, D. B., and Webster, M. 1977. Neonatal sound deprivation affects brainstem auditory nuclei. Archives of Otolaryngology 103:392–396.

Webster, D. B., and Webster, M. 1978a. Cochlear nerve projections following organ of Corti destruction. Otolaryngology 86:ORL 342–ORL 353.

Webster, D. B., and Webster, M. 1979a. Brainstem auditory nuclei following organ of Corti destruction: Preliminary report. Abstracts of the Second Midwinter Research Meeting, Association for Research in Otolaryngology, p. 27.

Webster, D. B., and Webster, M. 1979b. Effects of neonatal conductive hearing loss on brain stem auditory nuclei. Annals of Otology, Rhinology, and Laryngology 88:684–688.

Webster, D. B., and Webster, M. 1980. Mouse brainstem auditory nuclei development. Annals of Otology, Rhinology, and Laryngology 89 (Suppl. 68): 254–256.

Webster, D. B., and Webster, M. 1981a. Multipolar residual spiral ganglion neurons. (abstract). Journal of the Acoustical Society of America. In press.

Webster, M., and Webster, D. B. 1978b. Cochlear nuclear projections from outer hair cells. Neuroscience Abstracts 4:11.

Webster, M., and Webster, D. B. 1981b. Spiral ganglion neuron loss following organ of Corti loss: A quantitative study. Brain Research 212:17–30.

Wolf, A. 1943. The dynamics of selective inhibition of specific function in neurosis. Psychosomatic Medicine 5:27–38.

Zinkus, P. W., and Gottlieb, M. I. 1978. Chronic otitis media and auditory processing deficits: A preventable learning disability. Ohio Journal of Speech and Hearing 13:86–97.

Zinkus, P. W., Gottlieb, M. I., and Shapiro, M. 1978. Developmental and psychoeducational sequelae of chronic otitis media. American Journal of Diseases of Children 132:1100–1104.

Section **III**

Diagnosis and Treatment of Central Auditory Processing Disorders

Chapter 11

Selecting Tests of Auditory Function in Children

Charlotte Dempsey

INTRODUCTION

Tests of central auditory processing are used by a variety of professionals interested in assessing perceptual problems that may be related to learning disabilities in children. This chapter examines some of the more popular tests that are commercially available and discusses variables that may affect the results and the implications for listening abilities in the classroom.

SELECTING THE CHILD FOR TESTING

What kinds of problems may indicate CAP difficulty? The problem may be stated directly in auditory terms, such as, "He doesn't seem to hear me." Occasionally, however, the auditory problem may be obscured by complaints of "poor memory" or "poor word-attack skills" for reading. Most instruction in the home and classroom, especially in the early years, is presented verbally. The ability to receive a clear message and to attend amid distractions is critical to language learning.

Classroom learning of math, reading, and spelling also requires processing of auditory information (Dodd, 1980; Wiig & Semel, 1976). A child who is having unexpected difficulty attending to and comprehending information at home and in school may be a candidate for CAP testing. Fisher's Auditory Problems Checklist (Fisher, 1980) is a useful tool to identify children whose classroom behaviors may reflect hearing or listening problems. The checklist takes no more than a minute of a teacher's or parent's time, and results can be compared with normative data to reduce overreferrals.

PREPARING FOR TESTING

Purpose of Testing

Traditionally, the audiologist chooses tests to indicate site of lesion in the auditory pathway or to describe an individual's ability to understand speech in a social situation. Both of these objectives are reflected in tests of auditory processing given to children suspected of having CAP problems. The evaluation provides information regarding integrity of the peripheral and central auditory system. Results may also suggest the need for medical attention. These and other tests may aid educational specialists in planning remediation programs. Keith (1980) discussed problems the audiologist may face when site of lesion test results are used educationally.

Speech-language pathologists may have other purposes for testing children thought to have auditory processing difficulties. They might want to assess auditory abilities prior to speech or language therapy, or they may be seeking an explanation for classroom problems. Care must be taken in such cases to ensure that the test materials and the environment are controlled so that, after testing, an auditory problem can be ruled in or ruled out.

To provide a reasonably thorough evaluation of auditory abilities, more than one test must be given. There is no one test that samples the variety of functions the auditory system must perform in a learning situation. In selecting tests, each test should be examined for reliability, validity, and sensitivity to the presenting problem. A flexible procedure can also provide an opportunity to observe each individual's dynamic abilities within the task dimensions.

The tester must choose tests related to the person's complaint. Is the problem one of attention in noise? Is it related to poor abilities to "close" onto a message under difficult listening conditions? Does changing the rate of speech affect the child's difficulty? Is auditory sequencing a problem? Is the complaint so vague that all of these and more should be tested?

If a battery of tests is to be presented, the tester must be able to define auditory skills that he or she feels are necessary for classroom learning. These have been discussed under such diverse labels in the literature that making sense of them is sometimes difficult. Tests, however, do seem to organize themselves under labels that seem identifiable to professionals working with children. The labels include auditory attention, distorted speech, and auditory memory. The tests of auditory attention use language units in a background of competition. Tests of distorted speech use speech stimuli in which frequency and time constants have been altered. Tests of auditory memory use tasks that require retention of strings of items. A profile of function in each area can be obtained by careful selection of tests.

The test situation can provide opportunity to determine the child's strengths as well. The manual or literature should be examined to determine not only whether specific test results are related to classroom behaviors, but also whether the test can be modified to evaluate ways a child may be able to overcome problems related to the classroom environment.

Analyzing the Test Stimuli

The stimulus items should be examined for vocabulary level, complexity of sentence structure, and level of cognitive function required to encode and decode information. Is the vocabulary appropriate to the child's age and experience levels? Are sentences controlled for syntactic structure? Are some easily visualized items mixed with more abstract items, hampering interpretation of results? There should be internal consistency to the items presented; if some items can be decoded through visualization, the same should be true for all items in a set.

If the child is tired or has attentional lapses, the length of the test or subtest may affect results. Conversely, a sufficient number of items need to be presented to provide a reliable estimate of function. The tester should practice giving the test and be familiar with results from representative populations of normal and disabled children before using the results diagnostically.

Analyzing the Task

Some tests require repetition of the stimuli as the response, whereas others may ask the child to point to or manipulate an object. If the task is to repeat what was said, the articulatory ability of the child must be sufficiently clear to judge the response. If the response mode is nonverbal, the child's visual-motor system must be sufficiently intact so that variables are not added that may affect performance. As we cannot directly measure auditory input, we must make inferences about its reception by observing behavior. We may be testing very complex interhemispheric functions when we ask a child to point to a picture of a spoken word. Intrahemispheric function may be engaged when we ask the child to repeat an item. Although a say-back type of test seems to be less strenuous for the subject, the tester must hear and interpret the subject's speech accurately. The say-back response, therefore, also tests the tester's auditory skills.

Some tests may be given by live voice; some are recorded on tape. Taped tests have greater intrasubject and intertester reliability, because the child hears the stimuli with the same emphasis and at the same speed regardless of the tester. This tends to reduce the flexibility of the test to accommodate a particular child's rate of response. If tests are given by live voice, visual cues can be added. This is desirable if performance with and without lipreading is of interest, but the tester must be alert to the contribution of other cues such as stress and gestures that inadvertently trigger the correct response.

Test Equipment

If a tape player is to be used, attention must be paid to its reproductive quality. Some cassette recorders have little or no high frequency reproduction beyond 3000 or 4000 Hz. This effectively filters the signal. If the tests you select require analysis of high-frequency components of language, have the tape player checked electroacoustically. An electronic equipment repair company or a local speech science laboratory may help you do this. Unfortunately, you cannot check the tape's reproduction by listening to it. Linguistically experienced people tend to close on the presence of a sound because it *should* be there, not necessarily because it was heard.

The playback heads of the tape player should be cleaned frequently. Each time the tape pulls across the heads, a deposit is left that may add background noise. The mechanical noise the player makes when it is pulling tape also adds to interference levels.

Test Tape

When using recorded materials, inspect the physical condition of the tape carefully. Tapes vary in brittleness and in tendency to stretch, especially in extreme temperatures. If there is a calibration tone, pull gently on a section of the tape and listen again to see whether the pitch changed. Then inspect the relative intensity levels of the items on a VU meter. Is needle deflection approximately equal for all stimuli? Recording intensity should be consistent throughout. Finally, listen for extraneous background noise such as hum or hissing noises. Discard a poor tape rather than test with it.

Test Environment

Control of the environment is essential to the reliability of the test results. Because sound intensity decreases as the square of the distance from the source increases, the position of the child and tape recorder output is critical. As no room is absolutely quiet, earphones should be used to move the output closer to the ears of the child. Earphones help reduce effects of extraneous noise in the test room as well. Earphones have to be checked for frequency response characteristics. If earphones for your tape recorder are not available, follow the calibration instructions provided in the test manuals. Set the intensity at a louder than normal conversational level, and move the tape player as close to the child as possible. Keith (1981) observed that some children with impaired auditory perception require louder than average speech for good discrimination. Average sound levels in your testing area can be monitored with a sound level meter that may be borrowed from an audiologist or equipment salesperson.

Audiologists have the advantage of being able to control the acoustic environment by testing in sound-treated booths. The audiometer will compensate for hearing thresholds so that test levels can be monitored accurately.

Hearing Sensitivity

It is obvious that before the signal can be understood, it must be heard. Neglecting to test auditory thresholds prior to other testing may completely invalidate any findings. Even slight losses of 15 dB, especially in high frequencies, add filtering characteristics to the signal. If hearing thresholds are poorer than 25 dB in one or both ears, certain central test results cannot be interpreted. Therefore, audiometric screening should be done for frequencies of 1000 through 8000 Hz at 10 dB (if room conditions allow) in each ear before presenting any language stimuli. The effects of low-frequency hearing loss on language tests is not fully understood but must be compensated for by increased intensity. Thresholds for low frequencies are invalid if hearing testing is done in an open room.

Summary

The variables discussed in the foregoing section are only a few of those that may operate in a test situation. Experienced testers are also aware that time of day, health of the tester and testee, test-taking jitters, and so on are conditions that frequently cannot be controlled. If results seem inconsistent with your expectations or are inconsistent from item to item, retesting at another time is recommended.

AUDITORY SKILLS FOR CLASSROOM LEARNING

Attending to the Signal

A child must learn what to listen for in the classroom. Instructions may be given during periods of increased noise levels, and the child must identify the signal and ignore unwanted intrusions. The process of assigning relevance to one set of auditory patterns and suppressing attention to others requires certain neurologic and voluntary actions involving brainstem and cortex (see Protti, Chapter 7, this volume). This may be referred to as selective attention, auditory figure-ground, auditory vigilance, or "hearing what he wants to hear."

Background noise in a classroom may be constant or intermittent, loud or soft, or change in frequency spectrum from moment to moment. Most children, including those who are developing normally, may have difficulty with extraneous noise; in general, the younger the child, the greater the difficulty. Most tests that purport to test auditory attention use language stimuli in a background of environmental sounds or talking.

Some children also have difficulty concentrating on auditory language if visual, tactile, or kinesthetic distractions are present. We have few tests that control for multisensory input. If visual stimuli, such as pictures, are used, the visual system may be activated by the novelty of the stimulus, possibly blocking auditory input. If blocks are to be manipulated, tactile and kinesthetic cues may interfere with the listening activities required.

Determining whether a child has difficulty attending amid distractions is only the first step. Test results may explain certain behaviors but contribute little to remedial procedures in the classroom. Manipulating the signal and the background independently can tell us: What signal-to-distraction ratio allows the child to perform at near normal levels? What types of distractions most interfere with language reception? Must some language stimuli be presented in relative quiet for this child? What happens when the child is not told what to listen for? The dynamic nature of listening abilities is best assessed by an audiologist, who has the equipment available to present the signal in a variety of background sounds at different ratios, under earphones or in the sound field. Stimulus items may be mixed with competing backgrounds and presented to each ear individually, then to opposite ears. The signal and noise can be delivered through loudspeakers, to simulate the same direction or different directions. Many commercially available tests have the noise and signal mixed onto the same recording track, so that test flexibility is extremely limited. This recording method may also add acoustic distortion by wiping away part of the signal when tracks are combined. Test selection has to be done carefully, as no two tests are alike in stimulus or type of distractor. Each probably tests a different type of attentional ability. Some may be more sensitive to language abilities than to auditory function.

Tests of Auditory Attention

Competing Environmental Sounds (CES; Katz, 1977)

Stimuli   Different environmental sounds are presented simultaneously to the ears. Sounds are recorded on separate tracks of the tape and can be manipulated separately.

Equipment   Two-channel audiometer or stereo tape player with channel separation and earphones.

Age/Skill Requirement   Age 5 years and up; visual-motor skills.

Task   Point to the two pictures representing the sounds.

Comments   This test can be used diagnostically as part of the audiologist's site-of-lesion battery. This is one of the few tests that may be sensitive to auditory pattern-matching abilities in children. This may be a strength in some language-disordered children and help to define a skill the child can use efficiently. One track of the tape can be used in a sound field as a distractor when presenting linguistic materials because the environmental sounds seem to occur at random intervals.

Competing Sentence Test (Willeford, 1977)

Stimuli   Different sentences on the same subject, spoken by the same person (male), are presented simultaneously to the ears. Stimuli are recorded on separate tracks.

Equipment   Two-channel audiometer, tape player, and earphones.

Age/Skill Requirement   Age 6 years and up; clear speech.

Task   Repeat the sentence presented to one ear, then conditions are reversed.

Comments   Each ear can be tested individually. This test was designed to be part of the site-of-lesion battery for audiologists. These materials provide an opportunity to observe responses to contextual materials presented dichotically. The test is sensitive to neurologic development in children. Test difficulty may be increased by asking the child to repeat both sentences. This may add variables of rate of sampling and rules for syntax. The child may be allowed to pick the sentence to repeat. In a free recall situation, the child may consistently choose to report sentences from only one ear. Natural listening biases or attentional strategies can be monitored.

Flowers-Costello Test of Auditory Abilities:
Competing Message Subtest (Flowers & Costello, 1970)
Stimuli Fill-in-the-blank sentences are spoken by a female in the presence of a story told by the same person. Stimuli and story are recorded on the same track of the tape and cannot be manipulated separately.

Equipment Portable tape player and earphones. The manual gives calibration procedures.

Age/Skill Requirement Age 5 and up; visual-motor skills are required.

Task The child is to point to the picture of the thing that completes the sentence. Example: "With a net we catch _____."

Comments This seems to be a language test given in the background of distraction. If the child passes the test, auditory attentional problems cannot be ruled out; if the child fails the test, interpretation of poor auditory abilities does not necessarily follow. The authors give data correlating test results with reading problems in school-aged children. The test seems to be sensitive to a number of variables that are not clearly separated for the tester.

Flowers Auditory Test of Selective Attention
(FATSA; Flowers, 1972b)
Stimuli A series of words is presented and one or more of the words has the name "George" immediately preceding it. The tagged words may appear once or more than once within a group of words; "George" may also appear without a word following it.

Equipment Portable tape player.

Age/Skill Requirement Age 5 years and up; visual-motor skills are required.

Task The child, through a series of reinforced practice items, is instructed to mark a picture corresponding with the word following the name "George."

Comments This test requires a high degree of vigilance to the task over time. It stresses attentional abilities (auditory or other). The task is similar to the game "Simon Says," and specificity to auditory language skills is not clear. Flowers (1972b) recommends the test as a group screening device. Tests given in open rooms are subject to extraneous variables.

Goldman-Fristoe-Woodcock Auditory Skills Battery: Auditory
Selective Attention Subtest (Goldman, Fristoe, & Woodcock, 1977)
Stimuli Single-syllable words spoken by a male, with fanlike noise, cafeteria noise, and voice as background competition. The signal-

to-competition ratios get progressively more difficult. Both signal and competition are recorded on a single track.

Equipment Portable tape player. Calibration instruction is on tape.

Age/Skill Requirement Age 5 years and up; good visual-motor skills are required.

Comments Test results are to be compared with the score achieved for similar items in quiet. As the vocabulary is not easy, the child should probably be familiarized with the pictures and words in advance, but the effect on the results is not known. The noise subtests are attractive, as the sounds are realistic and might be easily generalized to school situations. However, as no two fans or cafeterias have exactly the same sound spectra, that assumption may be erroneous. When the test is given in an uncontrolled environment, room noise may interact with the background sound on the tape, making interpretation difficult.

Short-Term Auditory Retrieval and Storage Test (STARS; Flowers, 1972a)

Stimuli Single- and multisyllable words are presented simultaneously by a male speaker and mixed on one tape track.

Equipment Tape player.

Age/Skill Requirement Age 5 years and up; good visual-motor skills are required.

Task Child is asked to mark the pictures representing the two words. Numerous practice items are reinforced before presentation of test items.

Comments Test items seem to range from easy to difficult, depending upon the acoustic characteristics of the competing words. Flowers (1972a) calls this "overlapping" rather than "simultaneous" presentation. He suggests its use as a screening test for groups of children. When given in an open room, this test may be fraught with uncontrolled variables, especially when given as a group pencil-and-paper task, where visual cues may be available to some children.

Staggered Spondaic Word (SSW) Test (Katz, 1968)

Stimuli Competing spondaic words are staggered to the ears. A carrier phrase precedes each test item. Stimuli are spoken by a male and recorded on separate tape tracks.

Equipment Two-channel audiometer or stereo tape player with good channel separation and earphones.

Age/Skill Requirement Age 6 and up; clear speech.

Task Repeat both spondees.

Comments   Scoring this test is complicated because many factors are assessed independently. Order of recall of syllables is also noted and may relate to sequential skills. This test was designed as a site-of-lesion test for audiologists. In children the test offers an opportunity to observe different test-taking skills. The child must deal with the carrier phrase (a rhetorical question) and the unique semantic properties of compound words in which the syllables have been separated by a pause. The slow rate of speech may allow the child to rehearse items before responding.

Synthetic Sentence Index (SSI; Jerger, Speaks, & Trammel, 1968)

Stimuli   Nonsense sentences (third-order approximations) are presented in the background of a story read by the same male talker. Sentences and story are recorded on separate tape tracks.

Equipment   Two-channel audiometer, tape player, and earphones.

Age/Skill Requirement   Age 6 or 7 and up; some reading skills required, visual-motor skills needed.

Task   The child points to the test sentence from a list of 10 test sentences. The child must be familiarized with the stimuli and the task prior to testing.

Comments   This is a sensitive test with normative data for ipsilateral and contralateral competing message presentation modes. This test probably measures more than auditory function, as the child must match the spoken stimulus to the written one. The task may be modified by asking for verbal recall of the sentences. This seems to force the child to recall strings of words in a syntactic framework. Some children restructure the words into real sentences. The nonsense nature of the stimuli may stress sequential abilities.

Wepman Auditory Discrimination Test:
Noise Subtest (Wepman, 1958)

Stimuli   Single-syllable word pairs are presented in a background of thermal noise at a constant signal-to-noise ratio. The word pairs are either the same word presented twice or differ by one phoneme.

Equipment   Tape player.

Age/Skill Requirement   Age 6 and up; clear speech.

Task   The child indicates whether the words are the same or different.

Comments   As concepts of same versus different may not be developed in young children and in some language-disordered children, results can be questioned unless the concepts are pretested. The test is supposed to analyze the child's ability to "hear" phoneme elements in words, but the child may make judgments on the basis of merely matching two sound patterns. This may be a strength in some children. A forced-choice paradigm requires numerous trials to rule out guessing. This test may have nothing to do with auditory skills required for phoneme perception.

Resistance to Distortion

Persons speaking a foreign language often seem to "talk too fast." Similarly, a young child not yet totally familiar with his or her own language may have difficulty following adult rates of speech. The rate at which he or she can correctly identify rapidly changing acoustic signals may be related to the depth of analysis possible (Tallal & Piercy, 1974).

In a group of tests, frequency of the stimulus has been altered by filtering. In other tests, duration of the stimuli has been artificially altered to measure the effect of rate on processing. In low-pass filtered speech tests, low frequency elements of words or phrases are available to the listener. Acoustic cues are present but are limited to rapidly changing formant frequencies, voice onset times, and spectral cues for some vowels and consonants (Dempsey, 1977). These tests seem to challenge auditory areas of the cortex.

Time-altered or compressed speech provides a wide frequency band, but the overall duration of the signal is reduced. Temporal distortion is introduced by the compression process, which randomly deletes brief bits of information. The remaining bits are reassembled into a speeded message. The greater the speed (percent compression), the greater the deletion-to-retention ratio. Because the sampling process is random, it seems reasonable that formant duration, coarticulatory cues, and durational cues for analysis of elements may be abbreviated, eliminated, or distorted.

Compressed speech and filtered speech tests are tests of reduced redundancy. They are sensitive to the condition of the auditory pathway at all levels and are useful to the audiologist in site-of-lesion testing (Bocca and Calearo, 1963). For children with immature neurologic and language systems, interpretation of results is difficult. The responses of the child to distortion are interesting to observe and may be related to the real world of the classroom, where the child listens in a highly reverberant setting while the teacher talks to the chalkboard.

The tests in this section are limited in flexibility, since few of us have the equipment needed to vary the degree of filtering or compression ratios. It is difficult to determine whether the child could have performed the task if conditions were altered even slightly.

Distorted Speech Tests

Binaural Fusion Test (Willeford, 1977)

Stimuli Spondaic words, preceded by a carrier word, are filtered to retain only a narrow low-pass band that is presented to one ear and a high-pass band presented to the other ear.

Equipment Two-channel audiometer, tape player, and earphones.

Age/Skill Requirement Age 6 and up; clear speech.

Task Repeat the test word.

Comments The vocabulary was selected to withstand the filtering process and is very difficult for children. They should be familiarized with the words before testing. The two lists are not balanced in difficulty.

The carrier word closely precedes the test item, so that if children respond to it, they miss the test word. However, the test is useful to a limited extent for site-of-lesion assessment, as it may be sensitive to brainstem problems. Filtering is sensitive to problems at all levels of the auditory system, and low test scores must be validated by combining the bands for monaural or binaural presentation. Continued difficulty with the test is due to other than brainstem problems (Matzker, 1959).

Compressed Word List (Beasley, Schwimmer, & Rintlemann, 1977)

Stimuli Tape-recorded NU-6 lists of single-syllable words have been compressed to 0%, 30%, and 60% compression.

Equipment Single-channel tape player.

Age/Skill Requirement Age 6 and up; clear speech.

Task Repeat the word.

Comments The value of this test is not clearly stated (Rees, 1981). Normative data are available only for sound field presentation. Data by ear for children are necessary if this test is to monitor maturational development of the auditory system.

Filtered Speech Test (Willeford, 1977)

Stimuli Monosyllables, bandpass filtered to 500 Hz. Frequencies above 500 Hz are attenuated 19 dB per octave. Two 50-word lists of CVC words are read by a male speaker.

Equipment Single-channel tape player, audiometer, earphones.

Age/Skill Requirement Age 6 and up; clear speech.

Task Repeat the test word.

Comments This test is extremely difficult for young children. The carrier phrase preceding each word has also been filtered so that the item sounds like a phrase. No practice items are provided. All 50 words are given to each ear, making the test time-consuming. No information is given about list equivalence after filtering.

Filtered Word Identification by Picture Test (WIPI; Willeford, 1977)

Stimuli   Discrimination lists of monosyllables developed by Ross and Lerman (1971) have been filtered and are unpublished but available through J. Willeford at Colorado State University. A male speaker presents the test words.

Equipment   Single-channel tape player to earphones.

Age/Skill Requirements   The WIPI may be given to very young children, but age norms for filtered presentation are not available in print. Visual-motor skills are needed.

Task   Point to the picture of the test word.

Comments   The task seems much easier for children, and this test might replace the more difficult filtered speech test. Articulation-disordered or nonverbal children might be testable. More research is needed to evaluate this procedure.

Flowers-Costello Test of Auditory Abilities:
Filtered Speech Subtest (Flowers & Costello, 1970)

Stimuli   Fill-in-the-blank sentences have been low-pass filtered to 960 Hz.

Equipment   Portable tape player.

Age/Skill Requirement   Age 5 and up; good visual-motor skills.

Task   The child points to the picture that represents the missing word in the sentence.

Comments   Filter characteristics make this a less strenuous listening task than the Filtered Speech Test (Willeford, 1977). The test items, however, seem to test language rather than listening abilities. Reasons for failure might be difficult to explain in auditory terms.

Rapidly Alternating Speech Perception (Willeford, 1977)

Stimuli   Sentences presented at a rapid rate of speech are segmented so that brief bits are presented alternately to the ears.

Equipment   Two-channel audiometer, tape player, and earphones.

Age/Skill Requirement   Age 5 and up; clear speech.

Task   Repeat the sentence.

Comments   This test is probably more useful as a test of attention to rapidly presented information than as a site-of-lesion test. Scores for 5-year-old children are nearly as good as for adults (Keith, 1981). The sentences are spoken rapidly with little time for response between items. Error patterns reveal the extent to which the child is forced to paraphrase what he or she has heard at that speed, but as the complexity of the syntax is uncontrolled, interpretation of these errors is not possible.

Retention of the Signal

There are several different kinds of memory, and we should try to treat them as separate tasks when selecting tests. Immediate (echoic) memory lasts only a few seconds and may be likened to an afterimage of the stimulus. Short-term and long-term auditory memory seem to involve storage of the signal in other than its original state (Lindsay & Norman, 1972). Many auditory memory tests do not require much more than echoic memory, and items are usually sequential; they are probably better described as tests of sequencing abilities.

Oral language is not presented or received instantaneously. Bits of information come rapidly, but over time. The bits must be stored in the correct order for encoding. The ability to hold rote information in proper sequence seems to be important for many classroom tasks. Spelling, following instructions, and ordering phonemes to sound out words all seem to require sequencing skills (Stark & Tallal, 1981).

Too many tests are in this category to list them all. Rate of presentation of items must be controlled since rate interacts with ability to reproduce a sequence. The slower the speed, the greater the opportunity to use mnemonic devices to store the information (Rees, 1981). Many tests are given by live voice, and few manuals mention the need to prevent lipreading to isolate auditory abilities. The tester is encouraged to use tape-recorded materials to obtain consistency from test to test.

Tests of Sequencing Abilities

Denver Auditory Phoneme Sequencing Test (Aten, 1979)

Stimuli Items numbered 51 through 70 present progressively longer series of rhyming words. Tape recording by male talker.

Equipment Good-quality tape player.

Age/Skill Requirement Age 6 and up; good visual-motor skills.

Task The child listens to the series without looking at the pictures. Then the child is shown pictures representing the words and must indicate the order in which the corresponding words were heard.

Comments The rate of presentation does not allow time for rehearsal and therefore probably tests immediate recall. The test is difficult for the tester, because the child's order of recall must be recorded by picture number. The items may be presented by live voice, with or without lipreading, to evaluate the contribution of visual cues. A live voice presentation may follow the taped one to evaluate effects of slowing the rate. The child may be asked to verbalize the strategy he or she used to improve on this test.

Lindamood Auditory Conceptualization (LAC) Test
(Lindamood & Lindamood, 1971)

Stimuli Phonemes and nonsense stimuli are presented by live voice.

Equipment None needed, although if this test is to be used regularly, a tape recording of good quality should be made to eliminate visual cues.

Age/Skill Requirement Age 5 and up; good visual-motor system; understanding of same versus different.

Comments Although a useful test of the child's ability to analyze and sequence phonemes, the task requires translating sound symbols into colored block symbols which do not have a one-for-one correspondence. Any colored block may be used to represent a phoneme. Colors are used to designate the same or different phonemes, so training time is required. Normative data suggest that test scores may be used to predict reading or spelling problems.

Pitch Pattern Sequences (Pinheiro, 1977)

Stimuli Recorded tonal sequences of two pitches, in groups of three. Each ear is tested individually.

Equipment Audiometer, tape recorder, and earphones.

Age/Skill Requirement Age 5 and up; visual-motor skills needed.

Task The child manipulates blocks representing high and low tones, arranging them into the sequence heard.

Comments This is a helpful test of sequential abilities, as the stimuli are not contaminated with linguistic variables. The test is time-consuming because there are many practice items and a very long inter-stimulus interval is provided. Ear effects can be observed in young children.

Staggered Spondaic Word (SSW) Test (Katz, 1977) As mentioned before, this test is also scored in relation to the order of recall of four test syllables. Reversal in the order of the words is a useful indicator of the need for further testing of this skill. The lack of reversals does not rule out a sequencing problem.

Summary

The diversity of test formats available under the heading of auditory tests is nearly overwhelming. It should now be obvious that each test has its own strengths and weaknesses and task requirements. Each of us must decide which tests to include or exclude from a battery through the evaluation of many factors.

Screening for auditory problems related to language learning must include tests selected from the skill areas the tester has decided are important. If results from one test in each area are normal, an auditory problem still cannot be ruled out. Failure on any test only indicates that further, more extensive testing should be done.

If an audiologist is testing, tests should be selected so that neurologic and behavioral data are obtained in the shortest amount of time. The audiologist may modify the traditional use of recordings to evaluate effects of diverse listening conditions. The most flexible materials seem to have been prepared for audiologic tests while good control of the test conditions is maintained. The audiologist should become aware, however, of linguistic variables in these materials (Jerger, 1981). Rees (1981) has stressed the importance of extending test results to language learning situations.

Speech-language pathologists and learning specialists must recognize the influence of hearing sensitivity and test environment on results. Tests designed to be given in the schools offer little flexibility to modify performance to allow remediation procedures to be inferred.

Recommendations made based on these tests continue to be cautious and without prescription for remediation procedures. There are some common-sense statements that can be made to benefit the child with auditory problems and that are probably applicable to all children in the classroom as well.

TRANSLATING RESULTS INTO RECOMMENDATIONS

Reporting Test Results

The report writer should use caution in reporting actual test scores. Some results are given in age- or grade-equivalent scores, implying that the child's behavior is like that of a younger child. This may be misleading, suggesting that a year or two of going over the same material in the same way is all the child needs. Some children's problems may represent differences in neurologic organization rather than maturational lags (Witelson, 1977). If the child's intellectual abilities are within normal limits, the assumption of a lag or delay may lead to inappropriate remediation strategies. Results should be interpreted in lay terms for parents and teachers.

The tester can discuss the child's individual needs if materials have been presented under a variety of conditions. The response time required, the number of presentations before attention wanes, and the types of materials the child can handle should have been noted during the test. No two children seem to respond exactly alike to all parts of the test situation. The report should include specific references to the child's strengths.

Recommendations for Children with Auditory Attention Problems

Treat this child as if he or she is hard of hearing. Seat the child in the front of the classroom with the strong ear open to most of the conversation. Tap lightly on the shoulder to get the child's attention. Let the child see your face while you are speaking. Be sure there is little background noise if you have something important to say. Write things down or tape record them. Keep other visual distractions at a minimum. Allow the child to use a carrel or quiet place to read or study. Amplification of language by use of an auditory trainer or FM transmitter might help if levels are closely monitored. The best solution is to sound-treat the classroom (see Hart, Chapter 18, this volume). This can be done relatively inexpensively.

Recommendations for Children with a Low Resistance to Distortion

Seat the child preferentially in the classroom so that the child is close to the teacher. Speak slowly and distinctly, paraphrasing occasionally. Check on comprehension by asking questions concerning the subject matter. Avoid long, complex instructions or syntax, as this tends to force the speaker to speed production. Give the child time to process. Pause occasionally. Face the child, as he or she may have to augment auditory information with visual cues. Give frequent illustrations of concepts.

Recommendations for Children with Sequential Problems

Give directions and homework assignments one stage at a time. Repeat frequently. Speak slowly so that memory devices may be used to retain rote information. Use visual reinforcement for rote learning by writing information on the chalkboard. Visually present an outline of topics to be discussed so that the child can see the organization of the material. Pause frequently to give the child time to process. Allow the child to use a tape recorder in class to collect rote information. Analysis and synthesis of phonemes might be difficult, and the child's strengths should be used to attack this type of material.

Summary

The recommendations presented have been gleaned from a variety of sources and seem second nature to an audiologist, who will recognize them as those usually given for a child who has a hearing loss. The resemblance of the child with CAP problems to a hearing-impaired child is striking. The child with CAP problems is frequently referred for audiometric testing because the behaviors displayed could be due to a hearing loss. If we treat the child as if he or she is hearing impaired, adults will often adjust their speaking manner automatically. We must await further research to refine recommendations and to evaluate appropriate remediation strategies.

REFERENCES

Aten, J. 1979. The Denver Auditory Phoneme Sequencing Test, College-Hill Press, Houston.

Beasley, D., Schwimmer, S., and Rintlemann, W. 1977. Intelligibility of time-compressed CNC monosyllables. Journal of Speech and Hearing Research 20:108–115.

Bocca, E., and Calearo, C. 1963. Central hearing processes. In: J. Jerger (ed.), Modern Developments in Audiology. Academic Press, New York.

Dempsey, C. 1977. Some thoughts concerning alternate explanations of central auditory test results. In: R. Keith (ed.), Central Auditory Dysfunction. Grune & Stratton, New York.

Dodd, B. 1980. The spelling abilities of profoundly pre-lingually deaf children. In: U. Frith (ed.), Cognitive Processes in Spelling. Academic Press, New York.

Fisher, L. 1980. Fisher's Auditory Problems Checklist. Grant Wood, Cedar Rapids, Iowa.

Flowers, A. 1972a. Flowers Auditory Retrieval and Storage Test. Perceptual Learning Systems, Dearborn, Mich.

Flowers, A. 1972b. Flowers Auditory Test of Selective Attention. Perceptual Learning Systems, Dearborn, Mich.

Flowers, A., and Costello, M. 1970. Flowers-Costello Test of Auditory Abilities. Perceptual Learning Systems, Dearborn, Mich.

Goldman, R., Fristoe, M., and Woodcock, R. 1977. Auditory Skills Battery: Selective Attention Test. Perceptual Learning Systems, Circle Pines, Minn.

Jerger, J., Speaks, C., and Trammel, J. 1968. A new approach to speech audiometry. Journal of Speech and Hearing Disorders 33:318–328.

Jerger, S. 1981. Evaluation of central auditory function in children. In: R. Keith (ed.), Central Auditory and Language Disorders in Children. College-Hill Press, Houston.

Katz, J. 1968. The SSW test: An interim report. Journal of Speech and Hearing Disorders 33:132–146.

Katz, J. 1977. The Staggered Spondaic Word Test. In: R. Keith (ed.), Central Auditory Dysfunction. Grune & Stratton, New York.

Keith, R. 1980. Central hearing tests. In: N. Lass, L. McReynolds, J. Northern, and D. Yoder (eds.), Speech, Hearing, and Language. W.B. Saunders, Philadelphia.

Keith, R. 1981. Audiological and auditory-language tests of central auditory function. In: R. Keith (ed.), Central Auditory and Language Disorders in Children. College-Hill Press, Houston.

Lindamood, C., and Lindamood, P. 1971. L.A.C. Test. Teaching Resources Corp., Boston.

Lindsay, P., and Norman, D. 1972. Human Information Processing. Academic Press, New York.

Matzker, J. 1959. Two new methods for the assessment of central auditory functions in cases of brain disease. Annals of Otology 68:1185–1197.

Pinheiro, M. 1977. Tests of central auditory function in children with learning disabilities. In: R. Keith (ed.), Central Auditory Dysfunction, Grune & Stratton, New York.

Rees, N. 1981. Saying more than we know: Is auditory processing disorder a meaningful concept? In: R. Keith (ed.), Central Auditory and Language Disorders in Children. College-Hill Press, Houston.

Ross, M., and Lerman, J. 1971. Word Intelligibility by Picture Identification. Stanwix House, Pittsburgh.

Stark, R., and Tallal, P. 1981. Perceptual and motor deficits in language-impaired children. In: R. Keith (ed.), Central Auditory and Language Disorders in Children. College-Hill Press, Houston.

Tallal, P., and Piercy, M. 1974. Developmental aphasia: Rate of auditory processing and selective impairment of consonant perception. Neuropsychologia 12:83–93.

Wepman, J. 1958. Auditory Discrimination Test. Language Research Associates, Chicago.

Wiig, E., and Semel, E. 1976. Language Disabilities in Children and Adolescents, Charles E. Merrill, Columbus, Ohio.

Willeford, J. 1977. Assessing central auditory behavior in children: A test battery approach. In: R. Keith (ed.), Central Auditory Dysfunction. Grune & Stratton, New York.

Witelson, S. 1977. Developmental dyslexia: Two right hemispheres and none left. Science 21:309–311.

Chapter 12

A Multidisciplinary Approach to Central Auditory Evaluations

Noel D. Matkin and *Pamela E. Hook*

Within the last decade, a substantial body of literature on central auditory processing in children has accumulated. Audiologists have utilized as models for their studies with children the approaches used in site-of-lesion work with adults. These concepts have been discussed at some length in previous publications (Jerger, 1960; Bocca & Calearo, 1963). Attention has been directed toward specification both of the acoustic stimuli in CAP testing and the level of the central auditory system that is being assessed by each measure.

On the other hand, language and learning specialists have explored the auditory abilities and language/learning profiles of children by using an information processing approach (Table 1). Their primary focus has been task analysis to identify the level of breakdown in information processing. The relationship between processing at different levels has also been stressed.

In short, the approach and test materials utilized by the two groups of professionals has been quite different. Yet there does seem to be a common assumption underlying CAP testing of children, namely, that certain auditory abilities are prerequisites to auditory comprehension and subsequent language learning during childhood. Unfortunately, evidence is lacking that the auditory abilities traditionally

Table 1.   Auditory processing abilities

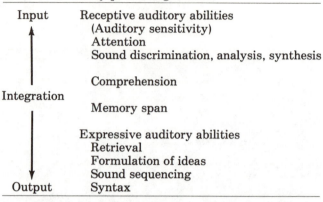

Input	Receptive auditory abilities
	(Auditory sensitivity)
	Attention
	Sound discrimination, analysis, synthesis
	Comprehension
Integration	
	Memory span
	Expressive auditory abilities
	Retrieval
	Formulation of ideas
	Sound sequencing
Output	Syntax

Adapted from Johnson (1977).

tested are prerequisites rather than correlates to the development of, for example, auditory comprehension of language (Rees, 1981). It is hypothesized, however, that such auditory abilities and receptive oral language skills, which begin developing during the early years, serve as the foundation for comprehending oral classroom instructions, for learning to read, and for academic achievement in language-based subjects once the child reaches school age. The language development hierarchy described by Myklebust (1960) is often cited in support of this viewpoint.

Investigations designed to test basic assumptions underlying CAP testing have been limited, and the results are inconclusive (Willeford, 1977). Two major clinical questions which merit careful study include: 1) Are audiologists and language/learning specialists measuring the same or different auditory abilities with their different approaches? 2) Are the scores from CAP testing predictive as to a child's reading abilities and/or general academic achievement? Obviously, these and numerous associated questions merit investigation as an increasing number of children are being referred to audiologists for central auditory testing. It is anticipated that referrals for a CAP evaluation will continue to increase for a number of reasons. First, there is a growing awareness in the professional community that audiologists are involved in the assessment of CAP function of children as well as adults. Second, many graduate training programs in audiology have added classroom instruction and clinical practicum relative to such testing. Further, there seems to be a shift of focus among special educators from visual to auditory processing deficits as the more common basis of academic (e.g., reading) problems among many learning-disabled children (Johnson & Myklebust, 1967; Mattingly, 1972; Vellutino, 1977). According to the present authors, a multidisciplinary research thrust is needed to understand better the influence of auditory disorder on learning. Such research will also clarify the advantages and limitations of the current approach to central audiologic testing of children.

The following discussion is based primarily on clinical experiences from a 3-year period during which the authors worked together in a multidisciplinary setting. A pilot study of approximately 100 school-age children was carried out. This was followed by a systematic clinical evaluation of a selected sample of children by professionals representing the disciplines of audiology, speech/language pathology, learning disabilities, and clinical psychology. By sharing our clinical observations and findings, it is hoped that new insights will be provided into this complex area.

SELECTION OF SUBJECTS

Initially, an open admission policy was maintained in our clinic, with referrals accepted from a variety of sources, including teachers, physicians, psychologists, and parents. After a 2-year period of following such a policy, a retrospective review of clinical records revealed that approximately one out of every four children seen for central auditory testing had been an inappropriate referral for one of several reasons. In this era of accountability of time and money expenditure, it is imperative that only those children who are likely to benefit from such testing be scheduled for assessment.

In our experience there are at least four categories of children who may not be reasonable candidates for CAP testing. First, a surprising number of children with average intelligence and average school performance from achievement-oriented families were referred to determine whether central auditory problems could account for their lack of superior achievement. Second, a substantial number of children with a history of chronic otitis media were referred before adequate medical treatment and resolution of a conductive hearing loss. A history of chronic middle ear problems has been reported as a common finding among children classified as language- and learning-disabled (see Webster, Chapter 10, this volume). Therefore, it was essential to ensure that the child had normal hearing sensitivity bilaterally before using those CAP tests normed on children with normal hearing. Third, a number of children with pervasive developmental delays, including mental abilities falling into the borderline or mild retardation range, were seen. A recent report by Stark and Tallal (1981) indicated that approximately 37% of the children referred from public school language programs to a special clinical project were subsequently found to have IQs on a performance scale below the normal range. A retarded child's scores on various central tests can be misinterpreted if the chronologic rather than the developmental age is considered. Finally, CAP testing by the audiologist may provide little useful information in one subtype of learning-disabled child. Eleven youngsters have been evaluated who had average scores on the verbal section of an intelligence test such as the WISC-R but marked deficits on the performance section. Such youngsters did not manifest any significant difficulty with the measures included in the central audiologic test battery. However, any generalization based on this small sample must be tentative, requiring further study.

On the basis of the preceding observations, it became apparent that admission criteria were needed to minimize the probability of over-referral. It therefore became our routine policy to screen all candidates referred for central auditory tests in the following manner. First, a pure tone audiogram and an impedance study indicating both normal peripheral hearing and middle ear function were required. Second, completion of the Pupil Rating Scale (Myklebust, 1971) by the child's teacher was required. With this instrument, the child's performance is rated on a 5-point scale across five areas of performance, including auditory comprehension, spoken language, orientation, motor coordination, and personal-social behavior. Finally, a school information form was requested before scheduling. This form provided current achievement test scores for the "three Rs" as well as teacher input about the child's strengths and limitations in the areas of cognition, motor development, and general classroom behavior. By utilizing this information, more insightful selection of subjects for central auditory testing was found to be possible.

In an attempt to answer several recurring questions, a systematic clinical investigation was initiated by the authors, one an audiologist and one a language/learning specialist, using a selected sample of children referred to our multidisciplinary center. Specifically, we were interested in determining which of the tests within our two measurement batteries were most sensitive in identifying the presence of auditory processing problems. To differentiate between the two sets of measures, the audiology battery was referred to as the Central Audiologic Test (CAT) Battery, whereas the language/learning specialist's battery was denoted as the Central Auditory Function (CAF) Battery. It should be noted that we tended to add additional measures to the central test battery once there was some evidence that the measures might yield additional information. Unfortunately, tests were not being deleted from the battery at the same rate, so CAP testing became extremely time-consuming and costly.

As stated, it seemed from personal experience and a review of the literature that the fields of audiology and language/learning disabilities had worked in parallel fashion, using different models and measurements to evaluate children at risk for auditory processing deficits. Thus, we wanted to explore the relationship among the tests included in the CAT and CAF batteries. We were interested in whether or not the two fields were duplicating such assessments or were testing related but different auditory processing abilities.

Although it may be beneficial to confirm that a particular youngster does have deficits in auditory processing, such labeling is of limited benefit unless the information can be utilized to modify educational and remedial programs in a meaningful way. Therefore, we also hoped to determine through a multidisciplinary approach whether or not scores on our measures predicted the child's academic difficulties.

All of the subjects included in our clinical study were selected from among those children seen at Boys Town Institute for Communication Disorders in Children, Omaha, Nebraska, for a multidisciplinary team evaluation. They had initially been referred because of concern by the parents and/or school personnel regarding possible learning disabilities. Initially, each child was examined by an ear, nose, and throat specialist and evaluated by an audiologist for hearing deficits. Each child also was screened for uncorrected deficits in vision.

An in-depth psychoeducational evaluation was then completed by a team of specialists. This evaluation included assessment of intellectual functioning, behavior, language, auditory and visual processing, memory, visual-motor coordination, and academic abilities including reading, written expression, spelling, and math. The reading scores for each child were of particular interest, because it appears that failure to learn to read efficiently is most often the basis for labeling a youngster as learning-disabled (Rampp, 1980).

The 29 children included in the study were selected on the basis of the following criteria: 1) normal peripheral hearing sensitivity and middle ear function; 2) corrected vision; 3) age 7–11 years; 4) English as the first and only language; 5) either a Verbal or a Performance intelligence score above 90; 6) no significant emotional problems; 7) no major gross motor deficit; and 8) classification as learning-disabled based on a significant discrepancy between IQ and ability in auditory and language areas, in nonverbal performance, and/or in academic achievement.

The final sample included in the study consisted of a somewhat heterogeneous group of learning-disabled children composed of 23 boys and six girls ranging in age from 7 years, 5 months, to 11 years, 7 months. The mean Verbal IQ for the group was 98 (range of 80–130), the mean Performance IQ was 107 (range of 77–136), and the mean full-scale IQ was 102 (range of 83–138). Although clinical impressions gained from testing a much larger sample of children will be shared, the specific findings from these 29 youngsters serve as the basis for attempting to answer the clinical questions that we had posed.

CENTRAL AUDIOLOGIC TEST BATTERY

Table 2 lists the tests included in the CAT battery. Each test was selected after a careful review of the literature and consideration of clinical findings for approximately 100 children obtained during the pilot study. An attempt was made to include measures purported to tap both brainstem and cortical auditory function while keeping the evaluation time to within 1 hour.

Discrimination of monosyllabic words in a quiet listening environment in the sound field was viewed as important in establishing a base of reference. Because references in the literature have been made to the difficulty that children with auditory processing deficits experience in a competing environment (Katz & Illmer, 1972; Siegenthaler & Barr, 1967), our subjects were tested with PBK-50 word lists in the presence

Table 2. The central audiologic test battery

Discrimination of Monosyllabic Words (50 dB SL)
  Sound Field: Quiet
  Sound Field: Speech Spectrum Noise (S/N ratio: +6 dB)
  Sound Field: Male Discourse (S/N ratio: +6 dB)
Filtered Speech (50 dB SL)
  (LP WIPI)
Binaural Fusion (40 dB SL)
  (Willeford tape)
Competing Sentences (35/50 dB SL)
  (Willeford tape)
Simultaneous Sentences (50/50 dB SL)
  (Willeford tape)
Dichotic Words (50 dB SL)
  Simultaneous
  Right ear lead (90 msec)
  Left ear lead (90 msec)
Masking level differences
  500 Hz
  Speech Reception Threshold

of both speech spectrum noise and a competing male talker at a signal-to-noise ratio of +6 dB. The ability to identify low-pass (500 Hz) monosyllabic words presented in the sound field at +50 dB sensation level (SL); the WIPI test materials and a picture pointing rather than a verbal response were used. Further, three taped tests from the battery developed by Willeford (1976) were utilized under earphones to examine binaural fusion, sentence repetition in the presence of a competing sentence in the nontest ear (Competing Sentences test), and repetition of two sentences presented simultaneously (Simultaneous Sentences test). A dichotic listening task was utilized which incorporated familiar consonant-vowel-consonant (CVC) words all beginning with the consonant /b/ (e.g., bed, ball, book). These taped materials were presented in a simultaneous mode, as well as in right ear lead and left ear lead (90 msec) modes. Again, a picture pointing rather than a verbal response was required. Finally, masking level differences (MLD) for both a 500-Hz pure tone and children's spondaic words were established. In general, the order of administration of these measures was randomized among subjects. Measures were obtained during two test sessions separated by a 15-minute rest period.

All audiologic testing was completed in a custom-designed double wall IAC booth which met American National Standards Institute standards for threshold measurements. A Grason-Stadler diagnostic audiometer (model 1701), a TEAC tape recorder (model 3300), and a custom-designed MLD unit were used to deliver the test stimuli.

CENTRAL AUDITORY FUNCTION BATTERY

With the limitations in testing time, language/learning specialists could not evaluate all abilities listed in Table 1. Through analysis of the data collected during the earlier pilot study, three general areas were considered to be the most promising for detailed analysis: sound processing, conceptual language, and memory. Table 3 lists the names of the specific tests employed. Within each of the three broad areas, several subareas were isolated. The following is a description of each area investigated:

1. Sound processing
    a. Discrimination: The task measured the child's ability to discriminate minimally contrasting pairs of words and required a picture pointing response.
    b. Sound analysis: The task involved isolating beginning, middle, and ending sounds in nonsense words and required a verbal response.

Table 3. The central auditory function battery

Sound processing
  Discrimination
    Goldman-Fristoe-Woodcock Diagnostic Auditory Discrimination Test,
    Part I
    (American Guidance Service, Inc., Circle Pines, Minn.)
  Sound Analysis
    Goldman-Fristoe-Woodcock Sound-Symbol Tests: Sound Analysis
    (American Guidance Service, Inc., Circle Pines, Minn.)
  Sound Blending
    Woodcock-Johnson Psycho-Educational Test Battery, Part I: Test of
    Cognitive Ability: Blending
    (Teaching Resources, Hingham, Mass.)
  Sound Manipulation
    Rosner and Simon Auditory Analysis Test
    (Learning Research and Development Center, University of Pittsburgh,
    Pittsburgh)
    Sound Manipulation Test
    (Pamela E. Hook, Unpublished doctoral dissertation, Northwestern Uni-
    versity, Evanston, Ill.)
  Auditory/Visual Integration
    Lindamood Auditory Conceptualization Test
    (Teaching Resources, Boston)
Conceptual language
  Vocabulary
    Wechsler Intelligence Scale for Children—Revised: Vocabulary
    (The Psychological Corporation, New York)
  Similarities
    Wechsler Intelligence Scale for Children—Revised: Similarities
    (The Psychological Corporation, New York)
  Comprehension
    Wechsler Intelligence Scale for Children—Revised: Comprehension
    (The Psychological Corporation, New York)
  Analogies
    Woodcock-Johnson Psycho-Educational Test Battery, Part I: Test of
    Cognitive Ability
    (Teaching Resources, Hingham, Mass.)
Memory
  Numbers
    Wechsler Intelligence Scale for Children—Revised: Digit Span
    (The Psychological Corporation, New York)
  Sentences
    Woodcock-Johnson Psycho-Educational Test Battery, Part I: Test of
    Cognitive Ability: Memory for Sentences
    (Teaching Resources, Hingham, Mass.)
  Retrieval
    Northwestern Word Latency Test
    (Elsa Telser, Unpublished doctoral dissertation, Northwestern University,
    Evanston, Ill.)

   c. Sound blending: The task involved blending isolated sounds to form real words and required a verbal response.
   d. Sound manipulation: The task measured ability to manipulate sounds in real words through omitting, adding, and/or reordering phonemes and required a verbal response.
   e. Auditory/visual integration: The task required creating a colored block pattern to match a sound pattern using nonsense words.
2. Conceptual language
   a. Vocabulary: The task involved defining orally presented single words and required a verbal response.
   b. Similarities: The task involved abstracting similarities between orally presented words and required a verbal response.
   c. Comprehension: The task measured ability to answer orally presented questions related to reasoning and judgment and required a verbal response.
   d. Analogies: The task involved ability to solve verbal analogies and required a verbal response.
3. Memory
   a. Short-term
       1) Numbers: Two tasks required repetition forward and backward of increasingly larger series of numbers.
       2) Sentences: The task involved repetition of increasingly longer sentences.
   b. Retrieval from long-term memory: The task involved rapid naming of pictures of 50 common objects over three trials.

READING BATTERY

The process of reading is complex; only certain reading abilities could be assessed within the limits of this study. Three areas were considered important for well rounded reading skills: 1) ability to apply phonic word attack skills, 2) ability to read words in isolation, and 3) ability to comprehend what is read. The specific tests were taken from the Woodcock-Johnson Psycho-Educational Test Battery, Part II: Tests of Achievement. A short description of each reading test follows:

  I. Word Attack (phonics): The task involved oral reading of single- and multisyllable nonsense words.
 II. Letter-Word Identification (single word identification): The task measured ability to read orally increasingly difficult real words in isolation.

III.   Passage Comprehension (sentence comprehension): The task involved use of context clues to fill in a word omitted from a
sentence and required a verbal response.

RESULTS

Results concerning which tests within the CAT and CAF batteries
identified the largest number of children in our sample with diagnosed
learning disabilities are found in Tables 4 and 5. Performance on tests
from the CAT battery was classified as pass or fail using available
norms from Willeford or data that had been systematically collected
in our clinics before the research study. On the CAF battery, scores
below the 16th percentile on nationally normed tests were considered
below average; a more arbitrary cutoff based on clinical experience was
used for tests without adequate national norms.

As indicated in Table 4, four of the 10 measures included in the
CAT battery identified more than half of the children in the sample.
These measures include the Simultaneous Sentence test and the Binaural Fusion test (Willeford, 1976), the low-pass Filtered Speech test, and
the Dichotic Words test.

Each of the tests is discussed individually. As would be anticipated, all 29 youngsters scored between 90% and 100% on the task re-

Table 4.   CAT measures rank-ordered by difficulty ($N=29$)

Test	Number of depressed scores
Simultaneous Sentences	22
Binaural Fusion	
Right ear	23
Left ear	20
Filtered Speech (LP WIPI)	20
Dichotic Words	
Simultaneous	19
Right ear lead	18
Left ear lead	16
Discrimination (Sound Field: Male Discourse)	10
Competing Sentences	
Right ear	8
Left ear	8
Discrimination: (Sound Field: Speech Spectrum Noise)	7
MLD	
Speech Reception Threshold	5
500 Hz	4
Discrimination (Sound Field: Quiet)	0

Table 5.   CAF tests rank-ordered by difficulty ($N=29$)

Test	Number of depressed scores
Sound processing	
Sound Manipulation	18
Auditory/Visual Integration	13
Blending	7
Sound Analysis	7
Discrimination	2
Conceptual language	
Analogies	13
Vocabulary	4
Similarities	3
Comprehension	2
Memory	
Sentences	18
Retrieval	13
Numbers	11

quiring discrimination of monosyllabic words from the PBK-50 word lists presented in a quiet listening environment. Auditory recognition of PBK-50 words presented in competition, in noise, or in the presence of a competing talker was not difficult for most children in our sample. Further, release from masking was seen for both a 500-Hz pure tone and spondaic words in most cases, despite an earlier report by Sweetow and Reddell (1977) regarding the sensitivity of these measures with a sample of dyslexic children. Finally, the competing sentence test did not seem to be sensitive in terms of identifying auditory processing problems among 21 of the 29 test subjects.

An analysis of the failure rate on the four most sensitive tests in the CAT battery (Simultaneous Sentences, Binaural Fusion, Filtered Speech, Dichotic Words) revealed that all children would have been identified with these measures. In contrast, only 80% of the children would have been identified with any combination of three of the four tests. Although it is important to limit the amount of clinical testing undertaken, it seems that all four of these tests were needed if the goal was 100% identification of the cases in our sample.

Examination of Table 5 indicates that tests from each area of CAF (sound processing, conceptual language, and memory) presented significant difficulties for a substantial number of the children. However, the two most sensitive tests in the CAF battery were the Sound Manipulation and Sentence Repetition tasks; each accounted for 18 failures of the 29 children studied. The three next most sensitive tests (Auditory/ Visual Integration, Analogies, and Retrieval) each created significant difficulties for 13 children. If the scores on these five most sensitive tests are considered together, however, 28 out of the 29 children would have been identified. The one child who did not have difficulty on any of these five tests was found to have a primarily visual rather than auditory-based learning disability. Importantly, however, no single test from any of the three areas of CAF identified more than two-thirds of the group, and it was necessary to consider a profile of results obtained on tests from each area.

If the goal is identification, it seems that a number of tests could be deleted from both the CAT and CAF batteries, reducing the amount of testing by approximately one-half without reducing the sensitivity of either battery. This statement is valid only for the specific tests and methods of presentation that were used here and only if our sample is representative of the learning disabilities population at large.

Relationships Among Tests

To explore relationships between tests in the CAT and CAF batteries, correlations were computed comparing each test with every other. Correlations for the discrimination tasks were not computed due to missing data. The entire correlation matrix is not included, but results for those tests that correlated at the 0.05 or 0.01 level of significance are found in Table 6. An analysis of the data permits comparison of possible relationships between measures in each battery as well as those between batteries.

Table 6 shows the tests in the CAT battery that correlated significantly with any other test in the CAT battery for this population. The number of significant correlations suggests a common core among the CAT tests. Table 6 also lists a number of significant correlations between tests within and then across the three subdivisions of the CAF battery. Although sound processing and memory were not significantly related to one another, they were both related to conceptual language; Vocabulary, Comprehension, and other factors in the conceptual language category were related to performance in sound processing and memory tasks.

The close relationships that were noted within the test batteries were not found between the CAP and CAF tests. Among the 52 possible comparisons between CAT tests and CAF sound processing tests, there was only one significant correlation. Relating CAT tests to CAF conceptual language tests, only the Analogies test showed any significant correlations; it was related to Binaural Fusion and to Simultane-

Table 6. Correlations among tests in CAT and CAF batteries

Significant correlations among measures of CAT

Simultaneous Sentences	Discrimination (Sound Field: Quiet)	0.409*
Competing Sentences-Left	Binaural Fusion-Right	0.386*
Competing Sentences-Left	Binaural Fusion-Left	0.448*
Simultaneous Sentences	Binaural Fusion-Right	0.563**
Simultaneous Sentences	Competing Sentences-Right	0.449*
Dichotic Words-Simultaneous (Errors)	Competing Sentences-Right	− 0.517**
Dichotic Words-Right (Errors)	Binaural Fusion-Right	− 0.485**
Dichotic Words-Right (Errors)	Competing Sentences-Right	− 0.729**
Dichotic Words-Right (Errors)	Simultaneous Sentences	− 0.449**
Dichotic Words-Right (Errors)	Dichotic Words-Simultaneous (Errors)	0.599**
Dichotic Words-Left (Errors)	Dichotic Words-Simultaneous (Errors)	0.568**
Dichotic Words-Left (Errors)	Dichotic Words-Right (Errors)	0.438*
Tone MLD	Dichotic Words-Left (Errors)	− 0.533**
Speech MLD	Binaural Fusion-Left	0.370*
Speech MLD	Competing Sentences-Left	0.413*
Speech MLD	Tone MLD	0.387*

Significant correlations among measures of CAF

Sound processing

Sound Blending	Sound Analysis	0.462*
Auditory/Visual Integration	Sound Blending	0.368*
Auditory/Visual Integration	Sound Analysis	0.570**
Auditory/Visual Integration	Sound Manipulation	0.398*

Conceptual language

Analogies	Similarities	0.408*
Analogies	Vocabulary	0.748**
Analogies	Comprehension	0.545**
Similarities	Vocabulary	0.508**
Similarities	Comprehension	0.457*
Vocabulary	Comprehension	0.737**

Memory

Sentences	Numbers	0.457*

Across the above three areas

Sound Blending	Vocabulary	0.422*
Auditory/Visual Integration	Similarities	0.367*
Auditory/Visual Integration	Vocabulary	0.476**
Auditory/Visual Integration	Comprehension	0.448**
Sound Analysis	Analogies	0.412*
Sound Analysis	Vocabulary	0.456*

Table 6—*continued*

Sentence Repetition	Analogies	0.637**
Sentence Repetition	Vocabulary	0.553**
Sentence Repetition	Comprehension	0.416*
Number Repetition	Analogies	0.405*
Number Repetition	Similarities	0.488**

Significant correlations between CAT and CAF measures

Sound Analysis	Discrimination (Sound Field: Competing)	−0.430*
Analogies	Binaural Fusion-Right	0.409*
Analogies	Simultaneous Sentences	0.381*
Sentence Repetition	Simultaneous Sentences	0.602**

*$p < 0.05$.
**$p < 0.01$

ous Sentences. Although we see no obvious connection between these procedures, these results suggest that the Analogies task is tapping somewhat different information than the other conceptual language tests. On comparing the CAT tests and CAF memory tasks, Simultaneous Sentences (CAT) and Sentence Repetition (CAF) were found to be significantly correlated. Memory may be an important factor in dealing with Simultaneous Sentences.

On the basis of these relationships, it appears that the audiologist and the language/learning specialist were investigating different functions with relatively little overlap. Overlap within each of the batteries might permit reduction in the CAT or CAF tests. In any case, the relationship between the CAF conceptual language abilities tests and the other CAF tests suggests an underlying relationship on tasks purporting to measure very different abilities.

Relationships between the CAT and CAF Batteries and Reading

Correlations were computed between all tests in the CAT and CAF batteries and the three measures of reading ability: Phonics, Single Word Identification, and Sentence Comprehension. The correlations significant at the 0.05 and 0.01 levels are found in Table 7. Analysis of the results for the CAT battery indicates that the only test that correlated significantly with all three reading areas was the Dichotic Words-Simultaneous task. These findings lend support to the hypothesized link between dichotic listening and reading found in studies reporting differences between good and poor reading groups on dichotic listening tasks (Bryden, 1970; Kimura, 1967; Zurif & Carson, 1970). None of the other tests included on the CAT battery correlated significantly with any of the reading tests. Therefore, the performance on the majority of

Table 7. Significant correlations of measures in
CAT and CAF batteries with measures in reading battery

CAT battery		
Phonics	Dichotic Words-Simultaneous	0.503**
Phonics	Dichotic Words-Left	0.384*
Single Word Identification	Dichotic Words-Simultaneous	0.478**
Sentence Comprehension	Dichotic Words-Simultaneous	0.386*
CAF battery		
Phonics	Sound Blending	0.442*
Phonics	Sound Manipulation	0.437*
Single Word Identification	Sound Manipulation	0.506**
Single Word Identification	Vocabulary	0.407*
Single Word Identification	Sentence Repetition	0.405*
Sentence Comprehension	Analogies	0.457*
Sentence Comprehension	Similarities	0.369*
Sentence Comprehension	Vocabulary	0.425*
Sentence Comprehension	Sentence Repetition	0.640**

*$p < 0.05$.
**$p < 0.01$.

the CAT tasks used in this study did not relate directly to achievement in reading.

Results of the comparison of the CAF battery with reading are reported separately for each area of reading. Relative to the ability to apply phonics (Table 7), two sound processing tests, Sound Blending and Sound Manipulation, were significantly correlated. Findings for the Sound Manipulation task are consistent with results reported earlier by Hook and Johnson (1978) indicating a high (0.87) correlation between the ability to manipulate sounds in words and apply phonic word attack skills to reading. None of the tests on the conceptual language or memory sections were significantly related to the ability to apply phonics in reading. The more mechanical aspects of reading correlated more highly with the auditory abilities involved in sound processing (see Katz, Chapter 14, this volume) than with language or memory abilities as measured here.

One test from each of the three areas on the CAF battery was found to be significantly correlated with single word identification. They were: Sound Manipulation, Vocabulary, and Sentences. Factors involving vocabulary knowledge, the ability to sequence sounds in words, and memory for linguistic information seem to be related to being able to identify single words in reading.

In the area of sentence comprehension, our results indicate three conceptual language tasks (Vocabulary, Similarities, and Analogies) that are significantly correlated with the ability to use context cues to fill in missing words in sentences. The Sentences test from the memory section also is significantly correlated with this particular reading skill. In contrast, no tests from the sound processing area were related significantly to comprehension of sentence-length materials. Thus, it seems that the auditory abilities involved in reading comprehension relate more to conceptual language skills and memory for linguistic information than skills in processing sounds.

These findings indicate a logical pattern of relationship between the different sections of the CAF battery and the different areas of reading assessed. The mechanics of reading, or the ability to read non-sense words where no meaning cues are available, are more related to sound processing abilities, whereas comprehension of sentences seems more related to conceptual language abilities. Single word reading, where no language context is available, is related to skills in both sound processing and conceptual language, specifically vocabulary knowledge. In addition, memory for linguistic material is related to both of the reading tasks which involve meaningful language.

Adequate Readers Compared to Poor Readers

Because the population chosen for this study was a heterogeneous group of learning-disabled children, it was decided that further information could be gained by dividing the children into two groups, those with all three reading scores falling above the 16th percentile (adequate readers) and those with two or more reading scores falling below the 16th percentile (poor readers). Nine children were included in the adequate readers (AR) group, and 16 children were included in the poor readers (PR) group. The scores for four youngsters were deleted because they did not fit either category (e.g., only two scores rather than all three fell above the cutoff percentile). A series of t-tests was then used to compare these groups on the variables contained in the CAT, CAF, and reading batteries as well as age and IQ. Because of the number of variables involved, only the results significant at the 0.05 and 0.01 levels are listed in Table 8.

As expected, results indicated that the AR and PR groups differed significantly in all three areas of reading. Mean scores for the three tests of reading in the AR group ranged from the 42nd to the 47th percentile, whereas those for the PR group ranged from the 11th to the 14th percentile. The two groups did not differ either in chronologic age (mean age was 8.8 years for the PR group and 9.2 years for the AR group) or Verbal IQ (mean Verbal IQ score was 96.5 for the PR group and 97.2 for the AR group). As seen in Table 8, however, scores on Performance IQ were significantly different between the groups (mean

Table 8.   Comparison of performance of AR and PR on CAT and CAF
batteries, reading battery, and intelligence test (significant differences only)

Measure	AR (mean)	PR (mean)	p value
Performance IQ	112.56	100.88	0.016
Reading			
Phonics	47.00	13.56	0.014
Single Word Identification	44.33	11.38	0.011
Sentence Comprehension	42.78	14.31	0.010
CAT battery			
Dichotic Words-Simultaneous	4.33	2.19	0.034
CAF battery			
Sound Manipulation	2.56	1.93	0.046
Retrieval	2.78	6.13	0.050

Performance IQ was 100.9 for the PR group and 112.5 for the AR
group). Among tests in the CAT battery, only the Dichotic Words-
Simultaneous subtest showed significant differences between the two
groups.

On the CAF battery, mean scores for the two groups on the conceptual language tasks were not significantly different, a finding consistent with the lack of difference in verbal intelligence scores. On the
sound processing section, only one test, Sound Manipulation, showed
statistically significant differences between the AR and PR groups.
Finally, on the memory section, retrieval scores were significantly different between the groups.

It is somewhat surprising that many of the scores were not significantly different. This could relate to the small sample size and the fact
that all of the children had learning disabilities. The similarity in verbal
intelligence scores between the poor and adequate readers with a significant difference in performance nonverbal intelligence scores is interesting. A possible explanation is that children with otherwise similar
auditory processing abilities may be better able to compensate for any
auditory disorders if they have strengths in the nonverbal performance
areas in conjunction with better dichotic listening, sound manipulation, and retrieval skills. These strengths found in the AR group may
have aided them in developing reading skills more appropriate to their
intellectual level.

DISCUSSION AND CONCLUSIONS

Any conclusions based on the data from our study must be considered
as tentative because of the limited number of subjects. However, our
findings highlight several important points that should be considered

both in future research projects and in the clinical application of central auditory tests with learning-disabled populations.

First, on the question of the most sensitive measures in the CAT and CAF test batteries, it is important that in the CAT battery, the three (of our eight) tests that were difficult for the largest number of learning-disabled children (Simultaneous Sentences, Binaural Fusion, and Filtered Word tests) did not correlate significantly with more than one or two of the tests on either the CAT or CAF batteries. Nor, most importantly, did they correlate with any of the tests of reading. Neither the exact meaning of depressed performance on these particular audiologic tests nor the exact nature of what these tests are measuring is clear at the present time. Thus, extreme caution should be used in interpreting the results from these tests. Further, the lack of relationship leads to significant questions concerning the appropriateness of specific remediation based on identified auditory processing deficits that are not shown to correspond to educational deficits. Certainly remedial training focused upon these tests does not seem warranted at the present time.

Second, the results concerning the relationship between the tests included in the CAT battery and those in the CAF battery indicated very few significant correlations. Although our sample of learning-disabled children had difficulty on many of the tests within each test battery, there does not seem to be a direct relationship between the measures included in the CAT and CAF batteries. It appears, therefore, that in our roles as audiologist and language/learning specialist we were *not* assessing the same auditory processing skills.

Third, concerning the relationship of the findings from the CAT and CAF batteries to reading scores, only a small number of the tests on each battery correlated significantly with the three areas of reading assessed here. In addition, when our sample was divided into two groups (AR and PR), significant differences between the groups on the auditory tests were found on only three tasks (Dichotic Words-Simultaneous, Sound Manipulation, and Retrieval). In fact, nonverbal intelligence appeared to play a greater role in differentiating the AR group from the PR group among the learning-disabled children than did any of the auditory tests. Caution, therefore, must be used in interpreting results from auditory test batteries when discussing relationships to reading. Generally, it appears that the auditory skills required for efficient reading are related to different auditory processing abilities than are tapped by a number of the measures in either test battery. Not only is CAP quite complex, but so are the processes involved in reading. The relationship between auditory processing skills and reading abilities needs to be explored more fully in carefully designed multidisciplinary efforts. The role of nonverbal intelligence in compensating for reading problems also merits further exploration. More in-depth understanding of these relationships must be gained to provide useful remedial programs.

It is obvious that more questions were generated than answered by our clinical project. A similar multidisciplinary thrust needs to be undertaken with a large but carefully described sample of children at risk for CAP dysfunction before definitive generic statements can be made. Ideally, the performance of a contrast sample of normal subjects, matched for age, intelligence, and socioeconomic level, should be assessed. With the labels of learning disability and CAP disorder used to categorize a very heterogeneous population of children, the importance of considering measures of intelligence, language, and academic achievement, as well as auditory processing, becomes apparent. Various specialists testing children and interpreting the results in isolation may lead to further confusion rather than clarification of the issues. The basic assumption underlying the administration of either the CAT or the CAF battery is that problems in auditory processing may contribute to or result in deficits in receptive language development and/or in limited academic achievement. It is therefore imperative that recommendations for educational and remedial management be made only after integrating the findings from audiology, language pathology, learning disabilities, education, and psychology. Otherwise, each specialist may be viewing only one facet of the disability, and, as a consequence, recommendations may result in a fragmented rather than a unified approach.

REFERENCES

Bocca, E., and Calearo, C. 1963. Central hearing processes. In: J. Jerger (ed.), Modern Developments in Audiology. Academic Press, New York.

Bryden, M. P. 1970. Laterality effects in dichotic listening: Relations with handedness and reading ability in children. Neuropsychologia 8:443–450.

Hammill, D. D., and Larsen, S. C. 1974. The effectiveness of psycholinguistic training. Exceptional Children 40:5–14.

Hook, P. E., and Johnson, D. J. 1978. Metalinguistic awareness and reading strategies. Bulletin of the Orton Society 28:62–78.

Jerger, J. 1960. Audiological manifestations of lesions in the auditory nervous system. Laryngoscope 70:417–425.

Johnson, D. 1977. Psycho-educational evaluation of children with learning disabilities: Study of auditory processes. In: G. Millichap (ed.), Learning Disabilities and Related Disorders. Year Book, Chicago.

Johnson, D. J., and Myklebust, H. R. 1967. Learning Disabilities: Educational Principles and Practices. Grune & Stratton, New York.

Katz, J., and Illmer, R. 1972. Auditory perception in children with learning disabilities. In: J. Katz (ed.), Handbook of Clinical Audiology. Williams & Wilkins, Baltimore.

Kimura, D. 1967. Functional asymmetry of the brain in dichotic listening. Cortex 3:163–178.

Mattingly, I. G. 1972. Reading, the linguistic process, and linguistic awareness. In: J. F. Kavanagh and I. G. Mattingly (eds.), Language by Ear and by Eye. MIT Press, Cambridge, Mass.

Myklebust, H. 1960. Psychology of Deafness. Grune & Stratton, New York.

Myklebust, H. R. 1971. The Pupil Rating Scale: Screening for Hearing Disabilities. Grune & Stratton, New York.

Rampp, D. W. 1980. Auditory Processing and Learning Disabilities. Cliff Notes, Lincoln, Nebr.

Rees, N. S. 1981. Saying more than we know: Is auditory processing disorder a meaningful concept? In: R. W. Keith (ed.), Central Auditory and Language Disorders in Children. College-Hill Press, Houston.

Siegenthaler, B., and Barr, C. 1967. Auditory figure-ground perception in normal children. Child Development 38:1163–1167.

Stark, R. E., and Tallal, P. 1981. Selection of children with specific language deficits. Journal of Speech and Language Disorders 46:114–122.

Sweetow, R. W., and Redell, R. C. 1977. Masking Level Differences for Children with Auditory Perceptual Problems. San Francisco Hearing and Speech Center, San Francisco.

Vellutino, F. 1977. Alternative conceptualizations of dyslexia: Evidence in support of a verbal-deficit hypothesis. Harvard Education Review 47:334–354.

Willeford, J. A. 1976. Central auditory function in children with learning disabilities. Audiology and Hearing Education 2:12–20.

Willeford, J. 1977. Assessing central auditory behavior in children: A test battery approach. In: R. W. Keith (ed.), Central Auditory Dysfunction. Grune & Stratton, New York.

Zurif, E. B., and Carson, G. 1970. Dyslexia in relation to cerebral dominance and temporal analysis. Neuropsychologia 8:351–360.

Chapter 13

Auditory Processing and Language Interaction

Evaluation and Intervention Strategies

Elaine Z. Lasky and *L. Clarke Cox*

Children with central auditory processing problems often have difficulties in comprehending, integrating, and remembering auditory information. They may have problems selecting and attending to auditory signals in the presence of distractions (Cohen & Schiller, 1981; Gerber, 1981; Willeford & Billger, 1978). These difficulties and the subsequent frustrations are most often observed when the child must process language in a teaching-learning environment. They seem to increase as the language becomes more complex and less familiar and as the task becomes more challenging.

Chapter 2 of this volume proposed a framework to analyze children's processing of auditory information. This framework considered the *s*ignal and its *p*resentation, the *e*nvironment, the *r*esponse required, and the *s*trategies the child uses (SPERS). In this chapter we discuss: 1) case history information useful in planning individualized programs, 2) intervention procedures derived from SPERS, and 3) the necessity of measuring and documenting the results of any procedure. No attempt is made to separate auditory from linguistic or cognitive processing, because perception, comprehension, learning, and memory are intimately related (Bransford et al., 1977; Jacoby & Craik, 1979). Our goal is to specify a protocol to help the child with CAP disorder use auditory information.

The main concern is processing information in a teaching-learning environment. Many children with CAP problems approach a listening-learning task confused or unaware of how to proceed. They do not seem to know how to listen, learn, or judge what they know. We can help them comprehend the language signal and improve their performance in clinic and classroom. Audiologists, speech-language pathologists, and other professionals need to recommend specific procedures to facilitate comprehension.

EVALUATION PROCEDURES

Leads from the Case History

Evaluation of a CAP disorder should define specific problem areas and direct intervention. Often a child is referred because of behavioral patterns such as difficulties in following directions, attending, comprehending, remembering vocabulary, sequencing phonemes or syllables, or relating sequential events (Costello, 1977). We need data describing the conditions under which the child succeeds and demonstrates learning, and when he or she begins having difficulty and what the difficulties are. A patient's description of how he or she feels and behaves, together with clinicians' observations, may be more valuable than any diagnostic instrument (Duane, 1977). Our questions and recording techniques, then, must be precise and explicit.

Conditions under Which the Child Comprehends and Learns Families, teachers, and specialists are probably aware of what works with the child—that is, which tasks the child can attend to, follow, remember, and comprehend. Ask them questions such as: What does the child listen to on television, radio, stereo? What does the child relate about a narrative after watching or listening to a television story, a movie, a story read out loud, or a sports event? Is the response more correct or complete at any time or for any activity? Are any events remembered and reported about school, interests, friends, or family? Are one- or two-line jokes understood? Is there laughter at the appropriate time? How is a joke retold? Does the child understand one individual better than others? Depending on age, we can determine the child's awareness or acceptance of the problem, and the child may serve as informant to these questions. To plan efficient intervention, begin with conditions in which the child has demonstrated attending, comprehension, or learning.

When Does the Child Seem to Have Difficulties? Parents and teachers are often keenly aware of the child's poor performance or problem behavior, such as hyperactivity, distractibility, or memory problems. Probe for changes in the problem with changes in topic, manner of presentation, environment, and task expectancies. What happens when the task becomes difficult? Does the child attempt to figure out meaning? stop attending? ask another student? What behaviors indicate frustration, confusion, or fatigue? Does the child realize when he or she isn't understanding a message or story? What does the child do when a response is correct? incorrect? when the child offers no response? Do problems decrease or increase with louder or softer speech? when several persons are talking? when visual stimuli are added?

These questions provide directions for the clinician to pursue. All data obtained should be recorded with other history and results of formal testing.

Selection and Interpretation of Evaluation Instruments

Pure tone and speech discrimination tests are always administered to verify integrity of the peripheral mechanism. However, persons with central nervous system lesions often show normal results. One approach to CAP assessment uses tests which purport to measure discrete auditory skills (e.g., discrimination, sequencing) by isolating components of the signal. At this time, however, we do not know whether discrete components operate or can be measured in isolation. These functions may not be separable or discrete but may overlap and operate in parallel rather than in series. We do not know the relationship between performance on these tests and processing of language. We urge caution in interpreting these tests.

Some tests to evaulate CAP distort, degrade, or use competition with the signal to make it less redundant and more difficult to process. Normal subjects show few problems, whereas those with disorders should show more difficulty and poorer scores. These tests were designed to assess problems related to space-occupying lesions, degenerative diseases, and vascular disorders (Bocca et al., 1955; Katz, 1962; Matzker, 1959; Smith & Resnick, 1972). They have been recently adapted to assess CAP in children (Willeford, 1977). One concern with these tests is that data obtained from normal children and those with CAP disorders are limited. Variables, including characteristics of the test and maturation level, should also be considered (Noffsinger & Kurdziel, 1979).

Electrophysiologic procedures are becoming more refined, and data reflecting structural integrity are increasing, particularly where auditory brainstem responses (ABR) are concerned (O'Donovan, Beagley, & Shaw, 1980; Jerger, Hayes, & Jordan, 1980; Cox, Hack, & Metz, 1981). These data may be used to corroborate results of other CAP tests and behavioral observations. Studies are beginning to document electrophysiologic responses from midbrain and cortical levels with tasks requiring higher levels of processing; clinical procedures, however, are not yet available.

Audiologists and other specialists recognize that no single test at any level can be used to determine disorder. Results of several procedures should be obtained and then compared to results following treatment.

Formal and Informal Testing Procedures for SPERS SPERS evaluation utilizes increasingly difficult signals, presentation, listening environment, and response requirements to analyze the strategies a child employs in listening and processing auditory information. Levels of difficulty in the teaching-learning classroom are simulated to determine factors that disrupt or enhance performance. The procedures presented here are examples which can be adapted to the age and functioning of any child. Records should be maintained of performance and any effects of altering parameters.

Altering the Language Signal and Presentation to Affect the Child Language processing is analyzed as signal complexity and presentation are altered. Factors varied include complexity of the phonologic, pragmatic, syntactic, and semantic segments; rate of presentation; redundancy; and availability of contextual cues. To evaluate processing of suprasegmental features, check the following: Does the child use stress patterns to interpret sentences? Present a sentence, then ask what it means. Alter the stress pattern and attempt to elicit a change in interpretation (e.g., *Neil* wanted a salad. Neil wanted a *salad*. *Neil?* [pause] *wanted* a salad?). Use different sentences with different stress patterns. Ask the child to paraphrase meaning or to role-play the event. Use obvious sarcasm (e.g., "Eric really wants to clean his room."). Is it comprehended? Does the child smile or laugh appropriately at one-, two-, or three-line jokes? Does the child retell a joke? Record stimuli and responses. A suggested format for recording data is shown in Figure 1.

Effects of syntactic complexity are evaluated by systematically increasing the complexity, with addition of adjectives, adverbs, embedded and conjoined sentences, and the like. Check logical conjunctions (and, or, nor, while, until, except, although, if . . . then, before, and after) which modify semantic meaning and increase syntactic complexity by conjoining clauses. Include constructions using deletions such as anaphora ("Pam went, too" ["to the zoo" is deleted]) and ellipses ("Where is Matthew?" [Matthew is] at school). Comprehension should be explicitly verified, such as by asking the child to paraphrase or follow with a logical next sentence. Does the complexity affect comprehension?

Semantic complexity increases for students throughout their

school years. Semantic concepts used for instruction in kindergarten and the first two grades are tested by the Boehm Test of Basic Concepts (BTBC; Boehm, 1971). This test is administered to classes or adapted for individual use. There is no similar standard set of required concepts for preschool or postprimary programs to use for evaluation, as curriculum at these levels varies from school system to school system. The speech-language pathologist, audiologist, or other specialist can, however, examine books and curricular material for listings of new words or concepts at the end of chapters, units, or texts. Comprehension of the concepts can be tested by asking the child to paraphrase or to explain concepts from current and earlier class material. Both the percent correct and concepts missed at each level should be listed.

Syntactic and semantic complexity interact to increase sentence difficulty and processing required. Standardized evaluation procedures in speech pathology and audiology frequently use simpler levels of syntax than are used in casual conversation or in classroom instruction. Semantic levels are also generally less demanding. If more difficult concepts are assessed, syntax is often shortened and simplified. To get a more complete picture of the child's processing of auditory information, stimuli should at times reflect classroom levels of semantic and syntactic complexity. For example, a typical question from a third-grade teachers' edition is, "Why do you think solar batteries are used instead of other batteries for such satellites?" (Blecha, Gega, & Green, 1979, p. 176). How does the child with CAP problems function when syntactic and semantic loads are increased?

To facilitate comprehension and remembering of auditory information, the presentation can incorporate techniques of slowing the rate, repeating a word or phrase, and/or using pictured or verbalized cues (Lasky, Chapter 2, this volume). Evaluate any changes in performance when repetition is used or when the rate is slowed by inserting pauses between phrases. Note the effects of adding contextual cues. The remediation section discusses these techniques in detail.

Evaluation procedures recommended in this section include:

1. Present sentences using different intonation. Can the child explain meanings and changes in meanings? Include sarcasm and joking.
2. Check comprehension of concepts of vocabulary words from classroom materials.
3. Check comprehension of these concepts in complex sentences (i.e., embedded sentences and sentences with logical conjunctions).
4. Note how performance is affected by slowing the rate.
5. Note how performance is affected by using redundancy.
6. Note how performance is affected by providing contextual cues.
7. Record results on a form as in Figure 1.

Figure 1. Suggested form for recording evaluative data.

Name	Birthdate	Grade Level	Dates of testing

Referred by _____ Complaint: _____

From case history: Conditions leading to success _____
Conditions leading to problems _____

Subject's remarks _____

Results of CAP procedures: Date _____ Remarks _____
Date _____ Remarks _____

Phonology (particularly suprasegmental features)

Level of task	Quiet	Competing message (1–2 talkers)	Slow rate (120 wpm)	Normal rate (150 wpm)	Immediate response	Delayed response (wait 5 sec)
I	S: ___ R: ___	S: ___ R: ___	S: ___ R: ___	S: ___ R: ___	S: ___ R: ___	S: ___ R: ___
II	S: ___ R: ___	S: ___ R: ___	S: ___ R: ___	S: ___ R: ___	S: ___ R: ___	S: ___ R: ___
III	S: ___ R: ___	S: ___ R: ___	S: ___ R: ___	S: ___ R: ___	S: ___ R: ___	S: ___ R: ___

IV S:_____ S:_____ S:_____ S:_____ S:_____
   R:_____ R:_____ R:_____ R:_____ R:_____

Pragmatics

I S:_____ S:_____ S:_____ S:_____ S:_____
   R:_____ R:_____ R:_____ R:_____ R:_____

II S:_____ S:_____ S:_____ S:_____ S:_____
   R:_____ R:_____ R:_____ R:_____ R:_____

III S:_____ S:_____ S:_____ S:_____ S:_____
    R:_____ R:_____ R:_____ R:_____ R:_____

IV S:_____ S:_____ S:_____ S:_____ S:_____
   R:_____ R:_____ R:_____ R:_____ R:_____

continued

Figure 1—*continued*

Syntax

Level of task	Quiet	Competing message (1–2 talkers)	Slow rate (120 wpm)	Normal rate (150 wpm)	Immediate response	Delayed response (wait 5 sec)
I	S: _____ R: _____	S: _____ R: _____	S: _____ R: _____	S: _____ R: _____	S: _____ R: _____	S: _____ R: _____
II	S: _____ R: _____	S: _____ R: _____	S: _____ R: _____	S: _____ R: _____	S: _____ R: _____	S: _____ R: _____
III	S: _____ R: _____	S: _____ R: _____	S: _____ R: _____	S: _____ R: _____	S: _____ R: _____	S: _____ R: _____
IV	S: _____ R: _____	S: _____ R: _____	S: _____ R: _____	S: _____ R: _____	S: _____ R: _____	S: _____ R: _____

Semantics

I   S: _____   S: _____   S: _____   S: _____   S: _____   S: _____
    R: _____   R: _____   R: _____   R: _____   R: _____   R: _____

II   S: _____   S: _____   S: _____   S: _____   S: _____   S: _____
    R: _____   R: _____   R: _____   R: _____   R: _____   R: _____

III   S: _____   S: _____   S: _____   S: _____   S: _____   S: _____
    R: _____   R: _____   R: _____   R: _____   R: _____   R: _____

IV   S: _____   S: _____   S: _____   S: _____   S: _____   S: _____
    R: _____   R: _____   R: _____   R: _____   R: _____   R: _____

Key: Describe stimulus (S) presented and response (R) obtained at increasing levels of difficulty (I–IV) and under varying presentation modes for each facet of the language signal.

The Environment Affects the Child's Performance   Performance may be affected by variables that operate differently in a classroom than in a one-to-one evaluation. For example: 1) competing auditory stimuli of one to three persons speaking simultaneously may disrupt the child's attention to relevant stimuli; 2) generally, a child in the classroom must wait to be called on, thus requiring a delayed response and use of memory; 3) the presence of other students in the classroom may create a more fearful social environment; 4) a speaker alters rate, intonation, redundancy, and other variables differently in a group than with one listener.

These effects may be evaluated in several ways. Administer materials suggested in the previous section and compare performance in quiet and with one, two, or three children as competing talkers. The competition can be from a few other children speaking or simulated through tape recordings placed at different locations. The quality of an immediate response can be compared to a response following a delay. A pause of 5–10 sec probably simulates the classroom and represents a sufficient delay.

Record changes in test performance and verbal and nonverbal behaviors in individual, small group, or classroom settings. Insights regarding reactions to anticipated peer group pressures and from changes in speaker interaction may emerge. The specialist can observe and test in the clinic and classroom. The teacher can also provide observations. Comparing these data may portray different problems and different operating styles and permit more effective intervention. We may see that progress observed in the clinic is not seen in the classroom, *not* because the child does not exert the effort but because the auditory processing demands are greater in the classroom.

The following are thus recommended:

1. Present stimuli in the quiet and then with one to three competing talkers. Observe behavior and performance. Ask the child about working while hearing the other talkers.
2. Compare immediate responses to responses delayed by 5–10 sec with questions that increase in semantic and syntactic difficulty and require more difficult responses.
3. Record changes in performance in different settings.

Difficulty of the Required Response Changes the Child's Performance   Many testing procedures utilized by audiologists and speech-language pathologists require the subject to repeat a stimulus—to imitate a word, phrase, or sentence or a degraded word, phrase, or sentence. Other procedures require a child to point to a picture to demonstrate comprehension. A child with CAP problems can often function adequately on these tasks.

What types of responses are required of a child outside of the clinic? A typical 4-year-old may hear, "Oh, Rachel! Daddy's just pulled into the driveway to take us to Grandma's and Christina's just spilled her milk. Hurry! run upstairs and get me clean overalls." Rachel's task is not to imitate this utterance or point to a picture. She must process complex syntax, remember semantic information, and heed the pragmatic intentions. Social interchange and questions and instructions from school are generally higher-level tasks than imitation or recognition (picking) of one of a set of pictures. Approximately 57% of questions asked by classroom teachers are recall questions; 30% require conjecture, explanation, or evaluation; whereas fewer than 14% are recognition questions (Guszak, 1967). A fourth-grader must synthesize information to answer a question such as: "What things are necessary for the development of a manufacturing region?" (Ahlshwede, 1977, p. 238). A specialist cannot depend exclusively on repetition or recognition tasks if the purpose is to evaluate a child's usual CAP and relate it to school. Begin the assessment with material of interest to the child and/or from the curriculum. Ask the child to use information presented to give a reason or explanation. Sample questions from the teacher or worksheets, textbooks, or achievement tests not currently used by the child's school can be used which demand comprehension, integration, and formulation of a response. Note effects when the level of response is changed.

Asking the child to explain a concept without contextual cues is a relatively easy way to assess comprehension. It is also a higher-level task than picture pointing. If the child has difficulty, make the task easier by providing cues or requiring recall, cued recall, or even recognition-level responses. For a recall paradigm, a definition is given and the child supplies a word as a fill-in response. Cued recall adds a cue to help retrieval. Recognition requires selection of one of from two to five alternatives. Is performance different if the response task is easier? Is comprehension shown at higher levels or just at a recognition level? Can the concept be applied in learning?

Assessment procedures in this section propose evaluating with tasks of varying difficulty. The following are suggested: 1) require the child to demonstrate comprehension by defining, explaining, making an inference, or adding a logical follow-up; 2) if that is too difficult, ask the child to recall a word you define; 3) if that is still too hard, use a cue to help (cued recall); 4) an easier task requires recognizing one of from three to five choices; 5) easier yet is discrimination of one of two alternatives or imitation of the stimulus; 6) record the type of task presented with the complexity of syntax and semantics. Indicate percent correct, items missed, types of errors, and changes in behavior.

Are Strategies Used to Listen, Understand, and Remember the Signal? When children enter school, they must acquire a set of operating procedures different from those they used at home. They must learn what to listen to and how to listen (Cook-Gumperz, 1975). They must learn to attend to what the teacher says, remember it, and learn how to ask and answer questions (Norman & Bobrow, 1977). They must learn to recognize what they know and do not know, what was said and what was meant (Bransford & Nitsch, 1978).

Most children develop these skills and various learning strategies spontaneously, as they need to learn and retain information, from about second to third grade on to ages 11 or 12 (Brown, 1977; Brown, 1979; Naus & Halasz, 1979). They learn to evaluate the demands of a task and use knowledge of narrative structure to comprehend and organize information (Brown, 1979). They learn to identify essential features, crucial elements, and central themes (Dent & Thorndyke, 1979; Hagen & Stanovich, 1977). They develop knowledge about memory (metamemory) which helps them determine whether and what strategies will be used (Brown & DeLoache, 1978; Flavell & Wellman, 1977).

Some children, even with increasing age, experience, and normal cognitive abilities, do not acquire these skills; they may not listen to and pick out relevant information or comprehend its organization and content. Listening problems may relate to failure to evaluate a task, select an appropriate plan, and use and modify a strategy (Brown, 1979; Naus & Halasz, 1979). Gerber (1981) suggested that learning-disabled children often do not recognize a need to develop learning strategies since they tend to regard what happens to them as unrelated to their own behavior and not within their control.

Children with CAP problems may need help in developing strategies for listening and knowing what they do or do not comprehend. We need to identify strategies a child uses and recommend strategies to aid listening, attending, comprehending, and remembering. This is discussed more fully under "Approaches to Remediation."

Interpreting Results of Testing Procedures One purpose of evaluation is to compare a child to others of the same chronologic age and/or grade level. Normative data exist for standardized CAP tests, but many CAP tests are informal or in process of development. There is not yet a reliable, valid, graded sequence to assess CAP difficulties.

A second purpose of evaluation is to develop an intervention program. Children with language or reading disorders, however, are not homogeneous subgroups but may represent different neurologic organizations not assigned to one diagnostic category and matched with one educational program (Galin, 1979). We need to look at facets of the processing that affect performance (Galin, 1979). Error analyses show positive or negative effects of altering the signal, its presentation, environment, or response task. Strategies used are documented. From these data a remediation program can be outlined.

APPROACHES TO REMEDIATION

Traditional Approaches to CAP Remediation

Traditional remediation has identified problems and provided training in skills such as discrimination, memory, attention, analysis/synthesis, localization, sequencing, and auditory-visual integration (Barr, 1976; Gerber & Mencher, 1980; Rampp, 1980; Wood, 1975). This assumes that CAP involves separate skills that must be isolated and remediated to improve or correct CAP disorders (Rampp, 1980). Books and commercial programs are available which describe techniques for training specific skills. The most frequently defined skills include the following:

Discrimination or differentiating between sounds; that is, are two stimuli the same or different? (Barr, 1976; Rampp, 1980). Remediation involves practice in discriminating nonlinguistic, linguistic, similar, dissimilar, meaningful, and nonmeaningful stimuli (Lindamood & Lindamood, 1969; Reagan, 1973; Willette, Jackson, & Peckins, 1970).

Memory and auditory sequencing activities involve remembering auditory images and sequential order of numbers, tonal and/or rhythmic patterns, environmental sounds, and components of speech such as phonemes, words, and phrases (Reagan, 1973).

Attention and figure-ground separation is directed toward the distractible child, with training in selecting and attending to the signal while disregarding irrelevant stimuli (Rampp, 1980).

Auditory analysis requires separating components of speech, that is, separating words into syllables or phonemes (Rosner, 1975).

Auditory synthesis or sound blending requires the opposite of auditory analysis, blending speech components into units, phonemes into syllables, syllables into words.

Localization requires determining the direction of a sound source and requires the participation of both ears (Gerber, 1974).

Auditory imagery or *auditory visual integration* provides practice in associating a sound with a graphic representation, and oral productions with printed symbols.

CAP components may exist but may not be discrete skills or operate in isolated, sequential fashion (Sanders, 1977). These processes may not be separable but interrelated and occur concomitantly, with completion of one process contingent upon another (Williamson & Alexander, 1975). Willeford and Billger (1978) reported little improvement with skills training and recommended a global approach to reduce emphasis on training the child and increase emphasis on modifying the environment. They listed the following guidelines: reduce extraneous auditory and visual stimuli during key instruction, present instructions in simple constructions with frequent repetitions, reduce the number of required written responses, gradually add academic material with constant review of previous information, control for classroom seating, and use sound-attenuating earmuffs or plugs and FM auditory training units. Other global approaches modify speech signals by increasing redundancy, using short, simple sentences and title headings before elaborating (Stark & Tallal, 1980). Although few programs document progress, McCroskey and Thompson (1973) and Peck (1977) reported improved performance among learning-disabled children when rate of speech is slowed. Because there are only limited data from studies showing improvement in CAP, language, or academic achievement after training in specific auditory skills, we urge caution in using these programs. Record progress and carefully evaluate effects on CAP, language, or academic performance.

Auditory SPERS Remediation

On the basis of the research discussed in Chapter 2, SPERS manipulates the signal, presentation, environment, and response levels, and teaches strategies to enhance listening and learning. Goals are to enable the child more effectively to select, comprehend, respond to, and remember auditory information. Organized and ongoing reports of progress from consultants, teachers, clinicians, and parents are critical and are obtained via circulation of short reports, questionnaires, meetings, or frequent telephone calls.

Altering the Signal to Aid CAP   Concepts a child knows and those he or she does not comprehend but needs are identified. Selected concepts are taught and used at home, school, or playground. Concepts are presented slowly at first, in simple constructions with contextual cues. Rate of speaking is slowed by inserting pauses between phrases for more time for processing—that is, between noun phrase and verb phrase, between verb and noun phrase, or in the verb phrase.

Contextual cues may be examples, key words, a main idea, pictures, graphs, diagrams, or an outline. When presenting new topics, list what will be talked about, talk about it, and summarize it. Use context to provide structure, order, and cohesiveness to the material (Moates & Schumacher, 1980). Instructions provide context by helping the listener focus on specific points.

Discussing how one comes to understand things not previously understood, or how one understands things in new ways, Bransford and Nitsch (1978) argued that examples relating new information to what is known improve comprehension. Listeners may hear what a speaker said, but one or more examples help them to understand it. Examples used should be dramatic (Gagné & White, 1978) and relevant to the listener's interests and experiences (Chapandy & Lasky, 1980). Personal examples (even if they are fanciful) are more meaningful and more readily comprehended. Familiar events and known names rather than unknown names for characters improve children's understanding of sentences (Olsen, 1974).

Present new concepts with redundancy, actually repeating both concept and definition. A key point can be repeated for listeners to hear again. The child should be actively involved and even supply part of the repetition. Classroom teachers can improve comprehension with these techniques (Lasky & Chapandy, 1976), and other listeners in class do not find the redundancy or pausing disturbing if the information is new. Presenting new concepts to a child before using them in class improves attending, listening, comprehension, and remembering. The child frequently reports that the teacher is easier to understand. Parents, siblings, peer tutors, and friends can be enlisted to teach new concepts before their use in class.

Some children perform better when they are closer to the signal source. Some are helped when the signal is more intense (louder) and find an auditory trainer valuable. Tape recording a lesson from a written script is helpful for initial exposure or for review. Use of a written script enables a speaker to control sentence complexity, rate, and redundancy.

With increasing familiarity of any concept, the rate can be increased to a normal rate, the concept can be used in sentences of increasing syntactic complexity, and contextual cues, examples, and redundancy are less necessary. Record any change in social or academic performance. Summarize progress for school personnel and family members.

Manipulate the Environment to Enhance Processing If performance with the audiologist, speech-language pathologist, or other specialist is better than performance in class, simulate class conditions gradually to desensitize the child to disrupting variables. Train maintaining attention by introducing actual or simulated competing messages. The signal-to-noise ratio (S/N) can be favorable at first (e.g., +20 dB S/N, that is, signal 20 dB greater than competing messages), with competition increasing as the child becomes desensitized and learns to focus. With easier, more familiar concepts, one should require a delay, not an immediate response. As strategies are acquired for remembering, introduce a delay even with unfamiliar concepts. Use an immediate/delayed response format with easier, then with progressively harder tasks. Work in groups to help a child recognize and control for social pressures and less individualization than in a dyad. If the child finds the disrupting effects of a group are greatest when information is new, he or she may be more willing to work with parents, peers, or tutors to gain familiarity with concepts prior to their use in a lesson. Document any progress seen after desensitization to competing messages, requiring delayed responses, and recognizing effects of a group environment.

Response Tasks Affect Processing Response requirements as part of remediation are discussed from two perspectives. First, the response affects processing and remembering of information. Second, if a child cannot respond at higher levels, easier responses are used with a buildup to harder tasks as material becomes meaningful.

If a response requires a decision based on superficial aspects of a word or phrase (sound or appearance), that response will not be remembered as well as if it were based on the meaning (Craik & Tulving, 1975; Nelson, 1979). Interpreting meaning encourages deeper levels of processing, with consequent longer retention in memory (Craik & Tulving, 1975; Jacoby & Craik, 1979; Kintsch, 1979). Progression is from shallow levels of processing (is the word in capital or small letters?) to slightly deeper levels (number of syllables, presence of one sound or letter), then to successively deeper levels, such as repetition of a word or sentence, then rhyming, then identifying a word's syntactic category. Still deeper levels go to paraphrasing, to indicating whether a sentence fits a context, to generating a sentence that can follow a given sentence.

Structure learning tasks so that information is processed more deeply and comprehension and memory are enhanced. A technique one of us uses is adapted from work showing that subjects who read aloud and had to supply the last word of a sentence remembered significantly more than subjects who merely read the entire sentence aloud (Anderson, Goldberg, & Hidde, 1971). Whether the last word was obvious from the semantic content, as in "Elevators stop at every _____" or not obvious, as in "Nathan bought a _____," performance was better for those who supplied a word than for those who just read the sentences aloud (Kane & Anderson, 1977). Active listening, processing, and attending with sentences structured to minimize errors aid comprehension and memory. Training subjects to ask themselves questions, verbalize answers, and make up new examples also helps.

The second aspect of structuring response tasks uses easier responses first and then builds to increased levels of difficulty. We may start with imitation but are aware that, in most circumstances, verbal responses tend to be summaries rather than verbatim reproductions— the meaning or gist of a message, not the exact words. If auditory information has been processed, what is repeated depends on what is known and deemed salient. Changes may reflect inferences the listener has drawn and elaborations based on his or her knowledge (Brewer, 1977) rather than inadequate CAP. We need to be cognizant of this when scoring imitation responses. We should also consider that, like shadowing, imitation does not reflect or provide practice in deep levels of processing auditory information. Imitation may be an easy starting point, but we need to move to more difficult tasks involving deeper levels of processing.

In recognition tasks, the more similar the items, the more difficult the task (Bahrick, 1979). Therefore, performance is developed with multiple-choice tasks with dissimilar items and then with similar items. We are careful to consider that a child can make a selection without fully comprehending the information presented (Anderson, Goldberg, & Hidde, 1971; Andre & Sola, 1976). A correct response can occur without comprehension through reaction to an unintended cue (Shipley & McFarlane, 1981). Recognition reflects a relatively passive process; we therefore progress up to cued recall and recall, which depend on active processing and use of organizing strategies (Bahrick, 1979; Naus & Halasz, 1979). We present concepts at easier levels early and quickly move on to cued recall. As a child gains greater comprehension, a response task makes increasingly greater demands: recall, paraphrasing, explaining, making inferences. The increased demands increase the level of processing and influence remembering. If the child has difficulty following directions and remembering, use materials relevant to the child's education and interests with tasks that increase in difficulty, simulating those in the classroom. Record progress observed in the clinic and in the classroom.

Teach Strategies for Auditory Processing and Remembering   Dansereau (1978) divided strategies into primary and support strategies. His primary strategies include imagery, networking, analysis of key words, and systematic retrieval. We added verbal mediation, rehearsal, paraphrasing, and learning how to follow directions, get the main idea, and draw conclusions. Support strategies include techniques for cognitive monitoring, maintaining concentration, and asking and answering questions. These strategies can help a child with CAP problems organize, comprehend, and remember auditory information.

Primary Strategies

Verbal Mediation   Speech can play a regulating role in mediation behavior (Luria, 1961). Both overt, speaking aloud to oneself and covert, inner speech can be useful in influencing perception, understanding, and problem solving (Blank, 1974; Kendler, 1963). We use verbal mediation when we tell ourselves how to organize or proceed on a project. Training in verbal mediation and self-direction can significantly improve performance of children with low language skills (Weithorn & Kagen, 1979). To use verbal mediation, what a child is or should be doing is described out loud, step by step. The child is taught to tell himself or herself what to do, how to listen, and how to respond. With success in overt verbalizing, covert verbal mediation is taught.

Rehearsal   Repeating to remember a telephone number or items to purchase are examples of rehearsal. Rehearsal is used to remember topics, items, or events. One cannot assume that a child spontaneously uses this or any other strategy. It may be helpful to teach active (aloud) rehearsal, then silent rehearsal, and to provide practice in each.

Paraphrasing   Putting something in our own words requires deeper levels of processing. A message is transformed into a child's language and integrated with information the child knows. Paraphrasing can help a child realize what he or she comprehends and what must be reviewed.

Imagery   A mental picture is drawn to represent material presented. Filling in details and organizing material to stimulate imagery can help in focusing and monitoring attention and remembering. Either imaging common scenes or imaging bizarre situations may be more effective for a child.

Networking An important concept is identified and related to familiar concepts—networks or bridges are built from stored ideas to new concepts. Networking places a concept in a context or outline. Teacher-prepared networks (outlines) orient listeners before a presentation and organize a review afterwards. Teachers can remind the student of relevant, related information they already know so as to relate the novel information to this prior familiar knowledge (Adams & Bruce, 1980; Schallert & Kleiman, 1979).

Analysis of Key Ideas The student learns to identify key ideas and to define, elaborate, and interrelate them (Dansereau, 1978).

Systematic Retrieval To help retrieve items from memory, a student learns to pick out the theme of a question and think through related ideas in a sequential, orderly manner (Dansereau, 1978; Lindsay & Norman, 1972). Related ideas often trigger a temporarily inaccessible item. A substrategy has students relax and imagine a situation in which they heard the information.

Following Directions At times a child seems to need help remembering directions. We also recognize that some children need to learn *how* to follow directions. Materials are available to work on this; for example, a direction is presented: "Put a line under the girl who is jumping." Questions follow which break down the task: "You are to find the girl who is _____ (A) jumping, (B) running, (C) talking. You are to make a line _____ (A) on her, (B) under her, (C) after her." A marked picture is presented and the child indicates whether it is correct (Boning, 1979). Levels of materials vary. We have adapted workbooks, used them for listening tasks, and found performance improved. Materials can be adapted to teach listening and learning how to get the main idea, use the context, locate an answer, and draw conclusions. A program for training memory strategies has been developed by Campione et al. (1980).

Support Strategies When support strategies are used to monitor concentration, progress, and attitude, primary strategies can have greater impact.

Cognitive Monitoring This strategy influences comprehension of auditory information, language acquisition, memory, attention, and reading comprehension (Flavell, 1979). Cognitive monitoring utilizes metacognition, or knowing about knowing. It includes metacognitive knowledge, experience, and strategies (Flavell, 1979). Metacognitive knowledge involves your observations that you learn better by listening than by reading, that you aren't as good in math as Neil or Pam, or that a task is too hard. Metacognitive experience accompanies cognitive activity, (e.g., your feeling that you learned something well or did not understand it). You select cognitive strategies for learning something. Some children and adolescents need to be taught to use cognitive monitoring to select and attend to the appropriate auditory signal, to check their comprehension and remembering of auditory information, and to check whether their progress or behavior is appropriate or needs to be altered. The experience of listening to a lecture, and suddenly realizing we weren't really processing, involves monitoring. Monitoring can be critical to children who have difficulty selecting and maintaining attention. They learn to identify areas of difficulty, how to ask for help, and when and where to seek more information. Teaching monitoring strategies to a child can:

1. Help the child be aware of what he or she knows and doesn't know. The child learns to evaluate what he or she remembers and doesn't remember, and when he or she is listening and when not.
2. Help the child learn how to listen and to anticipate. When some children have difficulty processing information, they retreat from listening and learn not to listen (Bryen, 1981). Some children need practice in identifying and anticipating narrative structure. Normally children recall a narrative in an orderly fashion: recalled information is central to the theme rather than tangential, and recall is greater from a normal story than from a scrambled story (Dent & Thorndyke, 1979). From stories, TV shows, and commercials good listeners anticipate a setting, a theme, a plot with episodes, and a resolution. Anticipation of this structure and practice with it facilitate processing of incoming information (Brown, 1975).
3. Help the child ask relevant questions. Learning to ask appropriate and relevant questions is critical (Bransford & Nitsch, 1978). One can provide practice by presenting a question and part of a story. The child paraphrases what he or she has heard and is helped to identify what he or she must find out and how to ask the question.
4. Help the child know how to answer questions. To answer a question one must know why the question was asked, have knowledge of what is being asked, and, often, have knowledge about the person who asked the question (Norman, 1973). Exercises for various ability levels are available to teach this strategy, such as the following level six exercise (Boning, 1979) that presents the question "Why does the speedboat move so fast?" The child selects what is being asked from: (A) time, (B) place, (C) reason, (D) degree, (E) number. Asked another example: "About how many stars are there in our

galaxy?" the child selects an answer from (A) type, (B) way, (C) person, (D) number, (E) place. We present these auditorily for practice in listening and comprehending what is asked and what is necessary to answer it.

Positive Learning Attitude   Students often indicate various attitudes about learning, including such negative emotions as anxiety, anger, guilt, fear, and frustration (Dansereau, 1978). Children experiencing difficulty in CAP may experience these feelings as well as confusion. To improve these attitudes, Dansereau (1978) combined desensitization and relaxation (Jacobsen, 1938), rational emotive therapy (Ellis, 1977), and therapies based on self-talk (Meichenbaum & Goodman, 1971; Meichenbaum & Turk, 1975). Students become aware of feelings and their self-talk. They learn to modify their images and self-talk, to image anxiety-producing events during relaxation, to image successful studying, to image distractions and overcoming them, and to use more positive self-talk (Dansereau, 1978). Similar approaches can be used with young children (Schultz, 1981; Wells, 1981).

Concentration or Coping with Internal and External Distractions   Many children with CAP problems are distracted by internal and external stimuli. Finding inability to concentrate the most common student complaint, awareness training helps the student determine when, how, why, and for how long he or she is distracted, and his or her reactions to the distraction (Dansereau, 1978). Use of awareness, relaxation, positive self-talk, and imagery facilitate development of appropriate learning states. We have found that even children in primary grades can learn to monitor their concentration.

Inclusion of these strategies in a chapter on CAP may elicit criticism. Our rationale is that in evaluating many children referred for CAP problems, we saw their confusion and frustration as they approached the auditory processing of language. Our approach has been to build from basic and clinical research reported in various fields to facilitate comprehension of the auditory signal. Techniques we adapted forced us to reevaluate and modify our clinical work, and then risk criticism in discussing it.

CONCLUSION

In this chapter, we have argued that many children with CAP problems are referred because of difficulties in comprehending, using, and remembering information presented auditorily in the teaching-learning environment. Our approach has been to modify the auditory SPERS.

We propose an evaluation and remediation program to enable these children to perform more effectively and efficiently by manipulating variables: 1) in the signal, 2) in its presentation, 3) in the environment, 4) in the response required, and 5) in the use of strategies. We also argue that results of any test procedure or treatment should be documented by recording changes in behaviors, test scores, or academic performance.

REFERENCES

Adams, M., and Bruce, B. 1980. Background knowledge and reading comprehension. Technical Report No. 13. Center for the Study of Reading, University of Illinois, Champaign, Ill. (Available from ERIC Document Reproduction Service, Arlington, Va., No. ED 181 431.)

Ahlschwede, B. F. 1977. Exploring Our World: Regions. Follett Publishing Co., Chicago.

Anderson, R. C., Goldberg, S. R., and Hidde, J. L. 1971. Meaningful processing of sentences. Journal of Educational Psychology 62:395–399.

Andre, T., and Sola, J. 1976. Imagery, verbatim and paraphrased questions, and retention of meaningful sentences. J. Educ. Psychol. 68:661–669.

Bahrick, H. 1979. Broader methods and narrower theories for memory research: Comments on the papers by Eysenck and Cermak. In: L. Cermak and F. Craik (eds.), Levels of Processing in Human Memory, pp. 141–158. Lawrence Erlbaum Associates, Hillsdale, N.J.

Barr, D. F. 1976. Auditory Perceptual Disorders. Charles C Thomas, Springfield, Ill.

Blank, M. 1974. Cognitive functions of language in the preschool years. Developmental Psychology 10:229–245.

Blecha, M. K., Gega, P. C., and Green, M. 1979. The Laidlow Exploring Science Program Red Book. Teacher's Edition. Laidlow Brothers, River Forest, Ill.

Bocca, E., Calearo, C., Cassinari, C., and Migliavacca, F. 1955. Testing "cortical" hearing in temporal lobe tumors. Acta Oto-laryngologica (Stockholm) 45:289–304.

Boehm, A. 1971. Boehm Test of Basic Concepts. Psychological Corporation, New York.

Boning, R. A. 1979. Specific Skill Series. Barnell Loft, Ltd., Baldwin, N.Y.

Bransford, J. D., and Nitsch, K. E. 1978. Coming to understand things we could not previously understand. In: J. F. Kavanagh and W. Strange (eds.), Speech and Language in the Laboratory, School and Clinic, pp. 267–307. MIT Press, Cambridge, Mass.

Bransford, J. D., McCarrell, N. S., Franks, J. J., and Nitsch, K. E. 1977. Toward unexplaining memory. In: R. Shaw and J. Bransford (eds.), Perceiving, Acting, and Knowing, pp. 431–466. Lawrence Erlbaum Associates, Hillsdale, N.J.

Brewer, W. F. 1977. Memory for the pragmatic implications of sentences. Memory and Cognition 5(6):673–678.

Brown, A. L. 1975. The development of memory: Knowing, knowing about knowing, and knowing how to know. In: H. W. Reese (ed.), Advances in Child Development and Behavior, Volume 10, pp. 104–152. Academic Press, New York.

Brown, A. L. 1977. Development, schooling and the acquisition of knowledge about knowledge. In: R. C. Anderson, R. J. Spiro, and W. E. Montague (eds.), Schooling and the Acquisition of Knowledge, pp. 241–253. Lawrence Erlbaum Associates, Hillsdale, N.J.

Brown, A. L. 1979. Theories of memory and the problems of development: Activity, growth, and knowledge. In: L. Cermak and F. Craik (eds.), Levels of Processing in Human Memory, pp. 225–258. Lawrence Erlbaum Associates, Hillsdale, N.J.

Brown, A. L., and DeLoache, J. S. 1978. Skills, plans, and self-regulation. In: R. Siegler (ed.), Children's Thinking: What Develops, pp. 3–35. Lawrence Erlbaum Associates, Hillsdale, N.J.

Bryen, D. N. 1981. Language and language problems. In: A. Gerber and D. N. Bryen (eds.), Language and Learning Disabilities, pp. 27–60. University Park Press, Baltimore.

Campione, J., Nitsch, K., Bray, N., and Brown, A. 1980. Improving Memory Skills in Mentally Retarded Children: Empirical Research and Strategies for Intervention. Technical Report No. 196. Center for the Study of Reading, University of Illinois, Champaign, Ill.

Chapandy, A., and Lasky, E. 1980. The effect of word familiarity on children's comprehension and memory. Ohio Journal of Speech and Hearing 15:1–11.

Cohen, C. K., and Schiller, J. S. 1981. Group training of auditory processing skills. In: A. Gerber and D. Bryen (eds.), Language and Learning Disabilities, pp. 295–324. University Park Press, Baltimore.

Cook-Gumperz, J. 1975. The child as a practical reasoner. In: M. Sanches and B. G. Blount (eds.), Language, Thought, and Culture, pp. 137–162. Academic Press, New York.

Costello, M. R. 1977. Evaluation of auditory behavior of children using the Flowers-Costello Test of Central Auditory Abilities. In: R. W. Keith (ed.), Central Auditory Dysfunction, pp. 257–276. Grune & Stratton, New York.

Cox, L. C., Hack, M., and Metz, D. A. 1981. Brainstem-evoked response audiometry: Normative data from the preterm infant. Audiology 20:53–64.

Craik, F. I. M., and Tulving, E. 1975. Depth of processing and the retention of words in episodic memory. Journal of Experimental Psychology: General 104:268–294.

Dansereau, D. 1978. The development of a learning strategies curriculum. In: H. F. O'Neil (ed.), Learning Strategies, pp. 1–29. Academic Press, New York.

Dent, C. H., and Thorndyke, P. W. 1979. Children's Use of Schemata in Comprehension and Recall of Narrative Texts. The Rand Corporation, Santa Monica, Calif.

Duane, D. 1977. A neurologic perspective of central auditory dysfunction. In: R. W. Keith (ed.), Central Auditory Dysfunction, pp. 1–42. Grune & Stratton, New York.

Ellis, A. 1963. Handbook of Rational Emotive Therapy. Springer, New York.

Flavell, J. H. 1979. Metacognition and cognitive monitoring: A new area of cognitive-developmental inquiry. American Psychologist 34:906–911.

Flavell, J. H., and Wellman, H. M. 1977. Metamemory. In: R. V. Kail, Jr., and J. W. Hagen (eds.), Perspectives on the Development of Memory and Cognition, pp. 3-33. Lawrence Erlbaum Associates, Hillsdale, N.J.

Gagné, R. M., and White, R. T. 1978. Memory structures and learning outcomes. Review of Educational Research 28:187-222.

Galin, D. 1979. EEG studies of lateralization of verbal processes. In: C. L. Ludlow and M. E. Doran-Quine (eds.), The Neurological Bases of Language Disorders in Children: Methods and Directions for Research, pp. 129-141. (NINCDS Monograph No. 22.) National Institutes of Health, Bethesda, Maryland.

Gerber, A. 1981. Problems in the processing and use of language in education. In: A. Gerber and D. N. Bryen (eds.), Language and Learning Disabilities, pp. 75-112. University Park Press, Baltimore.

Gerber, S. E., and Mencher, G. T. 1980. Auditory Dysfunction. College Hill Press, Houston.

Guszak, F. J. 1967. Teacher questions and reading. The Reading Teacher 67(21):227-234.

Hagen, J. W., and Stanovich, K. E. 1977. A memory: Strategies of acquisition. In: R. Kail and J. W. Hagen (eds.), Perspectives on the Development of Memory and Cognition, pp. 89-111. Lawrence Erlbaum Associates, Hillsdale, N.J.

Jacobsen, E. 1938. Progressive Relaxation. University of Chicago Press, Chicago.

Jacoby, L., and Craik, F. 1979. Effects of elaboration of processing at encoding and retrieval: Trace distinctiveness and recovery of initial context. In: L. Cermak and F. Craik (eds.), Levels of Processing in Human Memory, pp. 1-22. Lawrence Erlbaum Associates, Hillsdale, N.J.

Jerger, J., Hayes, D., and Jordan, C. 1980. Clinical experience with auditory brainstem response audiometry in pediatric assessment. Ear and Hearing 1:19-25.

Kane, J. H., and Anderson, R. C. 1977. Depth of processing and interference effects in the learning and remembering of sentences. Technical Report No. 21. Center for the Study of Reading. University of Illinois Press, Urbana, Ill.

Katz, J. 1962. The use of staggered spondaic words for assessing the integrity of the central auditory nervous system. Journal of Auditory Research 2:327-337.

Kendler, T. S. 1963. Development of mediating responses in children. In: J. C. Wright and J. Kagan (eds.), Basic Cognitive Processes in Children. Monographs of the Society for Research in Child Development 28:33-48.

Kintsch, W. 1979. Levels of processing language material: Discussion of the papers by Lachman and Lachman and Perfetti. In: L. Cermak and F. Craik (eds.), Levels of Processing in Human Memory, pp. 211-222. Lawrence Erlbaum Associates, Hillsdale, N.J.

Lasky, E. Z., and Chapandy, A. M. 1976. Factors affecting language comprehension. Language, Speech, and Hearing Services in Schools 7:159-168.

Lindamood, C., and Lindamood, P. 1969. A.D.D. Program (Auditory discrimination in depth). Teaching Resources, Boston.

Lindsay, P. H., and Norman, D. A. 1972. Human Informal Processing: An Introduction to Psychology. Academic Press, New York.

Luria, A. R. 1961. The Role of Speech in the Regulation of Normal and Abnormal Behavior. Liveright, New York.

Matzker, J. 1959. Two new methods for the assessment of central auditory functions in cases of brain disease. Annals of Otology 68:1185–1197.

McCroskey, R. L., and Thompson, N. W. 1973. Comprehension of rate controlled speech by children with specific learning disabilities. Journal of Learning Disabilities 6:621–627.

Meichenbaum, D. H., and Goodman, J. 1971. Training impulsive children to talk to themselves: A means of self-control. Journal of Abnormal Child Psychology 77:115–126.

Meichenbaum, D. H., and Turk, D. 1975. The cognitive-behavioral management of anxiety, anger, and pain. Paper presented at the Seventh Banff International Conference on Behavior Modification, Banff, Canada. (Cited in Dansereau, D. 1978. Learning Strategies, pp. 1–29. Academic Press, New York.)

Moates, D. R., and Schumacher, G. M. 1980. An Introduction to Cognitive Psychology. Wadsworth, Belmont, Calif.

Naus, M., and Halasz, F. 1979. Developmental perspectives on cognitive processing and semantic memory structure. In: L. Cermak and F. Craik (eds.), Levels of Processing in Human Memory, pp. 259–288. Lawrence Erlbaum Associates, Hillsdale, N.J.

Nelson, D. 1979. Remembering pictures and words: Appearance, significance, and name. In: L. Cermak and F. Craik (eds.), Levels of Processing in Human Memory, pp. 45–76. Lawrence Erlbaum Associates, Hillsdale, N.J.

Noffsinger, P. D., and Kurdziel, S. A. 1979. Assessment of central auditory lesions. In: W. F. Rintelmann (ed.), Hearing Assessment, pp. 351–377. University Park Press, Baltimore.

Norman, D. A. 1973. Memory, knowledge, and the answering of questions. In: R. Solso (ed.), The Loyola Symposium on Cognitive Psychology, pp. 135–165. Winston, Washington, D.C.

Norman, D. A., and Bobrow, D. G. 1977. Descriptions: A basis for memory acquisition and retrieval. Technical Report No. 74. Center for Human Information Processing, San Diego.

O'Donovan, C. A., Beagley, H. A., and Shaw, M. 1980. Latency of brainstem response in children. British Journal of Audiology 14:23–29.

Olsen, D. R. 1974. Towards a theory of instructional means. Invited address presented to the American Educational Research Association, Chicago, April 1974. (Cited in: J. F. Kavanagh and W. Strange (eds.), Speech and Language in the Laboratory, School and Clinic, p. 264. MIT Press, Cambridge, Mass.)

Peck, D. J. 1977. The effects of presentation rates on the auditory comprehension of learning-disabled children. Paper presented at the Annual Convention of the American Speech-Language-Hearing Association, Chicago.

Rampp, D. L. 1980. Auditory Processing and Learning Disabilities. Cliffs Notes, Lincoln, Nebr.

Reagan, C. L. 1973. Handbook of Auditory Perceptual Training. Charles C Thomas, Springfield, Ill.

Rosner, J. 1975. Helping Children Overcome Learning Difficulties. Walker and Company, New York.

Sanders, D. 1977. Auditory Perception of Speech. Prentice-Hall, Englewood Cliffs, N.J.

Schallert, D. L., and Kleiman, G. M. 1979. Some reasons why teachers are easier to understand than textbooks. (Available from ERIC Document Reproduction Service, Arlington, Va., No. ED 172 189.)

Schultz, E. D. 1981. Teaching coping skills for stress and anxiety. Teaching Exceptional Children. 13(4):12–17.

Shipley, K. G., and McFarlane, S. C. 1981. Facilitating reading development with speech- and language-impaired children. Language, Speech and Hearing Services in Schools 12(2):100–106.

Smith, B. S., and Resnick, D. A. 1972. An auditory test for assessing brainstem integrity: Preliminary report. Laryngoscope 82:414–424.

Stark, R., and Tallal, P. 1980. Perceptual and motor deficits in language impaired children. In: R. Keith (ed.), Central Auditory and Language Disorders in Children: Diagnosis and Remediation, pp. 121–144. College Hill Press, Houston.

Tulving, E., and Thompson, D. M. 1973. Encoding specificity and retrieval processes in episodic memory. Psychological Review 80:352–373.

Watts, G. H., and Anderson, R. C. 1971. Effects of three types of inserted questions on learning from prose. Journal of Educational Psychology 62:387–394.

Weithorn, C. J., and Kagen, E. 1979. Training first graders of high-activity level to improve performance through verbal self-direction. Journal of Learning Disabilities 12(2):23–29.

Wells, D. H. 1981. Breathing exercises for relaxation. Teaching Exceptional Children 14(2):87–88.

Willeford, J. 1977. Assessing central auditory behavior in children: A test battery approach. In: R. W. Keith (ed.), Central Auditory Dysfunction, pp. 43–72. Grune & Stratton, New York.

Willeford, J. A., and Billger, J. M. 1978. Auditory perception in children with learning disabilities. In: J. Katz (ed.), Handbook of Clinical Audiology, pp. 410–425. Williams & Wilkins, Baltimore.

Willette, R., Jackson, B., and Peckins, I. 1970. Auditory Perception Training (APT). Developmental Learning Materials, Chicago.

Williamson, D. G., and Alexander, R. 1975. Central auditory abilities. Maico Audiological Library Series 13(7).

Wood, N. 1975. Assessment of auditory processing dysfunctions. Acta Symbolica 7:113–124.

Chapter 14

Phonemic Synthesis

Jack Katz

As a group, children with learning and communicative problems perform more poorly on certain auditory tasks than do youngsters in the general population. Fifty years ago, Travis and Rasmus (1931) demonstrated that pupils with articulation problems had depressed speech-sound discrimination, and Monroe (1932) showed auditory synthesis skills to be reduced in a large group of reading-disabled children. Since that time there has been a considerable increase in the number and types of techniques available for evaluating children who might have auditory disabilities. All of these procedures are deserving of careful consideration and study, both from the standpoint of what they can and what they cannot do.

The chapters in this book point out that one can ignore the influence neither of peripheral nor of central auditory function in relation to communication and learning problems. It has been my experience that teachers and parents often correctly identify the auditory channel as being deficient in a particular child, yet they are not able to indicate consistently whether it is associated with a peripheral hearing loss, a central auditory impairment, or both. It would be prudent to rule out both factors in evaluating any child with suspected auditory disability. Indeed, we have found many children who were not specifically thought to have auditory disabilities to demonstrate important limitations in dealing with auditory information.

In selecting a battery of auditory tests, priority should be given to those procedures that have relevance to academic or communicative performance. Special attention should be given to tests that can be easily translated into appropriate therapeutic procedures. Our first obligation is to demonstrate that the disorder is not "simply" a function of peripheral hearing loss. However, the presence of such a loss does not indicate that the child does not also make inefficient use of the information that is heard.

The purpose of this chapter is to discuss phonemic synthesis. Briefly, phonemic synthesis (PS) is a type of sound blending task in which the individual phonemes of words are delivered to the listener one at a time. The child must then indicate the word that was presented. Included in this discussion is a neurologic model suggesting the relevance of PS to phonemic skills and thereby to articulation, language, spelling, and reading. PS is then considered as a diagnostic procedure, with a brief review of the literature indicating the relationship between it and both achievement in school and in communicative abilities. Finally, the therapeutic relevance of PS is presented, along with specific techniques that have been found useful in ameliorating PS difficulties and, importantly, having a positive influence on the presenting problems.

NEUROLOGIC REGIONS OF THE BRAIN

The eminent neuropsychologist A. R. Luria studied the effects of focal brain lesions on a wide variety of skills (Hatfield, 1981). Luria's subjects were soldiers who had sustained small cerebral lesions due to trauma, chiefly gunshot wounds. He made functional maps of important language, speech, reading, spelling, and other regions, by matching behavioral abnormalities with known loci of lesion. Luria's findings laid the groundwork for a better understanding of how the auditory system interrelates with articulation, reading, and other skills. One must bear in mind that there are no doubt important differences, both anatomical and physiologic, between the initial development of skills in children and the maintenance of these skills in adulthood. Despite this caution, however, it is inconceivable that the large regions associated with articulation or reading problems in adults are not also involved in the development and refinement of these skills in children.

We do *not* assume that children who have learning disabilities or communication problems have some type of brain damage. This interpretation is not intended, nor do we feel that it is justified (Duane, 1977). Although some children who have reduced auditory abilities might show evidence of brain damage due to trauma, stroke, or tumor, such observable etiologies are atypical in the population of learning- and speech-disabled children. Dysfunctions are more likely due to delayed maturation, biochemical imbalance (Gross & Wilson, 1974), or neurologic variations (Hier et al., 1978). It is logical to assume that it is the degree of regional involvement and the functions within those regions that have the major influence on the child's ability to learn and communicate.

Of particular interest in the work of Luria (1966, 1970) is his discussion of auditory processing, articulation, language, reading, and spelling disorders. He suggested that various functions are localized in certain areas of zones of the cortex. These areas (e.g., the phonemic, articulation, spelling, reading, and receptive language zones) seem to underlie or may have primary responsibility for specific functions. Although important functions are concentrated in these regions, no one region of the brain can account for all aspects of reading or receptive language skills. All such skills are complex abilities and are made up of numerous subskills. Dysfunction of the central nervous system is not a static process. During periods of great CNS plasticity, considerable reorganization may take place. It may also be possible to compensate for inadequacies in one particular function by means of related or complementary skills.

Phonemic Zone

The middle and posterior portions of the superior temporal gyrus are considered to constitute the auditory cortex (Celesia, 1976). It is made up primarily of the auditory association areas that surround the auditory reception center. Luria (1970) referred to this region as the "phonemic" zone, which primarily constitutes Brodmann's area 22 (Elliott, 1969) and is associated with three important functions: analysis, synthesis, and memory for phonemic information. One can assume that not only damage but immature development or faulty performance for any reason in this zone would affect auditory perception. If this important decoding center did not function adequately, one might observe impairment in discrimination, synthesizing, and remembering of speech sounds. Difficult discrimination material would require a much longer time to analyze, synthesize, and remember. Depressed performance would be noted when the subject listened to rapid, distorted, or less redundant speech. A logical consequence of these difficulties could be impaired ability in processing word endings (in longer or more difficult words) or in dealing with words and phrases that are embedded in long, complex sentences.

Luria (1970) did indeed note that lesions to the phonemic zone were associated with errors on word endings. Burns and Canter (1977) found similar results. They noted significantly more errors on the final as compared to the initial portions (phonemes and consonant clusters) of words in a group of aphasic patients with posterior cerebral involvement.

On the Staggered Spondaic Word (SSW) test, a procedure in which there is a dichotic presentation of paired spondaic words, there is a tendency for patients with posterior temporal lesions to have more errors on the second spondee (Katz, 1976, 1978). One explanation for these findings is that individuals with a dysfunctional auditory cortex are inefficient in the analysis of incoming information. Although slowed and somewhat less complete processing would take place for the first spondee, it is more likely to be correct than the second spondee. The last one or two monosyllables of the item might need to be held in a short-term or even a sensory memory store while the first spondee is processed. In the less efficient storage systems one can assume that phonemic information will tend to fade rapidly. By the time the sounds are analyzed they have become degraded, with a greater likelihood of error. This peculiarity on the SSW test is associated with posterior temporal disorders. Lesions limited to the frontal lobe or anterior temporal region do not show this tendency.

By utilizing Luria's findings we can anticipate disruption of decoding skills, with dysfunction in the region around the primary auditory reception center. If we can expect analysis, synthesis, and memory problems in adults who presumably have acquired normal communicative and academic skills when there is damage to the phonemic zone, what can we expect of children who lack age-appropriate development in this region? Such children would likely have faulty or incomplete perception of speech. Such approximations of the sounds of our language would then serve as models for the child in articulation and as the basis for sound-symbol associations in reading and spelling. Because of the high speed of naturally occurring speech, it would be particularly difficult for these children to alter their faulty notions even after further maturation or compensations took place. The relationship between phonemic synthesis and the phonemic zone is discussed in a later section.

Articulation Zone

Luria's (1970) articulation zone borders the phonemic zone superiorly, and overlaps it to some extent. Subjects with lesions to the frontopariɘtal and adjacent superior temporal regions demonstrated various types of articulation disorders. Functionally, this region seems well suited to serve articulation. It includes the portions of the sensorimotor strip that provide sensory information to the tongue, lips, and vocal folds as well as serving motor control for these same organs. The superior temporal portion of the articulation zone is also a part of the phonemic zone and no doubt contributes to our understanding of what the various speech sounds should sound like (Geschwind, 1970). These conceptions or engrams probably serve as the target sounds for purposes of production and are then used to check on the accuracy of the speech. The large somatosensory portion of the articulation zone might tend to explain how children with poor articulatory skills could compensate for an auditory deficiency. They could improve articulation by methods stressing tactile and proprioceptive senses. This then could allow a motor theory of speech perception explanation (Liberman et al., 1961) for improved auditory conceptualization.

Spelling and Reading Zones

Perhaps the most important area for spelling and reading skills is the angular gyrus (Orton, 1937). This auditory-visual integration area is situated in the parieto-occipital region (Luria, 1970). Pirozzolo and Rayner (1979) found that 42% of those classified as developmentally dyslexic had reversed asymmetries in the parieto-occipital region. An additional 25% showed essentially no asymmetry between the right and left hemispheres, leaving only about one-third of the subjects with the expected hemispheric relationship.

Lucker (1980) pointed out that behavioral central auditory signs, which are thought to be associated with the angular gyrus, are found in children with spelling and reading problems. Almost all of the children had spelling problems, whereas reading disorders were not quite as pervasive. Luria noted that there was significant overlap of the areas involved with spelling and reading difficulties.

Luria argued that spelling, in particular, is heavily based on auditory functions and that the spelling area is closely tied neurologically to the auditory cortex (phonemic zone). Because the phonemic zone and the angular gyrus are extensively interconnected neurologically, it should follow that disruption of function in the auditory cortex would reduce the quality of information available for auditory-visual integration and sound-symbol relationships.

Bannatyne and Wichiarajote (1969) demonstrated a close association between sound blending and written spelling ability in school children in regular classes. Hammill and Larsen (1974) reviewed many studies dealing with the relationship between reading and auditory skills. Although they tried to minimize the association between reading and auditory perception, they were not able to explain away sound blending.

Receptive Language Zone

The receptive language zone, or posterior language region, is situated in the posterior temporoparietal area of the left hemisphere in most people (Penfield & Roberts, 1959). A lesion to this zone tends to produce a disturbance in deriving meaning from spoken and written symbols.

The receptive language zone (Penfield & Roberts, 1959) almost completely encompasses the phonemic zone and covers a major portion of the spelling and reading zones as well as being adjacent to and overlapping part of the articulation zone. It would be very difficult to separate receptive language completely from phonemic analysis, synthesis, memory, and auditory-visual integration functionally or anatomically. Before a person can understand a spoken message, he or she must first have a basic appreciation of the incoming signal. It seems reasonable that the proper and efficient perception of speech requires a well functioning phonemic area. Without an efficient decoding system one is likely to be handicapped in developing age-appropriate skills in receptive language (e.g., receptive vocabulary). Such deficits may not be apparent in a child's early years when the parents use simple sentences, speak more slowly, limit the range of topics, and provide considerable redundancy and contextual cues. The receptive language disorder might become more obvious as the child gets older and his or her decoding as well as receptive language functions are more greatly challenged. If the child fails to develop a much more efficient decoding system as he or she gets older, the dysfunction may be compounded. With limited receptive language and inadequate auditory processing skills, the child's task in overcoming the deficit becomes greater.

In relating auditory processing to receptive language one should not imply that receptive language is exclusively a function of phonemic decoding. The reception of language incorporates syntactic, semantic, and other higher levels of knowledge. Rapid and accurate handling of the auditory signal is only one important aspect of the language process (Sloan, 1980). The case can also be made for the close functional relationship between reading and spelling abilities with language competence (Vellutino, 1977; Mattingly, 1972).

Application of the Functional-Anatomical Model

The monumental work by Luria and others provides us with concepts and information that can aid us in understanding certain auditory processing problems and how they relate to disorders of articulation, decoding, spelling, reading, and language. The four zones that were described and their relationships to one another should help us to: 1) better understand each of these individual communication and learning problems, 2) be able to conceptualize the cluster of symptoms and problems encountered in working with children who have auditory processing difficulties, 3) provide a rationale in the selection of diagnostic procedures, and 4) offer a basis from which we can understand current therapeutic procedures and develop new approaches.

PHONEMIC SYNTHESIS

The PS task is similar to the usual sound blending procedures (Roswell & Chall, 1963; Oliphant, 1971; Goldman, Fristoe, & Woodcock, 1974) in a number of ways. Words are broken up for the listener and presented one phoneme at a time. As in sound blending or auditory synthesis, a silent pause is inserted between each phoneme. PS incorporates additional features that may make it a more effective diagnostic tool and at the same time increase its usefulness as a therapeutic procedure. In sound blending, the rate of 2 phonemes per second is often suggested (Kirk, McCarthy, & Kirk, 1968). For PS a slower rate is used. The sounds are typically presented at a rate of 1 per second or slower. This provides for both a longer phoneme duration and a longer pause than at 2 phonemes per second. The increase in duration of signal and pause are considered to be the most important characteristics of PS. In addition, all phonemes are presented in their stressed form, and the speaker tries to present the prototype phoneme for each speech sound (attempting to neutralize the influences of coarticulation by delivering the "standard" form). Thus, the listener hears a more consistent target sound which differs least from the other variations of the sound.

The distortions of natural speech introduced by the PS procedure aid in the detection of processing problems. Later we point out that these same variations, when utilized as part of a therapeutic program, can aid in simplifying the auditory task and thereby enrich the child's knowledge of the individual sounds. The distortions come from elongating phonemes, inserting pauses between them, utilizing sounds with reduced contextual influences, decreasing formant transitions, greatly increasing the duration of the word, and forcing the listener to retain in storage rather unfamiliar and meaningless sounds. For those who do not have a clear notion of what certain phonemes truly sound like, those who have storage problems for phonemic information, and for those who have difficulty in being able to combine phonemes, the PS task is extremely difficult.

PS Test and Testing Considerations

Two types of PS tests that the author has constructed in recent years are described here. The first one is an open set procedure that can be used with first-graders up to adults. Two similar open set tests are discussed: List 2A (Metzl, 1969) and List 3A (Harmon, 1974). In these measures there are 25 items increasing in difficulty from two-phoneme words such as "shoe" to four-phoneme words such as "child" and "milk." The items are ordered in increasing levels of difficulty. All of the PS tests are recorded on tape to maintain consistency of phoneme production and timing. The listener is to repeat the words that are presented "in a funny way."

The open set tests may be analyzed in two ways. The standard procedure is to sum the number of correct responses and consult the norms for children at various grade levels. Harmon's (1974) results also give an indication of percentile rank. A supplementary scoring procedure might offer some further insights into the child's specific difficulties. One should be careful not to overinterpret simply on the basis of one or two items, except as indicated. Discrimination errors can be noted (i.e., substituting one phoneme for a similar one), as can memory errors (i.e., omitting one or more sounds), reversal errors (i.e., changing the order of the sounds), consonant blend errors, or difficulty with synthesis (i.e., repeating the sounds back without being able to fuse them). It is this last error type that could be significant even if noted only once on the test. Because the children are told that they are to give back a *word*, they are free to guess a word from whatever information they have gathered. Therefore, spurious interpretations of discrimination, memory, or reversals could be made if consistency is not sought. However, if a child is able to discriminate the sounds well enough, remember them, and maintain the proper order, but cannot say them as a word, it seems reasonable to assume that the child was simply unable to blend the phonemes together. Thus, for the word "stone", the child repeats the phonemes /s/ /t/ /o/ and /n/ (this is recorded on the answer form by showing dashes between the individual phonemes).

The second type of PS test utilizes a four-choice response format which can be used with kindergarten and first-grade children (Katz, 1971). The obvious advantage is that the child's speech will not interfere with performance on the test. In addition, it enables the testing of a lower level of ability, which is expected in young children (see Lasky, Chapter 2, this volume). The multiple-choice test that has been used in the research reported in this chapter contains 15 items in the first half. These same items are then repeated to see how much improvement is made on the second presentation. One correct test response and three foils (wrong answers) are pictured on a page. The response differs from each of the foils by one phoneme (i.e., the initial consonant, the vowel, or the final consonant). This test is preceded by word-picture familiarization and then training with the PS procedure. Results on the PS Picture (PS-P) test can be interpreted in two ways. The number of items correct out of 30 can be used to obtain a quantitative result. The normal range of scores for kindergarten children is 16–24 (Katz & Harmon, 1981). Qualitatively, we get insight into the child's responsiveness to therapy by noting whether the child is able to improve from the first to the second half of the test. In addition, there is a tendency for the least able children to make more errors on the final consonant as compared to more capable children. If children show less of a tendency to make errors on the final consonant on the second half of the test, this too is considered a positive sign.

Relationship of PS to Communication and Learning Disorders

Sound blending skills have been associated with reading and spelling for a long time. A number of studies have shown that children with reading disabilities, as a group, have poorer performance in sound blending skills than those achieving normally in reading (Mulder & Curtin, 1955; Chall, Roswell, & Blumenthal, 1963; Conners, Kramer, & Guerra, 1969; Sawyer, 1981). In a group of 50 normal achieving third-grade children, Bannatyne and Wichiarajote (1969) found auditory synthesis and spelling ability to be significantly correlated ($r = 0.40$ at the 0.01 level). This correlation was higher than for any of the other auditory or visual subtests on the Illinois Test of Psycholinguistic Ability (ITPA). When the 25 better spellers were compared to the 25 poorer ones in sound blending, the difference was significant at the 0.01 level of confidence.

A number of studies have noted the relationship between synthesis skills and articulation ability (Mange, 1953, 1955, 1960; Beasley et al., 1974; Stovall, Manning, & Shaw, 1977). The two latter studies were of particular interest because they dealt with the influence of the inter-phoneme interval (100–400 msec) in a sound blending procedure. Children with articulation problems had significantly more errors with longer interphoneme intervals than did children with normal articulation. In addition, those with more severe articulation problems demonstrated more errors on the test, particularly with the long intervals. This supports the use of the longer pause in the PS procedure.

Katz et al. (1969, 1970) evaluated a large group of learning-disabled children from a single school district. They ranged from kindergarten through junior high school level. A definition of learning disabilities (Katz & Illmer, 1972) and a list of specific characteristics to look for were given to each teacher, counselor, and school principal. The characteristics included inattentiveness, hyperactivity, trouble in following directions, and, of course, difficulty in one or more school subjects or in readiness skills for the younger children. Speech, language, or hearing disorders were not appropriate referral criteria by themselves. One study dealt primarily with children in the first grade and above (Katz et al., 1969) and the other with kindergarten youngsters (Katz et al., 1970). The children were tested on the 67-item Templin-Darley Test of Articulation (Templin & Darley, 1960), the Utah Test of Language Development (UTLD; Mecham, Jex, & Jones, 1967), and the Peabody Picture Vocabulary Test (PPVT; Dunn, 1965). The kindergarten children were given the PS-P, and the older children were administered the PS-2A, the Wechsler Intelligence Scale for Children (Wechsler, 1949) Verbal (WISC-V) and Performance (WISC-P) subtests, and the Draw-A-Person Test (DAP; Urban, 1963). The IQ data on these tests were courtesy of Dr. Arnold E. Moskowitz.

Table 1. Total group (N=110) means, standard deviations, and correlations with PS-P for chronologic age and four developmental measures

	CA	PPVT	UTLD	Artic	PS-P
Mean	6;0	6;4	6;2	5.8	14.3
Standard deviation	4.4	17.4	11.3	8.6	5.0
Correlation					
(r) with PS	0.14	0.33*	0.34*	0.39*	

Subjects were 110 kindergarten children referred for learning problems. CA, chronologic age; Artic, Templin-Darley Articulation Test.

*$p < 0.01$.

Complete data were available for 110 kindergarten children. Table 1 shows the means and standard deviations for chronologic age and each of the four measures, as well as correlations with PS-P. The language age-equivalent scores were slightly above chronologic age, suggesting that as a group these children were not deficient in their measured language skills. However, the mean number of articulation errors was almost 6, and the PS-P score of 14 was significantly depressed (normal range is 16–24). As a group they did not show difficulty in language but did in PS and had questionable performance in articulation. PS-P was significantly correlated (at the 0.01 level) with the speech and language measures but not with age.

Table 2. Performance of Low PS and High PS kindergarten groups on four developmental measures

	CA	PPVT	UTLD	Artic	PS-2A
Low PS Group					
Mean	6;0	6;0	5;11	8.2	10.8
Standard deviation	4.1	17.1	9.3	9.4	2.5
High PS Group					
Mean	6;0	6;10	6;6	2.7	18.9
Standard deviation	4.8	16.4	12.3	6.2	3.5
t	0.87	3.04	3.48	3.44	
Probability	NS	0.001	0.0004	0.0004	

CA, chronologic age; Artic, Templin-Darley Articulation Test; NS, not significant; t, result of t-test between groups.

The children were divided into two groups on the basis of their PS scores. The 62 children with PS-P scores below the mean comprised the Low PS group, and the 48 with scores above the mean constituted the High PS group. Table 2 shows their respective performance. The Low PS group had poorer performance on each measure than the High PS group, but there was no difference in mean age. On the language tests the differences between the groups were 10 months and 7 months, respectively, favoring the High PS group. The poor PS group had 8 articulation errors compared to 3 for those with better PS scores. All of the differences were significant beyond the 0.001 level of confidence.

A similar study had been carried out earlier with older children referred for learning disabilities. Children in grades two through six were studied because of the availability of PS norms (Metzl, 1969). Inclusion was also based on having an IQ of at least 90 (on WISC-V, WISC-P, or DAP) as well as results on PS-2A, the PPVT, and/or the UTLD. Although Templin-Darley data for 20 of the 67 subjects were not available, and almost two-thirds of the remaining pupils showed no errors on the test, their results are included for comparison. For the language tests a difference score (D) was computed to help neutralize the influence of age across the sample (a range of 71 months). Thus, PPVT-D and UTLD-D are the language ages subtracted from the chronologic age (i.e., a negative score indicates language age equivalent better and a positive score language age poorer than chronologic age).

Table 3 shows the means, standard deviations, number of children, and correlations with PS for age, DAP, WISC-P, WISC-V, PPVT-D, UTLD-D, Templin-Darley, and PS-2A. Although there was considerable scatter for each variable, the means were within the normal limits or better for each of the measures except PS (with a normal range of 13–18). The intelligence tests were within 3 points of the theoretical norm of 100, but PPVT-D was almost 7 months above chronologic age, and UTLD-D was at age level. The small number of articulation errors (1–2 per child) is perhaps more than would be expected for normally achieving children.

Correlations were not statistically significant for WISC-P, DAP, and Templin-Darley. It was expected that the former two tests would not be highly correlated with PS since they do not involve important auditory functions. It was of interest that the number of articulation errors was not significantly correlated either. This could be due to sampling error or, perhaps more likely, to the small number of positive scores (of one or more errors). Conceivably the older children might have compensated for their articulation problems by using tactile or proprioceptive skills without eliminating their auditory processing deficits. The correlation with age reached the 0.05 level of significance despite the lack of differences found in the normative study (Metzl, 1969). Whereas normal children may reach a plateau on the PS task at the second-grade level, children with problems in auditory processing seem to continue to improve with age. Sixty-two percent of the sixth-graders were within the range of normal, compared to only 27% of the second-graders.

The highest correlations with PS were seen with UTLD-D, PPVT-D, and WISC-V (all significant beyond the 0.01 level of confidence). The strong correlation with WISC-V and not WISC-P supports the notion that PS is related to verbal functions and not simply general intellectual skills. As in the previous studies a close relationship was found between language test scores and PS.

Table 4 provides separate information for the 33 children who scored below the group mean on the PS-2A (Low PS) and the 34 who scored above the mean (High PS). The number of subjects as well as

Table 3. Total group results on seven developmental measures and correlations with PS-2A

	CA	DAP	WISC-P	WISC-V	PPVT-D	UTLD-D	Artic	PS-2A
Mean	9;10	97.5	101.6	97.5	−6.0	−4.1	1.7	12.2
Standard deviation	16.9	13.4	10.9	12.2	23.5	23.0	3.4	5.3
N	67	63	43	43	65	53	47	67
Correlation (r) with PS	0.24*	0.18	0.22	0.42**	−0.44**	−0.48**	−0.10	

Subjects were children in grades 2–6 referred for learning disabilities. CA, chronologic age; Artic, Templin-Darley Articulation Test. See text for further explanation.
*$p < 0.05$.
**$p < 0.01$.

Table 4. Performance of Low PS and High PS school-age groups on seven developmental measures

	CA	DAP	WISC-P	WISC-V	PPVT-D	UTLD-D	ATIC	PS-2A
Low PS Group								
Mean	9;6	94.7	99.3	94.4	4.3	4.2	2.1	7.7
Standard deviation	15.7	14.1	9.8	11.2	16.7	16.0	4.4	3.3
N	33	32	23	23	32	26	23	33
High PS Group								
Mean	10;2	100.5	104.2	101.1	−15.9	−12.1	1.3	16.5
Standard deviation	17.4	12.2	11.8	12.7	25.1	26.0	1.97	2.5
N	34	31	20	20	33	27	24	34
t	1.92	1.74	1.50	1.82	3.81	2.74	0.76	
p	0.03	0.04	0.08	0.04	0.0002	0.004	0.23	

CA, chronologic age; Artic, Templin-Darley Articulation Test; t, result of t-test between groups. See text for further explanation.

t-test values and significance levels are shown. The difference on the WISC-P and DAP were not statistically significant. The most dramatic differences between the Low PS and High PS groups were on the two language measures. The subjects with poorer PS scores were 7 months below chronologic age on the PPVT-D, whereas the ones with the better PS scores were 19 months ahead of their chronologic age. The differences for the High PS and Low PS groups on the two language tests were significant beyond the 0.01 level. Age and WISC-V differed at the 0.05 level. This again suggests that children with PS difficulty may continue to show improvement in their scores with age. Because of the age corrections on each of the other tests, one can presume that the age difference in the two groups was not a significant factor. Grey Oral Reading test results were available for 37 children. The difference between the two PS groups was significant at the 0.05 level, favoring the High PS group.

This review relates sound blending to disorders of articulation, language, reading, spelling, and even verbal IQ. Other studies were discussed by Hammill and Larsen (1974) and Katz and Harmon (1981). Because of this relationship, it would be appropriate for the audiologist and the speech-language pathologist to evaluate this skill when concerned with such disorders.

THE THERAPEUTIC USE OF PHONEMIC SYNTHESIS

The relationship between auditory synthesis and communication skills and learning still requires a great deal of research and thought. However, from the point of view of the child, the family, and the school, the academic questions and theories are of little significance. The more important questions are whether this skill can be trained, and, if so, whether this training will lead to improved performance in the presenting disabilities and enable the child to benefit more from other therapies and learning experiences. Information on these questions is not yet available for PS nor most other procedures. There is, however, a body of information on PS training sufficient to encourage strongly its consideration.

Previous Therapeutic Use of PS and Related Techniques

Orton (1937) found phonetic synthesis to be an effective method in remediating the problems of disabled readers who had impaired speech perception. He indicated that such children should be referred for therapy to the speech specialist, who is knowledgeable in the manipulation of phonemic elements. Orton reported that children who were given this type of auditory training often made spontaneous gains in their speech despite the fact that no speech therapy was given.

McGinnis (1963) was an advocate of the sound blending approach. She worked with children who had severe language impairment, rather than those with lesser magnitude problems such as learning disabilities or language delay. The simplification offered by this method was found to be particularly helpful in the early phases of therapy. The reader will see that what was a distortion for the uninitiated child serves as a simplification for the youngster who is trained in this method.

By 1969, Katz had developed a series of programmed lessons in PS to aid children with learning problems. There were eight lessons that increased gradually in difficulty (to minimize errors) by controlling the phonetic content and the length of words and clues. Each lesson was kept under 10 min in length and often included a review of previous material. Two or three lessons were given at each 30-min session, once or twice a week. The materials were presented to the children in a quiet room, at a comfortable listening level, with the use of a high-quality reel-to-reel tape player and loudspeakers.

The initial lessons used two and three multiple-choice picture responses. Next the children were to respond to the same sounds without the pictures, and finally they were given new materials for which they had to generate their own answers. Because the children experienced a high level of success and the recordings were rather light and humorous, the lessons tended to be highly motivating.

Katz and Burge (1971) studied the results from 29 children who had received the PS training program. They ranged in age from 5 to 15 years, with a mean of 8–10 years. The youngest children who took the PS-P test improved from a mean score of 11 to one of 26. Because the normal range on the PS-P is 16–24, this represented a vast improvement and suggested at least normal PS skills following therapy. The older children took the PS-2A test, and their mean score improved from 11 to 18. This also demonstrated excellent improvement from a mean below the normal range to the upper limit of normal. No test of statistical significance was carried out in this initial study; however, all of the children improved by more than 2 points on retest. Metzl (1969) found an average improvement of 2 points on immediate retest.

The considerable gains noted following auditory training in the above study tended to support the notion that children who receive PS training do better in this skill. This helps to answer our first concern, namely, whether PS is teachable, but not whether it has a beneficial effect on the presenting complaint or problem. A great deal of anecdotal information was highly encouraging and beyond our expectations. We also noted spontaneous improvement in speech intelligibility in these children who were referred because of reading and spelling problems and not because of their articulation or speech clarity. Children who were getting PS and other auditory training programs were often reported to have improved listening skills and to be better in decoding auditory messages. Orton (1937) had made similar observations.

A study was carried out to determine the effect of PS training on articulation (Katz & Medol, 1972). The children were 25 pupils who were receiving speech therapy in the public schools. They were divided into two groups matched according to age, type, and extent of articulation difficulty as well as performance on the PPVT. The randomly chosen experimental group ($N=13$) was given PS therapy, live voice, based on the PS programmed instruction. These youngsters received no speech therapy. The control group ($N=12$) was given traditional speech therapy alone.

Five children did not complete the study for various reasons. The remaining nine youngsters in the control group improved by 4 points on PS-2A (2 points better than expected for immediate retest). On the Goldman-Fristoe Articulation Test (G-F; Goldman & Fristoe, 1969), they eliminated a mean of more than 6 articulation errors (significant at the 0.05 level). The PS group showed greater improvement than the controls on both measures. On the PS-2A they improved by 7 items to within the normal range of performance, whereas the controls remained below the normal range. On the G-F they improved by about 10 (from 13 to 3) articulation errors. This change was significant at the 0.01 level. The authors did not recommend PS training in lieu of speech therapy. Rather, they suggested that a combination of the two would probably lead to better results than either one alone.

The importance of this study is that it provided evidence that PS training could result in improved articulation. Because the children in that group received no speech therapy per se, one can assume that the change was at least partly due to the auditory training. This could suggest that the improved auditory skills may then be utilized in another activity (e.g., monitoring speech). It is of little importance at this time whether the improvement was associated with learning PS itself or some associated skills that were acquired in therapy.

In another study (Katz et al., 1971) 24 children were given auditory training in the public schools. The eight PS lessons were administered, as well as four speech-in-noise lessons. The speech-in-noise program was based on the same concepts as the PS materials for the purpose of helping the children to deal better with noisy environments. The children were seen in groups, not exceeding six per group.

The children improved from a pretest score of about 9 to a posttest score of 17.5 on the PS-2A. All of the children improved, and 22 of them improved by more than the expected 2 points for test-retest. The children also showed the equivalent of a 3-year gain on the SSW test.

This study pointed out that improved performance on auditory tests can be obtained following auditory training, and that the therapy sessions can be carried out in groups. It is felt that more than one type of therapy can be done in a session and that this is probably advantageous. A second therapy not only can provide complementary training but also helps to maintain interest. We have not seen direct effects of PS training on language test results. It is perhaps unreasonable to expect improved auditory skills to show up quickly and measurably in tests of reading and language, especially in the absence of specific training.

Recent Therapeutic Use of Phonemic Synthesis

A revised and refined PS program was developed by Katz and Harmon (1982). Importantly, children are found to be interested and motivated by the materials, which are easy to utilize and to monitor. It is of special importance that people appear to show improvement in PS, articulation, and other listening skills on follow-up testing.

The present program is made up of 15 lessons for the purpose of improving central auditory skills. The expansion of the program provides more therapy compared to the earlier program, as well as more gradual increments in difficulty level, a greater number of words in more diverse contexts, and more time on the difficult phonemes (e.g., semivowels) and concepts. More time is spent on synthesizing consonant blends than in the previous program. As in the past, the children plotted their own performance on charts and were therefore better able to evaluate their progress.

If the child did not get a specified number of items correct on each of the lessons, he or she had to take the lesson again at another time until the criterion level of proficiency was reached. Children who did particularly poorly on the first attempt at a lesson received great pleasure in watching their performance go up on subsequent attempts when they plotted their results.

A pilot study was carried out with 11 children who were enrolled in the public schools. Seven of them were trained with the PS program, whereas the four control children, from the same population, continued to receive language or reading therapy to aid them with their school problems. A Wallensak tape player (reel-to-reel at 7½ inches per second) was situated 1–2 feet in front of the child. The therapy was carried out in a quiet speech therapy room. The PS-3A and the Lindamood Auditory Conceptualization (LAC) test were administered to the children before and after training. The LAC (Lindamood & Lindamood, 1969) was administered to determine whether the PS training would generalize to a different but related auditory skill. Most of the children had normal articulation, and therefore this was not assessed in this study.

For the seven experimental group children the median PS score rose from 4, which is below the 5th percentile, to 23, at the 95th percentile (Harmon, 1974). On the LAC they showed improvement equivalent to about 3 years in the 6 months between test and retest. During this period the control youngsters showed no apparent improvement on either test.

After some modifications were made in the program, six clinicians from four states (Kansas, Louisiana, Missouri, and New York) took part in field testing the materials. Four of the field testers were speech-language pathologists, one an audiologist, and the last a reading specialist. Each clinician was supplied with a PS-3A test and the 15 programmed lessons on cassette. The picture materials were also supplied. Instructions were given regarding the program's objectives and procedures. The school system or the field testers themselves supplied the cassette players.

The clinicians were asked to choose at least 12 children with whom they work who might benefit from auditory training. At least six were to be experimental subjects receiving PS training and matched to at least six youngsters of the same sex and with similar ages, problems, and PS scores, who would serve as controls. Each child had an articulation problem, a reading problem, or both.

Because some of the clinicians began their work toward the end of the term or were forced to handle other assignments, some of the children received relatively little therapy. All of the available results were used regardless of the length of therapy. Fifty-four children comprised the experimental (PS) group, and 31 served as controls. Fourteen percent of the children took six or fewer lessons (completing no more than 40% of the program). The median number of lessons for the 54 children (including repeats of previous lessons) was 18, ranging from 5 to 32. Forty-six percent of the group completed the entire 15-lesson program. The median number of sessions (visits) required to complete the program was 11 (ranging from 5 to 26). One child was able to complete the entire program in five visits by reaching the criterion level for each of the three lessons given each visit.

For the PS group the mean PS-3A score before therapy was 7 (equivalent to the 6th percentile for second- and third-grade children), and 17 on the posttest (the mean score for normal second- and third-graders). The control subjects, who were retested at approximately the same time as the PS children, went from a mean of 10 on the first test to a score of 13 on the second. The improvement shown by the experimental group was significantly greater (at the 0.001 level) than that for the controls.

Results on the LAC test were available for 19 children in the PS group and 14 in the control group. The mean performance on test and retest for the children who got the PS training went from 50 to 76, respectively, whereas the controls went from 52 to 61 in the same period. The difference score showed a greater improvement for the experimentals over the controls, which was statistically significant at the 0.01 level. On the Arizona Articulation Proficiency Scale (AAPS), the 17 children who were tested in the PS group improved from 90 to 93 (out of 100), whereas the children who received their regular speech therapy went from almost 91 to 92. The difference in improvement between the two groups was significant at the 0.001 level. Unfortunately, the therapy period for some of the children in both groups was quite short, limiting the potential gains. Despite problems in carrying out clinical research, the results we have obtained thus far in field testing with the PS program have been most encouraging.

DISCUSSION

The PS Program as an Auditory Training Procedure

The most important feature of the PS program is that children who take it tend to show improvement on tests of articulation as well as on tests of auditory perception. Although the lessons are graded in difficulty from very easy at the beginning to very hard at the end, the children after mastering lessons six through eight tend to do much better on succeeding lessons rather than more poorly.

For each program there is a "target zone" that indicates sufficient skill to proceed to the next lesson. The "completion level" indicates that the child has shown sufficient skill that that particular lesson need not be repeated. This feature provided a convenient method of assess-

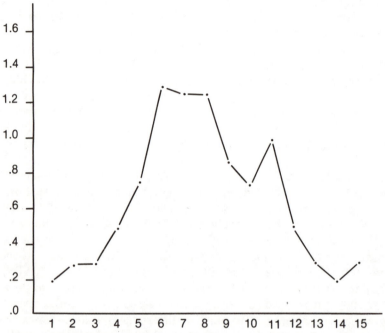

Figure 14.1 Mean number of times subjects retook each of the 15 lessons on the PS program (Katz & Harmon, 1981).

ing the relative difficulty levels of the various programs. The more difficult programs for the children are the ones that they had to repeat the most times.

Figure 1 shows the mean number of times that each lesson was repeated. A description of the materials will help to clarify the implications of the figure.

Figure 1 shows that it was quite unlikely that the children had to repeat any of the first three programs. These lessons begin with five simple key words (e.g., "eat" and "she"). For each of the key words there is a choice of two pictures (e.g., "eat" versus "pencil"). By the fourth lesson the child is weaned from the pictures, and four new words are added for which the child must generate his or her own answers. In lesson six all 15 of the words are new and contain the /l/ sound (e.g., "look" and "ball").

Given the progression of difficulty in the first six lessons it is not surprising to see the sharp increase in repetitions of the program for the average child. The lack of competence on lessons six through eight no doubt is a function of the difficulty these children have with perceiving the semivowels (Mange, 1953, 1955) and either no repetition of previous words or relatively few repetitions.

The lessons that follow contain even more difficult materials from the point of view of length and complexity. Lesson 8 has 16 new words and emphasizes consonant blends as well. Consonant blends are considered the most difficult PS task. Examples of the words are "spot" and "pink." Lesson 13 contains 30 new words such as "score," "trip," and "threw." In the final lesson many new words are introduced, such as "frost," "rifle," and "garage," and the hardest items from the previous lessons are reviewed.

One would think that the last half of the lessons would become progressively harder, just as was found with the first six lessons. The results were quite the contrary. Performance tended to improve rather than deteriorate, requiring fewer and fewer repetitions. The phenomenon is dramatized by the fact that the average number of repetitions for the first three lessons is the same as the last three. One can interpret these findings to suggest that the PS training in the first eight lessons not only facilitated the ability to blend but that the knowledge and familiarity of the speech sounds were sufficient to offset the increase in difficulty level.

Phonemic Synthesis and the Neurologic Model

In this chapter the close relationship between PS and the phonemic zone of the brain has been stressed. Luria (1970) indicated the three major features of the phonemic zone to be analysis, synthesis, and memory for phonemic material. The test of PS requires that each sound be analyzed without cues from the surrounding sounds and often without contextual cues. The child who is not clear about how the speech sounds actually sound is not aided by the added length of the sounds. In fact, for such a child it might serve as a further distortion. Calearo and Lazzaroni (1957) found that increasing the length of sounds could make speech more difficult for those with central auditory deficiencies. The pauses between the sounds and the overall duration of the item should create a strong challenge to the child's memory, especially if the child has poor blending skills. Good auditory conceptualization, as trained in the Lindamood program, should aid a child in fusing the succeeding sounds together. If, however, the child has not mastered this skill, then he or she is relegated to retain in memory relatively meaningless individual sounds. This, of course, increases the difficulty of the memory task, because meaningful material is easier to remember than nonmeaningful material. Thus, PS seems uniquely suited to challenge the functions of the phonemic zone.

The reader may be surprised that a child would have difficulty in identifying individual phonemes. We recently worked with an adult who had apparently had auditory processing deficits all her life. On hearing the sounds /i/ /t/ in an early PS lesson she correctly pointed to the picture of "eat," but showed amazement that the /t/ was even a human sound. She was incredulous to learn that /l/ was the "L" sound. She had the clinician repeat it for her and eventually tried to produce a similar sound herself. She was very pleased with her own production and commented, "That sounds just like everyone else." She indicated that the "L" sound sounded to her like /ɪdl/. This explained why her response to /b/ /ɔ/ /l/ was /bɔɪdl/ then *bottle* instead of *ball*. Although this is perhaps an extreme case, it is not an isolated problem.

How might dysfunction or inefficiency occur in the phonemic zone to produce limited PS performance and the associated communication and learning problems? Direct effects on phonemic zone function could result from genetic factors causing delayed or inferior levels of development. Trauma, infection, or allergy could be other etiologic factors. Even children who have normal or near normal anatomy and physiology for their ages could develop poor skills behaviorally linked to the middle and posterior temporal region. Fluctuating or inconsistent stimulation during periods of great CNS plasticity might cause the child to encode faulty, vague, or inconsistent engrams representing the sounds of the language. From the work of Webster (Chapter 10, this volume) and others one can infer that during periods of auditory plasticity faulty or rearranged CNS organization or development could occur (Beggs & Foreman, 1980; Coleman & O'Connor, 1979; Folsom, 1979; Henry & Haythorn, 1975; Tees, 1967). Studies in vision and other sensory modalities support and expand our knowledge about potential effects of early environmental influences on the structure and function of the brain and the subsequent behavior (Taylor & Taylor, 1979; Bennett et al., 1964; Freedman, 1971).

The studies cited above help to explain why a fluctuating conductive hearing loss could lead to poor PS ability. This was indeed observed by various investigators (Lewis, 1976; Katz & Illmer, 1972; Holm & Kunze, 1969).

Regardless of the specific cause of the problem, if a child's engrams are imprinted with somewhat vague, inconsistent, or inaccurate information, inefficiency in listening could result because of imprecise decoding. Even if the child subsequently obtains normal hearing and full maturation there may still be a problem of "listening through faulty engrams." The child might have difficulty in altering these inaccurate concepts because speech is generally too fast to focus on individual speech sounds, and these children require more than normal processing time (Tallal, 1980). The quicker the speech and the briefer the pauses, the more difficulty this child should have. If this is the case, it is little wonder that children who have PS difficulties tend to have problems in language skills even as they get older.

What does PS therapy provide that would help such a child? It would seem that the PS therapy, as described here, has the features that can break the failure cycle by helping the child to improve his or her engrams. Presenting each sound distinctly and independently gives the child an excellent opportunity to gain a greater appreciation of what the sound truly is. This is enhanced even when auditory processing is slow and inefficient by extending the duration of the sounds that can be lengthened. The long pauses that follow each phoneme provide ample time for the child to process the signal fully and to deal with it on a metalinguistic level (Rees, 1981) before the next sound arrives. Besides the most important features mentioned above, the use of the most standard production of the phoneme may help in two ways. First, there is less variation, which could have confused the child at the early stages. Once this standard production is learned, the child might then be better able to generalize from this sound because of its more neutral or medial position. Children who take the PS program might also benefit because they hear the sounds and see the pictures of the words they represent. Perhaps this helps to teach the child that a word is not an amorphous mass, but rather is composed of sounds that are blended together.

As the child begins to improve in his or her concept of what the sounds of the language actually sound like, the child slowly becomes more proficient in listening (decoding). With improved efficiency the child will have more time to analyze the sounds in conversation as well as strengthen his or her concepts of the various phonemes from the PS lessons. Once the child begins to improve, one could expect that having a clear notion of the sounds and needing less time to analyze speech could carry over into better listening, a better concept of the sounds for self-monitoring, and having better auditory information for use in spelling and reading therapy.

Many questions yet remain to be answered, and replication of the previous work would be in order. Nevertheless, the work with PS to date is very encouraging. Diagnostically, it seems to give us insight into problems of auditory decoding, articulation, language, spelling, and reading. Using PS as a therapeutic tool seems to produce important gains not only in the ability to sound-blend but also in other auditory skills and in articulation. It is helpful that when these factors are viewed from a model based primarily on the work of Luria, we are able to better understand why this skill should be such a valuable diagnostic and therapeutic aid.

REFERENCES

Bannatyne, A. D., and Wichiarajote, P. 1969. Relationship between written spelling, motor functioning and sequencing skills. Journal of Learning Disorders 2:6–18.

Beasley, D. S., Shriner, T. H., Manning, W. H., and Beasley, D. C. 1974. Auditory assembly of CVC's by children with normal and defective articulation. Journal of Communication Disorders 7:127–133.

Beggs, W. D. A., and Foreman, D. L. 1980. Sound localization and early binaural experience in the deaf. British Journal of Audiology 14:41–48.

Bennett, E. L., Diamond, M. C., Krech, D., and Rosenzweig, M. R. 1964. Chemical and anatomical plasticity of brain. Science 146:610–619.

Burns, M. S., and Canter, G. J. 1977. Phonemic behavior of aphasic patients with posterior cerebral lesions. Brain and Language 4:492–507.

Calearo, C., and Lazzaroni, A. 1957. Speech intelligibility in relation to the speed of the message. Laryngoscope 67:410–419.

Celesia, G. G. 1976. Organization of auditory cortical areas in man. Brain 99:403–414.

Chall, J. S., Roswell, F. G., and Blumenthal, S. 1963. Auditory blending ability: A factor in success in early reading. Reading Teacher 17:113–120.

Coleman, J. R., and O'Connor, P. 1979. Effects of monaural and binaural sound deprivation on cell development in the anteroventral cochlear nucleus of rats. Experimental Neurology 64:553–566.

Conners, C. K., Kramer, K., and Guerra, F. 1969. Auditory synthesis and dichotic listening in children with learning disabilities. Journal of Special Education 3:163–169.

Duane, D. 1977. A neurologic perspective of central auditory dysfunction. In: R. W. Keith (ed.), Central Auditory Dysfunction, pp. 1–42. Grune & Stratton, New York.

Dunn, L. M. 1965. Peabody Picture Vocabulary Test. American Guidance Service, Circle Pines, Minn.

Elliott, H. C. 1969. Textbook of Neuroanatomy, 2nd Edition. J. B. Lippincott, Philadelphia.

Folsom, R. C. 1979. Auditory brainstem responses in children with early recurrent middle ear disease. Unpublished doctoral dissertation, University of Washington, Seattle.

Freedman, D. A. 1971. Congenital and perinatal sensory deprivation: Some studies in early development. American Journal of Psychiatry 127:115–121.

Geschwind, N. 1970. The organization of language and the brain. Science 170:940–944.

Goldman, R., and Fristoe, M. 1969. Goldman-Fristoe Test of Articulation. American Guidance Service, Circle Pines, Minn.

Goldman, R., Fristoe, M., and Woodcock, M. 1974. GFB perceptual training drills. American Guidance Service, Circle Pines, Minn.

Gross, M. B., and Wilson, W. C. 1974. Minimal Brain Dysfunction. Brunner/ Mazel, New York.

Hammill, D. D., and Larsen, S. C. 1974. The relationship of selected auditory perceptual skills and reading ability. Journal of Learning Disorders 7:40–46.

Harmon, C. H. 1974. Collection and analysis of normative data on two tests of auditory perception: Phonemic synthesis #3, and same/different discrimination #4. Unpublished master's thesis, Central Missouri State University, Warrensburg, Mo.

Hatfield, F. M. 1981. Analysis and remediation of aphasia in the U.S.S.R.: The contribution of A. R. Luria. Journal of Speech and Hearing Disorders 46:338–347.

Henry, K. R., and Haythorn, M. M. 1975. Auditory similarities associated with genetic and experimental acoustic deprivation. Journal of Comparative and Physiological Psychology 89:213–218.

Hier, D. B., LeMay, M., Rosenberger, P. B., and Perlo, V. P. 1978. Developmental dyslexia: Evidence for a subgroup with reversal of cerebral asymmetry. Archives of Neurology 35:90–92.

Holm, V. A., and Kunze, L. H. 1969. Effect of chronic otitis media on language and speech development. Pediatrics 43:833–839.

Katz, J. 1971. Kindergarten Auditory Screening Test. Follett Educational Corporation, Chicago.

Katz, J. 1976. Localizing auditory disorders of the brain and brainstem. Short course presented at the American Speech and Hearing Association Convention, November 23, 1976, Houston, Texas.

Katz, J. 1978. SSW Workshop Manual. Allentown Industries, Buffalo, N.Y.

Katz, J., and Burge, C. 1971. Auditory perception training for children with learning disabilities. Menorah Medical Journal 2:18–29.

Katz, J., and Harmon, C. H. 1981. Phonemic synthesis: Testing and training. In: R. Keith (ed.), Central Auditory and Language Disorders, pp. 145–157. College-Hill Press, Houston.

Katz, J., and Harmon, C. H. 1982. Phonemic synthesis: Blending sounds into words. Developmental Learning Materials, Allen, Tx.

Katz, J., and Illmer, R. 1972. Auditory perception in children with language disabilities. In: J. Katz (ed.), Handbook of Clinical Audiology. Williams & Wilkins, Baltimore.

Katz, J., and Medol, I. 1972. The use of phonemic synthesis in speech therapy. Menorah Medical Journal 3:10–18.

Katz, J., Beyers, V., Illmer, R., et al. 1971. Implementation of a comprehensive educational program for children with learning disabilities. Grandview Consolidated School District No. 4, Grandview, Mo.

Katz, J., Chubrich, R. C., Davis, R. E., Gallaway, K. C., and Illmer, R. 1969. Speech, hearing, language and auditory perceptual function in children with learning disabilities. Grandview Consolidated School District No. 4, Grandview, Mo.

Katz, J., Davis, R. E., Johnson, M. G., Struckmann, S., and Illmer, R. 1970. Early identification of exceptional children. Grandview Consolidated School District No. 4, Grandview, Mo.

Kirk, S. A., McCarthy, J. J., and Kirk, W. D. 1968. Illinois Test of Psycholinguistic Ability. University of Illinois Press, Urbana, Ill.

Lewis, N. 1976. Otitis media and linguistic incompetence. Archives of Otolaryngology 102:387–390.

Liberman, A. M., Harris, K. S., Kinney, J. A., and Lane, H. 1961. The discrimination of relative onset-time of the components of certain speech and nonspeech patterns. Journal of Experimental Psychology 61:379–388.

Lindamood, C. H., and Lindamood, P. C. 1969. Auditory discrimination in depth. Teaching Resources, Boston.

Lucker, J. R. 1980. Diagnostic significance of the type A pattern of the Staggered Spondaic Word (SSW) test. Audiology and Hearing Education 6:21–23.

Luria, A. R. 1966. Higher Cortical Functions in Man. Basic Books, New York.

Luria, A. R. 1970. Traumatic Aphasia: Its Syndromes, Psychology and Treatment. Mouton, The Hague.

Mange, C. 1953. A study of speech sound discrimination within words and within sentences. Unpublished master's thesis, Pennsylvania State University, University Park, Pa.

Mange, C. 1955. Relationships between selected auditory factors and articulation ability. Unpublished doctoral dissertation, Pennsylvania State University, University Park, Pa.

Mange, C. 1960. Relationships between selected auditory perceptual factors and articulatory ability. Journal of Speech and Hearing Research 3:367–374.

Mattingly, I. G. 1972. Reading the linguistic process, and linguistic awareness. In: J. F. Kavanaugh and I. G. Mattingly (eds.), Language by Ear and by Eye. MIT Press, Cambridge, Mass.

McGinnis, M. A. 1963. Aphasic Children: Identification and Training by the Association Method. Alexander Graham Bell Association for the Deaf, Washington, D.C.

Mecham, M. J., Jex, J. L., and Jones, J. D. 1967. Utah Test of Language Development. Woodruff Printing and Litho, Salt Lake City, Utah.

Metzl, M. N. 1969. Measurements of sound synthesis ability in second, fourth, and sixth grade children and adults. Unpublished master's thesis, Hunter College, New York.

Monroe, M. 1932. Children Who Cannot Read. University of Chicago Press, Chicago.

Mulder, R. L. and Curtin, J. 1955. Vocal phonic ability and silent reading achievement: A first report. Elementary School Journal 56:121–123.

Oliphant, G. 1971. Oliphant Auditory Synthesizing Test. Educators Publishing Service, Cambridge, Mass.

Orton, S. T. 1937. Reading, Writing, and Speech Problems in Children. Norton, New York.

Penfield, W., and Roberts, L. 1959. Speech and Brain Mechanisms. Princeton University Press, Princeton, N.J.

Pirozzolo, F., and Rayner, K. 1979. Cerebral organization and reading disability. Neuropsychologica 17:485–491.

Rees, N. S. 1981. Saying more than we know: Is auditory processing disorder a meaningful concept? In: R. Keith (ed.), Central Auditory and Language Disorders in Children. College-Hill Press, Houston.

Roswell, F. G., and Chall, J. S. 1963. Roswell-Chall Auditory Blending Test. Essay Press, New York.

Sawyer, D. J. 1981. The relationship between selected auditory abilities and beginning reading achievement. Language, Speech and Hearing Services in Schools 12:95–99.

Sloan, C. 1980. Auditory processing disorders and language development. In:
P. Levinson and C. Sloan (eds.), Auditory Processing and Language: Clinical
and Research Perspectives pp. 101–116. Grune & Stratton, New York.

Stovall, J. V., Manning, W. H., and Shaw, C. K. 1977. Auditory assembly of
children with mild and severe misarticulations. Folia Phoniatrica
29:162–172.

Tallal, P. 1980. Auditory processing disorders in children. In: P. Levinson and
C. Sloan (eds.), Auditory Processing and Language pp.81–100. Grune &
Stratton, New York.

Taylor, V., and Taylor, D. 1979. Critical period for deprivation amblyopia in
children. Transactions of the Ophthalmological Societies of the United
Kingdom 99:432–439.

Tees, R. C. 1967. Effects of early auditory restriction in the rat on adult pattern
discrimination. Journal of Comparative Physiological Psychology 63:
389–393.

Templin, M. C., and Darley, F. L. 1960. The Templin-Darley Test of Articulation. Bureau of Educational Research, Iowa City, Iowa.

Travis, L. E., and Rasmus, B. 1931. The speech sound discrimination ability of
cases with functional disorders of articulation. Quarterly Journal of Speech
17:217–226.

Urban, D. H. 1963. Draw-A-Person test. Western Psychological Services,
Los Angeles.

Vellutino, F. 1977. Alternative conceptualizations of dyslexia: Evidence in support of a verbal-deficit hypothesis. Harvard Education Review 47:334–354.

Wechsler, D. 1949. Wechsler Intelligence Scale for Children. Psychological
Corporation, New York.

Wiig, E. H., and Semel, E. M. 1976. Language Disabilities in Children and
Adolescents. Charles E. Merrill, Columbus, Ohio.

Chapter 15

Language Processing

Selective Attention and Mnemonic Strategies

Katharine G. Butler

This chapter addresses auditory language processing, with specific emphasis on attention and cognition. Although various attributes such as attention and efforts and memory strategies are discussed separately, as components of the language processing act, it is not to be inferred that they occur as isolated or as separate and sequential events. The intent is not to suggest that language processing involves sequential and conscious "skills," each of which is amenable to direct instruction. As Norman (1979) noted, it is difficult to believe the "human mind is divided up into little compartments" (p. 121); rather, humans tend to respond in an integrated fashion. The current research efforts to analyze the ability to function holistically in a complex environment might seem of only esoteric interest to clinicians who must daily devise intervention strategies for language-disordered individuals. Discussions of schemas, structures, and memory pools may seem to provide little practical guidance. Although this research in cognitive processing may not provide all the answers as yet, there are some fascinating clues and emerging data which can be helpful to the clinician. Clinical techniques based on these notions are, however, experiments at this time.

AUDITORY LANGUAGE PROCESSING: A DEFINITION

Auditory language processing is considered as a psychologic process within an information processing model. Such a model delineates component processes which occur between the time a language stimulus is provided and the time a "meaning" response is given (Massaro, 1975). Language processing has been defined as "the abstraction of meaning from an acoustic signal or from printed text" (Massaro, 1975, p. 5). Thus, the term *auditory language processing* for this discussion is limited to "the abstraction of meaning from an acoustic signal and the retrieval of that meaning." In many ways, this is how speech-language pathologists and audiologists have viewed language; comprehension of oral language and expression have long been primary areas to be evaluated. What is added, perhaps, is the attempt to analyze language as a series of intertwined events, each necessary but not sufficient to account for the way individuals identify, extract, and utilize linguistic information. Here, language is analyzed with regard to such mechanisms as attention, perception, and memory, with the recognition that each of these mechanisms is related not only to each other but to the use of language (Gerber, 1981). Language-processing testing procedures do assess mental representations and memorial strategies used in performing language tasks (Sternberg, 1981). Therefore, in assessing language and its disorders we must recognize the basic relationships among attention, perception, and memory. Each is presumed to be controlled by internal cognitive functions or "central control processes" (Blumenthal, 1977) (Table 1).

The next section reviews some current and sometimes conflicting evidence regarding attention, particularly selective attention. There are a number of attention models in cognitive psychology, including those by Klatzky (1979), Lindsay and Norman (1977), Rumelhart (1977), and Wickelgren (1979). We will, however, consider primarily the work of Kahneman (1973), Massaro (1975), Norman (1979), and Anderson (1980).

SELECTIVE ATTENTION

Although we often speak of attention as if it were a single and conscious thing, it is really a multiprocess construct (Sexton & Geffen , 1979). Attention can be viewed in many ways: one can speak of attention span, of attention switching, of focused and divided attention, of thresholds of attention, and of intensive attention, either individually or in various combinations. Most importantly, we know attention is limited, or finite.

The role of attention and effort in processing has important implications for the speech-language pathologist and the audiologist. All individuals have limited attention and effort, and even normals find that some concurrent activities which require attention interfere with each other. It may be important to use such evaluation procedures as competing messages, dichotic listening tasks, and auditory figure-ground tests. *All* auditory information may enter sensory memory; however, because attention is limited, not all information can be attended to, and some is lost (Anderson, 1980).

Interest has increased in measuring the developmental interaction between attention and perception among normal and language-disordered children. Young children use relatively inefficient strategies in attending and perceiving (Kinsbourne & Caplan, 1979). Lack of experience rather than age per se may account for this. Young children (particularly language-disordered children) tend to pay more attention to meaningful items, that is, those represented in long-term memory (Gerber, 1981), but the store of items in long-term memory may be limited by a comparatively small repertoire of semantic and episodic memories.

Let us identify some terms. *Selective attention* implies attending to some mental activities in preference to others (Kahneman, 1973). Selective attention may be *divided,* as in dichotic listening tasks when more than one input may provide relevant information, or *focused,* as in competing message tasks where the subject is asked to listen to one message and exclude others. When one is unable to ignore irrelevant information, and performance suffers, an attentional limitation exists (Shiffrin, 1976).

One way to identify auditory attentional difficulties is to measure interference among concurrent auditory events. In so doing, we need to consider the subject's familiarity with information. Well known information requires less attention than novel information and is processed accurately and rapidly. When items (linguistic or otherwise) are practiced they become *automatic* and require a minimum of attention. Novel stimuli, however, require considerable conscious attention, and processing novel or unknown stimuli requires *deliberate* attention and more time. When reviewing current dichotic, competing messages and auditory figure-ground tests, the examiner needs not only to compare performance against existent norms but to measure reaction time *quantitatively* and estimate the familiarity of the stimuli presented *qualitatively*. This calls for the combined skills of the speech-language pathologist and the audiologist, because most of the assessment may be conducted by the audiologist, but interpretation requires knowledge of linguistic and semantic variables.

Normal children as young as 7 years are known to have developed differentiated strategies for focusing and dividing attention, and these attentional strategies become increasingly sophisticated with age. Geffen and Sexton (1978) note that resistance to distraction does not improve with age for focused attention tasks: children are unable to ignore irrelevant stimuli when asked to do so in the presence of relevant stimuli, but they are increasingly able to resist distraction for divided attention tasks, for example, when they are asked to listen to two relevant messages at the same time. It is not clear whether the increased ability to resist auditory distraction between the ages of 7 and 10 is due to increased attentional control or to the simultaneous development of more sophisticated memory and retrieval strategies (Butler, 1981a), discussed later in this chapter.

We have said that attention is not a single act or entity. Most of us can attend to two tasks simultaneously, but only when such tasks do not make excessive demands. We encounter difficulty when we are asked to perform two demanding tasks at the same time. In attending to auditory information, Bregman (1978) pointed out that "We are built to pay attention to auditory sources, not to acoustic components, [and the manner in which we] build auditory descriptions . . . out of complex acoustic input [places] strong constraints on the process of attention" (p. 74). Whereas many aspects of comprehending auditory language seem to be automatic in normal subjects (Anderson, 1980), at least some language-disordered individuals may be unable to attend and process auditory information with the same degree of automaticity.

Effort and Attention

The educator and the clinician frequently deal with so-called unmotivated children who do not "put forth sufficient effort." Professionals feel that if they can assist children to "attend," learning will be increased. Those of us who deal clinically with children and adults who "can't seem to remember directions," or "don't listen," or "can't comprehend instructions," tend to say that our clients are not putting forth enough *effort*. Effort (as well as attention), however, is limited. There is a finite amount of effort that may be expended which cannot be increased (Kahneman, 1973). You cannot try harder if you are giving full effort to a task.

Effort is a momentary matter, varying continuously and depending upon the load imposed by the task demands. Tasks with different levels of complexity require varying amounts of both attention and effort. Some attention and effort are usually expended on perceptual monitoring of the environment. This is called *spare capacity* (Kahneman, 1973), but such spare capacity diminishes when effort is put forward to answer task demands, thereby being withdrawn from perceptual monitoring.

Individuals can allocate their effort and in some respects their attention. This allocation is highly flexible among normal individuals. We know little about such allocation among the language-disordered. We do know, however, that task difficulty and time pressure both create differing demands on attention and effort. Thus, speech-language pathologists and audiologists may wish to examine their assessment instruments with an eye to the role played by task difficulty and time pressure. Certainly, attention, effort, and short-term memory are affected by the complexity of the auditory task and the temporal aspects of processing.

Attending and Emotion

Bower (1981) hypothesized a link between emotions and attention. He noted that subjects actively and selectively attend to material that is consistent with their feelings. Bower stated that emotions may even cause "congruent" words to "pop out" at the perceiver. It is interesting to speculate the degree to which emotional states impact upon attending and memory. Bower argued that emotion powerfully influences certain cognitive processes. Certainly we should be aware that emotions, moods, and motivation may be important to our allocation of effort and attention to incoming stimuli, as well as to how we process, retain, and recall information.

Physiologic Correlates of Effort and Attention

Although few practitioners measure the physiologic correlates of attention, some authorities have reported (again from adult research) that "arousal and effort are usually not determined prior to the action: they vary continuously, depending on the load which is imposed by what one does at any instant of time" (Kahneman, 1973, p. 16). The demands of the task are thought to control the mobilization of effort. Obviously, then, the level of complexity of the task is related to the degree of physiologic arousal and the amount of effort and attention devoted to the task. You need only think of the last time you were required to take a difficult written or oral examination for which you were ill prepared, to recall both your emotional and cognitive response.

A Review: Implications for Evaluation of Auditory Processing

We stated that auditory language is processed by abstracting meaning from an acoustic signal. "Listening" is complex and involves attention, perception, and memory. We identified the importance of attention, particularly selective attention. Attention is limited—we cannot attend to all the auditory information we may perceive. We must, and do, selectively attend. Through the use of focused and divided attention tasks we gain some understanding of an individual's ability to attend to relevant messages, ignore irrelevant stimuli, and resist auditory distractions. We need to consider the listener's familiarity with the auditory information. Well known items require little attention and effort to process; items that are novel or unknown require greater attention and effort. Consider these two instructions: 1) say the first three letters of the alphabet; 2) say "Popocatepetl." Comprehending and responding to instruction 1 is relatively simple; instruction 2 probably requires greater attention and effort to give the correct response.

Linked closely with attention is effort. The difficulty of the task affects our capacity to attend. Complex tasks might include situations such as attempting to understand what is said in a congested airport under particularly noisy conditions, listening to a lecturer explaining a conceptual model unfamiliar to you, assigning meaning to nonsense words, and the like.

We noted that emotion can affect how closely we attend and how much effort we put forth. Intuitively we may know that mood and motivation play an important role. Rarely, however, do we consider these factors in administering language processing tasks. Unless the child or adult is demonstrably upset or is unwilling to continue with testing, we tend to assume that he or she is putting forth effort and attention to complete the listening task successfully. Such may not be the case, and thus we might consider several testing periods.

Finally, we suggested that the amount of effort required may vary at any single moment. The level of task complexity, the *processing load*, may dictate the level of effort required. We need to examine our language testing instruments with their potential for *overload*, that is, for linguistic, perceptual, or cognitive requirements beyond the attentional capacity of our clients.

We considered only a portion of the factors relevant to evaluating attention. We also need to assess attention relative to the *kind* and *quality* of the auditory stimuli in our test instruments and intervention procedures. Does the child attend to the stimuli presented? Are multiple stimuli presented? Are such stimuli sequential or concurrent? Does the time permitted for response (reaction time) vary according to the complexity of the stimuli? Are multiple responses required? Is time for rehearsal of the incoming information provided? As we shall see, strategies for placing items in memory require rehearsal.

To place attention, perception, and cognition in perspective, two models of processing are briefly reviewed. One's inclination toward one or the other model, whether the data-driven, bottom-up model or the cognitive, top-down model, may dictate the assessment instruments selected and the intervention methods devised.

MODELS OF PROCESSING

There is considerable discussion as to whether information processing is primarily perceptual or primarily cognitive. Does information move in a sequential fashion or in a more fluid fashion, beginning with "shallow" sensory processing and moving to deeper levels of semantic and cognitive functioning?

The sequential or *multistore* model hypothesizes that information moves step by step through a series of memory stores. Information is received at the sense organ. Perceptually relevant features are derived, then pieced together and interpreted. Data which "drive" the processing act are incoming auditory stimuli which are then analyzed and assigned meaning. This bottom-up model is summarized only briefly here and in Table 1. It is the approach used by speech-language pathologists and audiologists when they measure processing via tests of speech discrimination, auditory closure, analysis and synthesis, auditory fusion, and the like. Intervention which stresses such "auditory skills" is presumed to be in keeping with such a model.

Whereas the multistore model proposed that information is held in short-term memory in an auditory-verbal-linguistic code and held in long-term memory in semantic and episodic memory, the depth-of-processing model stresses that information is retained based upon how deeply it is processed. Essentially, sensory processing of the stimuli is thought to be "shallow," and semantic processing is thought to be "deep," involving higher-order cognitive structures.

There is experimental evidence for both a perceptual and a cognitive model; there is considerable research to support both directions of processing (Norman, 1979). In either case, the concept of memory, both short- and long-term, is essential, although how information gets to short-term and long-term memory is seen differently in the different models.

Each model poses certain problems for those who must translate models into evaluation and remediation procedures. The multistore model may be adopted more easily, because it provides a framework to examine such things as rehearsal strategies, coding strategies, short- and long-term memory, episodic and semantic memory, and search pro-

Table 1.   Alternate models of processing: Multistore and depth-of-processing
models

Multistore model[a]	Depth-of-processing[b]

Three types of memory storage:
  Sensory registers
  Short-term memory (STM)
  Long-term memory (LTM)
Information flows through component stores, moving from sensory to STM to LTM.
	Initial levels of processing involve sensory processing (physical features) and stimulus properties: shallow processing, progressing to deeper abstract and semantic levels.

STM is limited in capacity; LTM is essentially unlimited.	Retention of information related to "depth" of processing
Information in STM is in auditory-verbal-linguistic code.	Information in STM may be coded in auditory-verbal-linguistic form but may also be in semantic-visual code
Information lost in STM is due to decay or displacement.	Information is encoded at various depths; nature of activity is primary determinant of retention.
Information is held in LTM in semantic and episodic memory; information lost from LTM is due to interference or temporary irretrievability.	Various encoding conditions have an effect on what is stored in memory; nature of activity is primary determinant of retention or loss.
Storage and retrieval (control processes) change according to task, are subject to individual's control, and include rehearsal, coding and search plans.	Recall is a by-product of the type of processing carried out on the material; mnemonic processing is deliberate, automatic processing is not.

[a]Based on Atkinson and Shiffrin (1968) and Ornstein (1978).
[b]Based on Craik and Lockhart (1972) and Ornstein (1978).

cedures for recognizing and recalling information. Because central control processes are thought to be under conscious control, it is possible to devise assessment tasks to measure at least a portion of these processes. We recognize, however, that changes in the complexity of the task directly affect storage and retrieval of that information. A format for evaluating performance across tasks is provided later in this discussion.

Perhaps more difficult to conceptualize are the depth-of-processing models wherein information is thought to be encoded at various depths. How well information is retained has to do with the depth of processing. Here, too, the conditions surrounding the moment of encoding have an effect on what is stored in memory. We may need to examine auditory assessment procedures through new questions. We require that instruments be valid, reliable, well normed, and technically excellent, but we should also ask ourselves what they require at the moment of processing and what kind of memory strategies may be required.

The levels-of-processing models emphasize the continuity between perception and memory. They stress the importance of the manner in which to-be-remembered material is studied prior to its retrieval and assist in the analysis of processes underlying learning (Tulving, 1979).

MEMORY SCHEMA ANALYSIS

Readers who wish to pursue recent permutations of the models presented here may find Norman (1979) helpful. He combined features of the multistore and depth-of-processing models to hypothesize that perceptual analysis is guided by an overall goal of integrating our interpretation of events. Perceptual events are recognized and interpreted within the context of past events. This requires a match between the information being processed and that stored in memory. Perceptual information and memory information must match, or the discrepancies must be accounted for. Past experiences create a large number of memory structures, or schemas, which are used to organize knowledge and serve as an interface between perception and memory. In Norman's view, bottom-up and top-down models of processing are both necessary, but neither is sufficient. I frequently refer to this approach as the "halfway up the down staircase" model.

To summarize, Norman (1979) proposed a model that requires perceptual analysis guided by stored memory schemas and a need for integrated interpretation. Thus, both bottom-up and top-down processing concepts coexist in his model. A match is sought between the sound pattern held in short-term memory and the representation or schema in long-term memory. With this model, evaluation of the sound pattern held in short-term memory is still relevant, but we must add measures of information held in long-term memory. A number of procedures can be borrowed from investigations of cognitive processing and memory strategies. In the next section, we look briefly at memory processing for clues of how to evaluate memory and the strategies used in storing and retrieving information.

MEMORY PROCESSING

No matter which model we use as a rationale for evaluation of auditory language processing, we need to assess how information is represented in memory and how it is retrieved from memory. To do so, we can borrow from literature on memory development and adapt experimental tasks to our needs. We can see such tests as short-term memory for digits with new eyes and recognize that one of the things measured by digit recall is "maintenance rehearsal."

In dealing with infants and young children, one can adapt tasks that require various levels of episodic and semantic memory (Naus, Ornstein, & Hoving, 1978), memory strategies of young children (Perlmutter, 1980) and of infants (Nelson & Ross, 1980), as well as the assessment of cognitive development (Roberts, 1981). From their work and the work of researchers in communicative disorders (Keith, 1981), we can devise assessment procedures which begin to answer some of our questions and provide initial guidelines for intervention.

In evaluating memory processing we may look at the distinction made between *episodic* and *semantic memory*. Asking a 9-year-old, "What happened on your fifth birthday?" is a very different kind of question than, "What happens on birthdays?" The first question requires recall of a specific, dated event, whereas the second requires a merging of many such episodes into a semantically based memory. Episodic memory is stored as an autobiographical reference and is susceptible to loss or transformation. (Anyone who has witnessed a car accident and been asked to give the police a report some days later knows the difficulty of accurate recall.) Semantic memory is much less susceptible to transformation and loss, because it reflects generalized knowledge and a language-based organization freed from specific experiences (Tulving, 1972; Nelson & Brown, 1978). Language tasks that require a child to "name four things in your living room" are quite different from those that require a child to "name as many wild animals as you can in the next 30 seconds." Not only are the types of memory involved different, but the time constraint also differs. Both the type of memory sought and the time allotted for response may affect the outcome.

New areas of inquiry include metacognition and cognitive monitoring (Flavell, 1979). How children think about their own thought processes and memory strategies and how they monitor those strategies is of increasing interest. It is not yet clear, however, how we can apply research on "thinking about thinking" to the children with language processing disorders. Attempts to teach handicapped children metacognitive strategies have met with limited success (Kauffman, 1980). Over the next few years we may begin to see procedures for training metacognitive strategies developed for the language-disordered and learning-disabled child.

ASSESSMENT

Wallach (1981) proposed at least three general categories to be assessed when evaluating language skills. These include:

1. Language components or levels, i.e., phonologic, syntactic, semantic, and pragmatic;
2. Information load, i.e., type and content of information provided, including analysis of the stimuli, the quantity of the stimuli and the context in which the stimuli are provided;
3. Strategies required by the stimuli presented, e.g., analysis of the linguistic-semantic problem-solving nature of the response.

It has been suggested (Butler, 1981b) that language tasks (or tests) be presented in a variety of assessment contexts, including the presentation of linguistic stimuli:

1. At differing rates of speed;
2. At differing levels of linguistic complexity;
3. Under variable background noise conditions;
4. Utilizing varying kinds of interruptions of an auditory nature, and at different rates;
5. At differing levels of familiarity (known, partially known, unknown);
6. At differing levels of concreteness and abstractness.

By varying conditions and systematically varying the response time required, estimates can be made of language processing abilities or disabilities. Differences in performance may be noted when a child is permitted to respond immediately as opposed to when the examiner requires that the child delay or postpone the response, thus noting short-term and long-term memory storage and retrieval strategies.

Visual processing has not been discussed, but it may be worthwhile to measure the individual's ability to resist auditory and visual distraction separately as well as together. The ability to focus upon relevant information and filter out irrelevant information is important to attending, processing, and retrieval.

A number of the items suggested above will permit analysis of a listener's performance on temporal and sequential language tasks and will provide insight into the automaticity and speed with which such tasks are processed. Information on facilitating children's performance on memory tasks is seen in Myers and Perlmutter's (1978) work with 2- to 5-year-olds and Paris's (1978) review in the same text. When analyzing task responses, consider whether the task requires simply recognition or whether it requires recall, as these procedures may require different "steps" (Perlmutter & Lange, 1978). Recall involves self-generated representations matched to memory representations, and requires encoding, searching, and decision making. Recognition requires that presented information be examined to decide which items are actually the to-be-remembered items. Recognition is considered relatively nonstrategic, whereas recall requires a higher level of mnemonic strategies. Recognition tasks frequently call for no more than *maintenance* rehearsal (i.e., holding items in short-term memory to pick out a to-be-remembered item from a set of items), whereas recall tasks require *coding* rehearsal (i.e., the active relating of items to other items in context and in long-term memory). For a fascinating review of rehearsal processes in children's memory, the reader is referred to Ornstein (1978) and Naus et al. (1978). Perlmutter (1980) provides a review of work in episodic and semantic memory that the clinician can adapt to evaluate children's memory.

Clinicians who analyze language tasks noting the rehearsal strategies inherent in the tasks will be better prepared to evaluate test responses. Asking a child to describe an elephant is a recall task which requires coding rehearsal. Asking a child to imitate the sentence, "I saw an elephant," is a recognition task requiring minimal maintenance rehearsal. The clinician might modify a short-term memory task by converting it to a long-term memory task. For example, the speech-language pathologist could say: "Listen carefully. I am going to say a sentence. I want you to remember it and repeat it exactly as I say it. But you must wait until you see me raise my hand over my head. Listen and repeat it when I raise my hand: I saw an elephant." (The length of delay depends upon the child's age and processing abilities.) This latter task is made more difficult by adding intervening stimuli, for example: "Mary, while you are waiting for me to raise my hand over my head, can you point to the window and the door?" The examiner's intervening language stimulus and the child's processing of that stimulus, motor response, and return to repetition of the original sentence task provide an opportunity to observe performance on focused and divided attention tasks as well as on recall and recognition tasks.

Assessment should also include an evaluation of *memory search* procedures through observing response time. *Automatic* search procedures occur when stimuli are sufficiently well learned. *Controlled* search procedures require a number of comparisons across a number of memory representations, each comparison taking time and tending to decrease performance. Controlled search procedures may be required when targets and distractors are of approximately equal strength or when the wanted message is the ground in a figure-ground task. For example, a task requiring automatic search may ask the subject to "Raise your hand every time you hear the name of an animal. Do not pay attention to anything else you hear—only to the names of animals." If the word or sound is well esconced in memory, the memory search response should be rapid. An example of controlled search is: "I'm going to say the names of many animals. Some are farm animals; some are wild animals. Raise your hand *only* when I say the names of wild animals." Responses are considered in terms of recall and retrieval mechanisms, semantic categories, reaction time, type of search procedure displayed, and so forth.

Selected instruments for assessing performance of 3-, 4-, and 5-year-olds on tasks which attempt to measure selective attention, auditory vigilance, and auditory figure-ground abilities among normal and high-risk children are reported elsewhere by Butler (1981c) and Shigezumi (1976). Those authors concluded that high-risk children demonstrate significantly lower scores and a concomitantly greater degree of vulnerability to some but not all processing tasks that require selective attention. However, "the degree to which information overloading occurs, or the degree to which auditory distractibility and auditory fatigue play a part is open to speculation" (Butler, 1981c, p. 315).

In summary, it is suggested that assessment be conducted in a number of *contexts* and measure *language components or levels* and the individual's *language processing strategies*. Suggested areas of evaluation are listed in Figure 1. The parameters measured for any task are identified by an X in the appropriate row of the table. Evaluation is informal. The same task is utilized under varying conditions, for example, speeded and nonspeeded. Various question forms require different degrees of memory processing and place different levels of demand on children. For example, wh-questions require the retrieval of a specific piece of information (a recall task), whereas yes-no questions require recognition responses only (Ratner, 1980). For some specific language screening suggestions, the reader is referred to Wallach and Lee (1981) and Blank, Rose, and Berlin (1978). Measuring information processing components as well as "mental representations" and task strategies is presently possible but requires expensive equipment such as computers or tachistoscopes (Sternberg, 1981). Eventually, access to such technology should provide the speech-language pathologist with instruments to assess higher-order skills, including cognitive strategies.

AREA	PERFORMANCE ACROSS TASKS AS IDENTIFIED				
	Task 1	Task 2	Task 3	Task 4	Task 5

ATTENTION
  Involuntary
  Voluntary
    Focused
    Divided

EFFORT
  Deliberate
  Nondeliberate

TIME PRESSURE
  Speeded task
  Unspeeded task

PROCESSING LOAD
  Well known information
  Partially known information
  Unknown information

PERCEPTUAL PROCESSING
  Auditory modality
  Visual modality
  Other modality
  Crossmodality
  Phonemic/phonetic
  Match/mismatched units

SHORT-TERM MEMORY (to 2 min)
  Maintenance rehearsal
    Auditory/visual
  Coding rehearsal
    Auditory/visual

LONG-TERM MEMORY
  Episodic
  Semantic
    Categorical
    Attributes

SEARCH PROCEDURES
  Automatic
  Controlled

RETRIEVAL
  STS/LTS
  Recognition
  Recall

Figure 1. Language processing: areas of evaluation.

INTERVENTION STRATEGIES

A few "training programs" utilizing information processing now exist. Feuerstein (1979, a and b) developed an intervention program known as "Instrumental Enrichment" and an assessment procedure designed to assess learning potential. Most such programs have been developed to assist children or adults who are mentally retarded, and these programs can be adapted in part for use with children with language processing problems.

An individual plan for a child with language processing disorders should provide instruction in those areas that will increase the efficiency of the processing act. If attentional deficits are noted, consider training to resist distractors. Determine distractors through observation of reactions to auditory stimuli (in particular, linguistic stimuli) or visual stimuli. Is the child less distractible if the instruction is one-to-one or if it is in a large group? What kinds and levels of language seem to cause difficulty? When asked to focus attention on a task for a specified length of time, can the child accomplish it? Does the child need you to provide attentional control or can you teach self-monitoring and self-instructional strategies? For example, does the child covertly instruct himself or herself by saying, "Do not pay attention to John when he whispers," or "Keep listening to the tape until the page is finished." The clinician can assist by providing external activities and reinforcement for successful performance. An auditory vigilance task might be: "Listen for the little word 'to' . . . I'm going *to* the store. I am going *to* be eight years old. I want *to* go swimming. When you hear "to," let me know by making a mark with your pencil." This kind of activity not only calls for vigilance, but requires a motoric response while continuing with the attending task. Such a task would have an added semantic component if the clinician then said, "Now I want you to listen for a different kind of meaning. Whenever you hear a *different* /tu/, draw a circle around your mark. [Provide examples.] It is *too* hot here. I want to go, *too*. I have more than *two* friends." It should be apparent that much more than attention is involved in such a task. Successful comprehension requires not only attentional and perceptual skills but higher-order processing as well.

Instruction may be of value in rehearsal training for short-term memory tasks or in coding rehearsal for long-term memory. Teaching strategies for storing information in memory has again become fashionable and is important.

Rehearsal assists in maintaining an item in short-term memory and facilitating movement to long-term memory (within a multistore model, at least). Ornstein (1978) reported that rehearsal type or quality, not just quantity, is critical. It is not enough to rehearse or repeat items over and over, either silently or aloud. "Active" rather than rote rehearsal is necessary. This implies that the child is monitoring the manner of rehearsal and is attempting to organize it. Active rehearsal can be assisted by instructing, "How can you group these 13 states so that you will say them and remember them all?" If necessary, assist the child to form subgroups to repeat together. For more information on rehearsal instructions, processing time, and how and why recall is affected by rehearsal training, see Ornstein (1978) and Naus et al. (1978).

The enhancement of other cognitive strategies may be sought through the use of overt labeling, maintenance and coding rehearsal, chunking, paired-associate recall, serial recall, free recall, mnemonics, and visual imaging and load-reducing techniques. Such procedures have proved helpful to language and learning-disordered children. Significant differences in memory performance have been found with very young children when they are provided with questions which ask them to talk about the use of objects in the context of the past, rather than the present, on a consistent basis (Ratner, 1980). Recalling from the past provides for retrieving information within a different context and increases memory performance.

Children with language and learning disorders are frequently inefficient in their use of strategies and often yield test scores that might be expected from younger children. They do not seem to use verbal rehearsal spontaneously, to organize information efficiently, or to use memory cues unless reminded to do so. Some may not reveal sufficient flexibility and may use similar strategies for different tasks where such strategies may not be appropriate.

For years speech-language pathologists have been providing training in "vocabulary." We may ask how object attributes are taught and how semantic meaning is achieved and stored. Much of what we know may not be easily accessible to us—whatever we know *about* things (declarative knowledge) may be embedded in *how* we do things (procedural knowledge) (Norman, 1979). How we assess such semantic concepts, when the child is only dimly aware of the difference between what he can "do" and what he can report that he "knows," creates some knotty questions for both assessment and intervention.

Slowly, practitioners are evolving procedures to look at memory storage and retrieval, conscious control structures, and complex information processing. Until we are all able to carry a microcomputer in our back pocket—a time which may not be so far away—and to have a packet of software floppy disks which will permit us to analyze language processing more directly, we will need to utilize what is available. As usual, we have the cart of remediation before the horse of theory, a state of events which should surprise neither clinicians nor researchers.

REFERENCES

Anderson, J. R. 1980. Cognitive Psychology and Its Implications. W. H. Freeman, San Francisco.

Atkinson, R. C., and Shiffrin, R. M. 1968. Human memory: A proposed system and its control processes. In: K. W. Spence and J. T. Spence (eds.), The Psychology of Learning and Motivation, Volume 2, pp. 89–195. Academic Press, New York.

Blank, M., Rose, S., and Berlin, L. 1978. The Language of Learning: The Preschool Years. Grune & Stratton, New York.

Blumenthal, A. L. 1977. The Process of Cognition. Prentice-Hall, Englewood Cliffs, N.J.

Bower, G. H. 1981. Mood and memory. American Psychologist 36(2):129–148.

Bregman, A. S. 1978. The formation of auditory streams. In: J. Requin (ed.), Attention and Performance, Volume VII, pp. 63–76. Lawrence Erlbaum Associates, Hillsdale, N.J.

Butler, K. G. 1981a. Language processing disorders: Factors in diagnosis and remediation. In: R. W. Keith (ed.), Central Auditory and Language Disorders in Children, pp. 160–174. College-Hill Press, Houston.

Butler, K. G. 1981b. Language disorders: Assessment of certain comprehension factors. Paper presented at the Sixth World Congress of the International Association of Applied Linguistics, August 8–14, 1981, University of Lund, Sweden.

Butler, K. G. 1981c. Language processing and its disorders. In: P. S. Dale and D. Ingram (eds.), Child Language—An International Perspective, pp. 307–318. University Park Press, Baltimore.

Craik, F. I. M., and Lockhart, R. S. 1972. Levels of processing: A framework for memory research. Journal of Verbal Learning and Verbal Behavior 11:671–684.

Feuerstein, R. 1979a. Instrumental Enrichment: An Intervention Program for Cognitive Modifiability. University Park Press, Baltimore.

Feuerstein, R. 1979b. The Dynamic Assessment of Retarded Performers: The Learning Potential Assessment Device, Theory, Instruments and Techniques. University Park Press, Baltimore.

Flavell, J. 1979. Metacognition and cognitive monitoring: A new area of cognitive developmental inquiry. American Psychologist 3:906–911.

Flavell, J. H., and Wohlwill, J. F. 1969. Formal and functional aspects of cognitive development. In: D. Elkind and J. H. Flavell (eds.), Studies in Cognitive Development: Essays in Honor of Jean Piaget. Oxford University Press, Oxford.

Geffen, G., and Sexton, M. A. 1978. The development of auditory strategies of attention. Developmental Psychology 14:11–17.

Gerber, A. 1981. Problems in the processing and use of language in education. In: A. Gerber and D. N. Bryen (eds.), Language and Learning Disabilities, pp. 75–112. University Park Press, Baltimore.

Kahneman, D. 1973. Attention and Effort. Prentice-Hall, Englewood Cliffs, N.J.

Kauffman, J. 1980. Teaching exceptional children to use cognitive strategies. Exceptional Education Quarterly 1(1):ix–xiii.

Keith, R. W. (ed.) 1981. Central Auditory and Language Disorders in Children. College-Hill Press, Houston.

Kinsbourne, M., and Caplan, P. K. 1979. Children's Learning and Attention Problems. Little, Brown, Boston.

Klatzky, R. L. 1979. Human Memory. W. H. Freeman, San Francisco.

Lindsay, P., and Norman, D. A. 1977. Human Information Processing. Academic Press, New York.

Massaro, D. W. 1975. Understanding Language. Academic Press, New York.

Myers, N., and Perlmutter, M. 1978. Memory in the years from two to five. In: P. Ornstein (ed.), Memory Development in Children, pp. 191–218. Lawrence Erlbaum Associates, Hillsdale, N.J.

Naus, M. L., Ornstein, P. A., and Hoving, K. L. 1978. Developmental implications of multistore and depth-of-processing models of memory. In: P. Ornstein (ed.), Memory Development in Children, pp. 210–231. Lawrence Erlbaum Associates, Hillsdale, N.J.

Nelson, K., and Brown, A. 1978. The semantic-episodic distinction in memory development. In: P. A. Ornstein (ed.), Memory Development in Children, pp. 233–242. Lawrence Erlbaum Associates, Hillsdale, N.J.

Nelson, K., and Ross, G. 1980. The generalities and specifics of long-term memory in infants and young children. In: M. Perlmutter (ed.), Children's Memory. New Directions for Child Development, Volume 19, pp. 87–101. Jossey-Bass, San Francisco.

Norman, D. A. 1979. Perception, memory and mental processes. In: L. Nilsson (ed.), Perspectives on Memory Research, pp. 121–144. Lawrence Erlbaum Associates, Hillsdale, N.J.

Ornstein, P. A. 1978. The study of children's memory. In: P. A. Ornstein (ed.), Memory Development in Children, pp. 1–20. Lawrence Erlbaum Associates, Hillsdale, N.J.

Paris, S. G. 1978. The development of inference and transformation as memory operations. In: P. A. Ornstein (ed.), Memory Development in Children, pp. 129–156. Lawrence Erlbaum Associates, Hillsdale, N.J.

Perlmutter, M. 1980. Children's Memory. New Directions for Child Development, Volume 10. Jossey-Bass, San Francisco.

Perlmutter, M., and Lange, G. 1978. A developmental analysis of recall-recognition distinctions. In: P. A. Ornstein (ed.), Memory Development in Children, pp. 243–258. Lawrence Erlbaum Associates, Hillsdale, N.J.

Ratner, H. H. 1980. The role of social context in memory development. In: M. Perlmutter (ed.), Children's Memory. New Directions for Child Development, Volume 10. Jossey-Bass, San Francisco.

Roberts, R. J. 1981. Errors and the assessment of cognitive development. In: K. W. Fischer (ed.), Cognitive Development. New Directions for Child Development, Volume 12. Jossey-Bass, San Francisco.

Rumelhart, D. E. 1977. An Introduction to Human Information Processing. John Wiley & Sons, New York.

Sexton, M., and Geffen, G. 1979. The development of three strategies of attention. Developmental Psychology 15(3):299–310.

Shiffrin, R. M. 1976. Capacity limitations in information processing, attention and memory. In: W. K. Estes (ed.), Handbook of Learning and Cognitive Processes, Volume 4, pp. 177–236. Lawrence Erlbaum Associates, Hillsdale, N.J.

Shigezumi, K. 1976. Auditory processing and language development in preschool children. Unpublished master's thesis, San Jose State University, San Jose, Calif.

Sternberg, R. 1981. Testing and cognitive psychology. American Psychologist 36(10):1181–1189.

Tulving, E. 1972. Episodic and semantic memory. In: E. Tulving and W. Donaldson (eds.), Organization of Memory. Academic Press, New York.

Tulving, E. 1979. Memory research: What kind of progress? In: L. Nilsson (ed.), Perspectives on Memory Research, pp. 19–34. Halsted Press, New York.

Wallach, G. 1981. Too Late, Too Early, Didn't Test the Right Things Anyway—Current Issues in Assessment. Unpublished paper presented at the Interdisciplinary Institute on Language and Learning, School of Health Sciences, City University of New York, New York.

Wallach, G. P., and Lee, A. D. L. 1981. Language screening in the schools. Seminars in Speech Language and Hearing 2(1):53–69.

Wickelgren, W. 1979. Cognitive Psychology. Prentice-Hall, Englewood Cliffs, N.J.

Other Forms
of Management

Psychological Interventions for the Child with Central Auditory Processing Disorder

Mark Hoffman

The child with a central auditory processing disorder is confronted with a confusing and frustrating world. Unable to process and organize verbal information clearly, the child may not be able to keep up with classroom instruction and may miss important directions and misunderstand questions. Faced with frustration, failure, and criticism, the child may lack a secure basis for learning. This primary disability may lead to secondary emotional and behavioral disorders.

This chapter presents a model for identification and treatment of emotional/behavioral problems encountered in the child with CAP disorder. A systems orientation is used to follow the child in family, school, and social environments. The etiology of emotional disorders, through the interaction of the individual with the social environment, is reviewed in conjunction with appropriate therapeutic procedures. Case studies drawn from clinical practice are presented.

IDENTIFICATION OF EMOTIONAL CORRELATES

Referral of a child with a CAP disorder for treatment to the mental health practitioner is often occasioned by disruptive behavior or poor school adjustment. Identification of the problem, therefore, is made after the cycle of frustration and failure has been established. The conditions that initially triggered the negative emotional reaction are often obscured by secondary habits and patterns of maladjustment. Failure to recognize early symptoms of emotional maladjustment and to intervene may necessitate a later, more urgent call for help. Often the intent of the referral is to change or manage the disturbing behavior without considering the emotional trauma and environmental factors that led to the problem.

It is useful to analyze the child in his or her social system to isolate sources of anxiety and stress. The child who has been labeled as hyperactive, when viewed in his or her milieu, is seen as easily distracted by conversation of peers or outside noise. The aggressive child may act out in response to teasing by peers. The disruptive child, frustrated with a problem, may misbehave to attract attention. Similar patterns can emerge in the home. Homework, as a source of frustration and failure, may lead to a conflict between parent and child. Oppositional behavior may surface as the child vies with siblings for attention and approval of parents.

Observational data is particularly relevant to analyzing the interplay between the child's CAP disorder, any resultant learning disability, and subsequent affective responses. Family members, teachers, and peers may be included in this evaluation process. Three methods may be utilized:

Classroom Observation

Observation of the child in the classroom may provide a rich source of information for therapy. Entering the child's school environment, the therapist may observe conditions producing emotional trauma. A firsthand impression can be gained of the child's reactions to criticism, rejection, frustration, and failure. The therapist may see efforts of the child with CAP disorder to cope with verbal information. The child's strengths and weaknesses may be noted as well as coping efforts and emotional needs.

Family Evaluation

Meeting with the family enables the therapist to observe the sources of conflict and the capacity for support. The therapist can determine the dynamic interplay between family members and the impact the child with a CAP disorder places on this system. Understanding of such forces and how they influence the child can provide data to generate therapeutic strategies.

Play Activity

Structured game-playing activities help define sources of emotional trauma. In this procedure the therapist is able to manipulate game activity to elicit a particular emotional response. The therapist may vary the difficulty of a task and assess the child's level of frustration. Using this technique, the therapist may be able to assess: 1) how the child processes verbal directions; 2) how the child solves problems; 3) how the child handles frustration; 4) the child's degree of impulse control; and 5) the child's level of anxiety.

CLINICAL PICTURE OF THE CHILD WITH CAP DISORDER

CAP disorder presents a disruptive influence to the emotional stability and social adaptation of the child. Information obtained from clinical evaluation using standard psychometric instruments and from the therapeutic assessments described can be used to construct a profile of the child's emotional functioning. The extent to which the difficulty leads to emotional disorder depends heavily upon the strengths of the child and the support provided by the family. Where these strengths and supports are weak or not present, a variety of maladaptive emotional/behavioral patterns may emerge. Types of disorders encountered in clinical practice with children diagnosed as having CAP disorder include hyperactivity, phobic reactions, aggressive behavior, and depressive withdrawal.

Hyperactivity

Ongoing emotional trauma associated with frustration and failure may affect a child's emotional stability and internal control. A pattern of disruptive, hyperactive behavior may result. In the classroom, the child becomes restless in the presence of distracting sounds, which further reduce his or her ability to function. In the home, the child may have difficulty delaying impulses and complying with parental guidelines. Unable to work independently, the child may act out and become disruptive.

Phobic Reactions

The lack of emotional security aggravated by CAP difficulties may erupt into fearful withdrawal from threatening situations. In the extreme case, these feelings may develop into phobias. School phobia, separation anxiety, and fear of failure are some of the emotional responses observed. The child may feel overwhelmed by these fears. When placed on a task, the child may become tense and immobilized, further inhibiting maximum performance. A pattern of avoidance of school may follow. Overdependency on parents at this point may provide a much needed sense of security; unfortunately, the eventual separation may become an even more fearful experience. Going out then produces tantrums, panic, or acting out behaviors.

Aggressive Behavior

The ongoing sense of frustration can also find expression in aggressive, belligerent behavior. The child may demonstrate negative behavior, such as verbally refusing to follow directions that may confuse him. Peer interactions, a source of teasing and rejection, may elicit aggressive antisocial responses. This child can become a management problem at home and at school, instilling further frustration and feelings of rejection. A cycle may develop which alienates the child further.

Depressive Withdrawal

Repeated exposure to failure situations may lead to emotional withdrawal and depression. When frustrated, the child may easily become upset and cry. The child, as a consequence, may lose interest in competitive activities and social interactions. A negative self-concept may emerge, leading to further depression and withdrawal. The child may set lower academic goals, avoid setting goals, or avoid any activity that may lead to failure.

Each of these clinical profiles demonstrates emotional responses that the child with a CAP disorder may experience. Although effective remedial education exists to help the child overcome his or her academic difficulties, the emotional overlay is at times overlooked or left unattended. Therapeutic techniques exist to reverse such patterns, particularly if introduced early.

THERAPEUTIC TECHNIQUES

Family Therapy

Family intervention can teach positive, supportive interactions within the home. Parents of children with any type of learning difficulty often feel frustrated and confused in attempting to meet their child's needs. As a result, they may react inconsistently, adding to the child's confusion with the world. Ineffective parental efforts at managing these problems and their ensuing frustrations threaten the stability of the family system. The anxiety level of family members may increase, followed by withdrawal and conflict avoidance. The child may become the scapegoat for other underlying family problems.

To provide a supportive and consistent environment for a child with CAP disorder, the therapist first may attempt to change the family dynamics and mobilize the emotional resources. Specific strategies are available to attain these goals (Haley, 1973). The therapist, serving as both educator and facilitator, may confront the style the family uses to make decisions, resolve conflicts, and reduce tensions. Problem solving training (Spivak & Shure, 1974) provides a model for the family to identify problems, define goals, and arrive at realistic solutions. Schoolwork may become a source of conflict in the family, with parental expectations clashing with the child's fears. By role-playing typical family problems and generating changes in the problem solving process, the therapist may enable the family to reduce tension levels.

Communication is a second focal point for the family therapist. Discussing the nature of CAP problems and the expectations held by both parents can produce healthy coping responses. Opening lines of communication within the family often helps the child vent frustration and anxiety while receiving support and acceptance. By training parents in communicating openly about their own fears and concerns, the child can learn to feel comfortable about his or her feelings and express them more directly. Maladaptive modes of expression, such as aggressive behavior, tantruming, or acting out, can be identified for family members, and more productive alternatives introduced. The child may be taught to verbalize anger or frustration directly to the parents. The child can learn to request the parents' support instead of throwing a tantrum.

Parent training in behavior management techniques (Patterson, 1968) is a third area for family intervention. By learning the impact of positive and negative consequences on behavior, parents can provide a consistent home environment in which the child works toward specific goals. Problem behaviors can be broken down into smaller, definable, and attainable behaviors. Parents can observe immediate, positive results and begin to feel more competent in assisting their child. To overcome the child's avoidance of school work, parents can reinforce small but increasing amounts of time on task. Attainment of positive results allows the child to reverse a pattern of failure. As the child increases time on-task and achieves more success, he or she begins to develop a positive self-concept. Charts and daily record keeping provide a visible display for assessing progress.

Therapeutic Guidelines for Working with the Child Individually

To break the cycle of failure and frustration, the child may need to develop specific skills to handle emotions differently and respond to the environment in a more effective manner. To accomplish these goals, the therapist may have several sessions of individual therapy with the child. Individual therapy can be highly effective in reducing the child's anxiety responses, developing self-control, and learning alternate forms of self-expression.

Relaxation Training   Relaxation training can be useful in counteracting negative emotional responses in children identified as anxious, emotionally labile, or hyperactive. Used in conjunction with other techniques, such as systematic densensitization, relaxation can help overcome anxious emotional reactions to events in school or at home. Relaxation can also be used to place the child in a state more conducive to learning positive approach behaviors such as responding in class and interacting with peers.

A variety of methods currently exist for developing states of deep relaxation. Jacobson (1964) presented a system of muscular exercises that are easily acquired and generalized to the daily environment. Used primarily with adults, these exercises can be modified for children (Putre et al., 1977). Children are receptive to relaxation training when it is introduced as a game-playing activity.

Instructions are given to "Make your body feel like jello." The therapist points out how relaxed muscles feel. Images can be utilized to enhance the relaxation response (Rosenthal & Scott, 1977). The child can be taught to focus on the sensation of the body becoming rubbery. Lazarus (1971) presented a detailed account of images used with children to counter anxiety in phobic situations.

Once the child has learned to modify these emotional responses, the technique can be utilized in situations associated with anxiety (Graziano et al., 1979). The child can learn to relax in school before the teacher passes out a test or asks a question. The child may relax himself or herself after experiencing an upsetting or frustrating situation.

Systematic Desensitization   In conjunction with relaxation training, desensitization can be used to decondition the child's phobic anxiety associated with school or home (Wolpe, 1973). Through the use of imaging or role-playing activities, the child is taught to associate the sensations of relaxation with fearful situations (VanHasselt et al., 1979). The child imagines working on test problems while in a relaxed state. Game activities are particularly useful in presenting stressful material in a less threatening way. The child with a fear of making mistakes may be encouraged to play a game with the therapist in which the child purposely gives incorrect answers. The child comes to feel less threatened when called on in class to give a response. By graduated exposure, situations associated with higher degrees of anxiety can be dealt with in the same manner. Imaginal desensitization is followed with practice in the actual situation. In this way, the child reduces the anxiety experienced in the real-life event. Through systematic desensitization, the child can learn to react more comfortably or with less anxiety to situations associated with failure, criticism, and rejection.

Assertiveness Training   Training in alternate styles of self-expression can assist the child in handling conflicts with peers, family, and teachers. The aggressive child can substitute conflict resolution for conflict initiation. Assertive skills resulting in reduction of emotional distress eliminate the use of aggressive responses.

The inhibited child can attain a sense of effectiveness in social situations by producing an appropriate assertive response. The child who is perpetually teased may learn to defend himself or herself more effectively rather than responding with an emotional outburst or tantrum.

Assertiveness training (Phillips & Groves, 1979) can be instrumental in helping the child attain a sense of competence and mastery. By developing a repertoire of social skills, the child can manage situations formerly viewed with apprehension.

Use of assertiveness may help the child reduce tension in this situation. Instead of acting out when angry, the child can learn to identify and to verbalize anger. The child may also learn to evaluate and express his or her own positive attributes.

Self-Control Training   Self-control training (Karoly & Dirks, 1977; Snyder & White, 1979) provides a variety of coping skills to apply when anxious or emotionally upset. For the hyperactive child, this training is a means of establishing impulse control. By utilizing self-administered prompts (e.g., "Slow down. One step at a time") and muscular tension exercises (e.g., standing with arms pressed against the body) the child may begin to bring stability to his or her emotional world. Self-control training can be incorporated into game activity (e.g., Simple Simon) to appeal to children. Games that require fine motor precision, such as a pegboard task, are also useful in developing such internal control. As the child learns to maintain control over behavior and focus attention for increasing periods of time, he or she may be better able to cope with the demands of the classroom.

CASE STUDIES

The utilization of the above techniques can best be understood through consideration of treatment protocols with learning-disabled children. These cases were seen at the Delaware County Memorial Hospital Hearing, Speech and Learning Center, an outpatient multidisciplinary treatment center. Two representative cases are presented.

Case 1

The first child, David, was 9 years, 8 months old when first seen in therapy. David was referred to the Center because of a history of underachievement and reading difficulties. A strong emotional overlay including anxiety and emotional lability was observed clinically. On the basis of the emotional component and pattern of underachievement, David was referred for psychotherapy. Psychologic testing performed before treatment indicated a child of very superior intellect, as measured on the Wechsler Intelligence Scale for Children—Revised, with marked impairment in auditory attention and memory.

David and his mother were seen for the initial therapy evaluation. The child was highly anxious and demonstrated a poor self-image. David tended to withdraw from social interactions when intimidated by family members or peers. His high degree of emotional reactivity, particularly within the classroom, caused David to become the object of rejection and teasing by peers. Having repeatedly experienced failure in the classroom, David had developed a phobia to tests and questions. On such occasions, he would panic, would lose track of his thoughts, and would break out crying. The family network was characterized by its avoidance of resolving tension and conflict. David's father often expressed high expectations to him for academic competence.

A multimodal treatment approach was adopted comprised of assertive training, desensitization, and self-relaxation exercises. Desensitization and self-control techniques were utilized in anxiety reduction to overcome test phobia. Because David enjoyed game playing, we role-played making mistakes. Imaginal rehearsal of test-taking situations effectively reduced David's apprehension of failure and mistakes. He was trained in managing stress in the classroom. Information for the therapeutic programs was drawn from David's teacher during initial telephone communication. David's teacher was also consulted to provide feedback concerning his use of the therapeutic procedures in class.

Social skill training was introduced. David was taught to use different strategies to solve problems with his peers. One approach he adopted was to ignore distracting classroom conversation and teasing from peers. We role-played expressing feelings of frustration and anger to his teacher as a substitute for the previous outbursts of crying. Assertiveness was also generalized to relationships at home by rehearsing expressing feelings of anger to his father and siblings.

David was seen in individual therapy for a period of 6 months. During this time, his anxiety diminished significantly and classroom adjustment improved as indicated by a decrease in frequency of disruptive behavior. Review with his teacher substantiated the clinical impressions. David's teacher reported a quantitative change in acting out as well as a qualitative change in test behavior. David no longer tensed during exams, nor did he burst into tears when frustrated. Peer relations improved, and David began to increase his involvement in social and recreational activities. Improvement was seen not only in reduction of anxiety but in improved adjustment to academic situations. David performed accordingly, and grade levels improved by the end of the school year. A 6-month follow-up indicated that David had maintained a positive adjustment into the next school year with no recurrence of anxiety.

Case 2

Judy, age 7, was referred to the Center for an evaluation because of poor school adjustment. Judy had difficulty following classroom instruction, was reading poorly, and displayed immature speech. She was described by her parents as easily upset, highly active, and showing occasional outbursts of emotion. The results of evaluation by the learning center team indicated low average intelligence as measured by the Wechsler Intelligence Scale for Children—Revised, with difficulties in intake and expression of information, both visually and aurally.

CAP evaluation indicated that Judy had problems in picking out, attending to, and remembering speech messages. A high degree of disruptive emotional behavior was observed during testing. Judy and her family were referred for therapeutic intervention of Judy's emotional disorder.

Therapy was initiated with the entire family unit. Judy's mother had divorced and remarried during the previous year, a situation that was felt to contribute to Judy's emotional instability. Contact with her natural father seemed to be a disruptive influence on Judy. Another unsettling factor appeared to be the recent birth of her stepsister. Judy seemed hyperactive and emotionally out of control. Her emotional state would swing wildly from joy to anger to sadness over the course of a few minutes. Her emotional reactions tended to be extreme and inappropriate to surrounding events. Social behavior was several years behind her chronologic age. Judy's mother reported that Judy had displayed severe tantrums both at home and at school. Judy showed little ability to relate to peers, at times being excessively demanding or emotionally volatile.

Judy was seen individually and with her family. In conjunction with psychotherapy, speech and language therapy was conducted. Educational recommendations were given to her teacher. From the onset of treatment, the parents were taught specific behavior management skills with which to attend to Judy's erratic outbursts. Conditions that triggered or increased such outbursts were identified for the parents and alternative responses were suggested. Time out, which required Judy to sit on a chair in a corner of the room, was used not only as a consequence for disruptive behavior but also as a means of developing self-control. To reduce rivalry with her sister for parental attention, Judy's parents were taught to involve her in activities, specifically those helpful to her stepsister.

Individual therapy focused on developing control over emotional outbursts. Through game-playing activities, Judy was taught to control impulses when confronted with frustration and failure. As she acted out, therapeutic interventions were directed to teaching self-control and appropriate emotional expression. Desensitization training was used in real-life situations to decrease her sensitivity to upsetting environmental events. Role playing and social skill building were frequently utilized to help Judy relate more appropriately to family and friends. Options other than tantrums were practiced in the context of home and school situations. Judy's teacher was frequently consulted to monitor use of coping skills. Conversational skills were repeatedly rehearsed to help Judy attend and respond appropriately to others' verbal cues.

Therapeutic involvement lasted approximately 1 year. Over that period, Judy's general level of activity and emotionality became more manageable and eventually fell within normal limits. Coordination of therapeutic goals by the therapist with Judy's parents and teacher provided a more consistent environment to promote behavioral control. Judy's parents became much more comfortable and effective in working with her. As this occurred, Judy felt more secure regarding her need for attention within the family. Although Judy is still prone to react in the extreme when frustrated, this occurs less frequently and is of shorter duration than in the past. Her adjustment within the classroom, as assessed through teacher reports on the frequency and severity of outbursts, also improved. As a result of therapeutic intervention, Judy was able to benefit to a greater extent from remedial education programs. Although Judy continued to display academic problems, she was able to keep up with her classmates and began to enjoy school.

CONCLUSION

The impact of CAP difficulty leading to a learning disorder in the young child can extend far beyond the academic environment. Early recognition of and sensitivity for the plight of the child can provide the support necessary to form a stable and secure emotional base. The mental health practitioner, as part of the team of learning specialists, can work within the child's social network to identify and modify sources of emotional trauma. In this manner, the child learns to cope with his or her environment while the environment learns to cope with a child with a problem. By establishing a flexible and responsive system, the therapist may not only produce changes in the current emotional/behavioral disturbances but may set up a mechanism that reduces the likelihood of its recurrence.

REFERENCES

Graziano, A. M., Mooney, K. D., Huber, C., and Ignasiak, D. 1979. Self-control instruction for children's fear reduction. Journal of Behavior Therapy and Experimental Psychiatry 10:221–227.

Haley, J. 1973. Strategic therapy when a child is presented as the problem. Journal of the American Academy of Child Psychiatry 12:641–659.

Jacobson, E. 1964. Anxiety and Tension Control. J. B. Lippincott, Philadelphia.

Karoly, P., and Dirks, M. J. 1977. Developing self-control in pre-school children through correspondence training. Behavior Therapy 8:398–405.

Lazarus, A. 1971. Behavior Therapy and Beyond. McGraw-Hill, New York.

Patterson, G. 1968. Living with Children. Research Press, Champaign, Ill.

Phillips, D. R., and Groves, G. A. 1979. Assertive training with children. Psychotherapy: Theory, Research and Practice 16:171–177.

Putre, W., Loffio, K., Chorost, S., Marx, V., and Gilbert, C. 1977. An effectiveness study of a relaxation tape with hyperactive children. Behavior Therapy 8:355–359.

Rosenthal, A. K., and Scott, D. S. 1977. Four considerations in using imagery with children. Journal of Behavior Therapy and Experimental Psychiatry 8:287–290.

Snyder, J. J., and White, M. J. 1979. The use of cognitive self-instruction in the treatment of behaviorally disturbed adolescents. Behavior Therapy 10:227–235.

Spivak, G., and Shure, M. B. 1974. Social Adjustment of Young Children: A Cognitive Approach to Solving Real-Life Problems. Jossey-Bass, San Francisco.

VanHasselt, V. B., Hersen, M., Bellack, A. S., Rosenblum, N. D., and Lamparski, D. 1979. Tripartite assessment of the effects of systematic desensitization in a multi-phobic child: An experimental analysis. Journal of Behavior Therapy and Experimental Psychiatry 10:51–55.

Wolpe, J. 1973. The Practice of Behavior Therapy. Pergamon Press, New York.

Chapter 17

Psychoeducational Correlates of Central Auditory Processing Dysfunction

Patricia Byrne and *Lanny Lester*

Auditory processing skills are related to school success and should be considered in the assessment and instruction of children who are learning to read (Harber, 1980). A major problem for educators has been developing diagnostic procedures. Educators variously have described auditory processing skills as closure, memory, sound blending, and sequencing and have tested these skills in settings that are unlike normal classroom listening conditions.

In audiology, strides in the development of auditory processing tests have been made since Dandy (1928) and Bunch (1928) observed that qualitative hearing disorders could occur in patients with normal hearing acuity. Today, the central auditory processing tests that are used by audiologists reflect neuromaturational development. Some of the tests attempt to approximate certain classroom listening conditions. Appropriate programs of intervention for children with auditorily based learning problems depend on the cooperation of educators, who are responsible for the psychoeducational aspects of assessment, and audiologists, who are best able to evaluate the auditory processing system.

The purpose of this chapter is to foster interdisciplinary cooperation in working with children with CAP disorders. We wish to find procedures for teachers to identify children who should be referred for CAP testing. Specifically, the performance of children with CAP problems was examined in terms of intellectual functioning, learning aptitude, laterality, and achievement. Because a clinical population was employed, direct comparisons with normal children were not possible. Expectancy levels based on normative data or a conventional grade expectancy formula were used. In addition, all variables were examined to identify those that would discriminate between mildly and severely CAP-disordered children.

REVIEW OF THE LITERATURE

Reading disability in children results from different etiologies (Myklebust, 1965; Tallal, 1976). Both visual and auditory dyslexics have been described (Orton, 1937). The latter are children whose poor reading performance may be due to a CAP disorder (Bateman, 1968).

The role of auditory perception in reading, largely ignored in early research, has become the focus of investigations into the correlates of learning disorders. Flowers (1964) compared the auditory processing abilities of third-graders on a CAP battery consisting of tests of low-pass filtered speech, accelerated speech, and competing messages. He found significant differences between the performance of good and poor readers ($p < 0.01$). Another study comparing the performance of normal and learning-disabled students was performed by Stubblefield and Young (1975) using Katz's (1962) Staggered Spondaic Word (SSW) Test. Statistically significant differences were noted for the learning-disabled group, which had more errors and more reversals ($p < 0.01$).

Studies that compared performance of learning-disabled children with the normative data on standardized tests also supported the diagnostic value of CAP testing. Pinheiro (1977) tested 33 dyslexic children on seven tests from the Willeford, Katz, and Pinheiro battery and found performance was below that of normals on tests of binaural fusion, filtered speech, and pitch patterns. In a large, well designed study, Angelo (1980) administered Willeford's (1978) CAP test battery to 60 randomly selected learning-disabled students 8–10 years old. The results suggested that learning-disabled students experienced auditory perceptual dysfunction at all tested levels of the central auditory system. In addition, CAP tests differentiated those students who were classified as learning-disabled due to medically confirmed neurologic impairment from those with no observable organic impairment.

METHODOLOGY

To identify a screening procedure for CAP disorders, the records of 36 CAP-disordered children (seen at Delaware County Memorial Hospital Hearing, Speech and Learning Center) with full-scale IQs of 90 or over were examined. The children were referred initially for suspected hearing problems possibly contributing to their academic difficulties; all were subsequently found to have normal peripheral hearing. By means of a CAP test battery consisting of five tests adapted by Willeford (1978) and Katz (1962), performance was categorized as mildly or severely CAP-disordered. Mild disorder was defined as below age expectancy on one or two subtests; severe referred to poor performance on three to five subtests. Performance on a battery of standardized and informal psychoeducational tests commonly administered within a school setting was analyzed to select instruments that would identify the children with CAP dysfunction. The psychoeducational battery consisted of the Wechsler Intelligence Scale for Children—Revised (WISC-R; Wechsler, 1974) or the Slosson Intelligence Test (SIT; Slosson, 1974); subtests of the Detroit Test of Learning Aptitude (DTLA; Baker & Leland, 1967); subjective evaluation of laterality, including eye, hand, and foot preference; the Daniels Informal Word Recognition Inventory (IWRI; Daniels, 1963); the Temple University Informal Spelling Inventory (ISI; Johnson & Kress, 1965); the Informal Reading Inventory (IRI; Johnson & Kress, 1965); the Informal Listening Inventory (ILI; Johnson & Kress, 1965); and the Stanford Achievement Test (SAT; Madden et al., 1972).

The CAP battery administered to all subjects included measures of Binaural Fusion (BF) and Rapidly Alternating Speech (RAS) as well as tests of Binaural Separation (BS) and Filtered Speech (FS), all from Willeford (1978). The BS and the SSW tests are competing sentence tests played simultaneously in the listener's left and right ears (for a more complete discussion of these tests see Protti, Chapter 7, this volume). This test measures the child's ability to attend to conversation in the presence of competing noise. The FS test presents low-frequency filtered speech to each ear monaurally. The FS test measures the ability of the student to understand conversation when the high frequencies are lost, as for instance when the teacher turns to face the blackboard.

The WISC-R was used as a measure of intellectual functioning for 30 subjects, and the SIT for six subjects. The SIT has a correlation of $r=0.75$ with the full-scale WISC IQ for reading-disabled children (Pekulski, 1973).

Discrepancies between Verbal and Performance IQs on the WISC-R were studied to determine whether they could be used to identify the CAP-disordered child. Poor CAP performance has been associated with low Verbal IQ (Wellman, 1980; Orlando, 1971). Rourke, Young, and Flewelling (1971) indicated that low Verbal, high Performance WISC scores are associated with audiophonic difficulties.

Modality strength and its relationship to CAP performance were assessed. Although identification of a deficit auditory modality is a major goal in designing a reading program for a CAP-disordered child, an equally important objective is the identification of comparative modality strength. The importance of teaching to a child's modality strength has been demonstrated with first-graders whose preferred modality was tactile-kinesthetic (Abrams, 1976). When the instructional approach was consistent with this modality preference, the student's word recognition scores were significantly higher than when instruction stressed the auditory mode. The presence of a deficit auditory modality should not lead a clinician to design a program that is based on a presumably stronger modality without comparative testing of all modalities. An evaluation of the visual and auditory channels as well as these modalities in combination with the haptic modality should be conducted. An instrument such as the DTLA was used to provide a profile of modality strength.

Subtests from the DTLA were used to assess the comparative sensory modalities of children with CAP disorders. The visual subtests included visual attention span for objects and visual attention span for letters. In the former, an increasing number (two to eight) of pictured objects were presented on cards. The child was given 1 sec to memorize each object presented. The visual attention span for letters subtest was similar, but the stimuli were more abstract. This test used six sets of letters with four trials in each set. The auditory subtests included auditory attention span for unrelated words and attention span for related syllables. On the former, series of two to eight words of one syllable were read to the student, who was to recall as many words as possible. The related syllables subtest consisted of sentences ranging from five words totaling six syllables to 22 words with 27 syllables. The oral directions subtest of the DTLA measured the child's ability to integrate the visual and auditory modalities (Banas & Willis, 1979). In this subtest, the child was to respond to instructions presented aurally by making an appropriate motor response on a referent sheet of pictures, numbers, and letters. Test performance on all subtests of the DTLA was reported as an equivalent mental age.

Complete data on informal laterality assessments were available on 20 subjects. Laterality assessments consisted of tests of eye, hand, and foot dominance. Preferences for hand (writing, catching, and tossing), foot (kicking, hopping), and eye (telescope use and a convergence task) were obtained. Performance was considered normal when unilateral preference for eye, hand, and foot were noted. Crossed, mixed, or incomplete dominance was classified as abnormal. Preference for eye, hand, and foot was considered established when use was consistent on all of three trials. During the 1930s and 1940s researchers assumed that eye and hand dominance were clear indications of brain dominance and that abnormalities in establishment of unilateral dominance were correlated with an increased incidence of learning disabilities. This assumption has not been supported in studies of total school populations, but when clinical populations were investigated, significant relationships were observed (Vernon, 1971).

To measure academic achievement, the Temple IRI (Temple University, 1953), IRWI, and a grade-appropriate level of the SAT, Form A, were administered. The IRI is based on a series of graded passages. Performance on the IRWI, recognition of words in the context of sentences, and comprehension of passages read aloud and silently at each level of difficulty were the criteria used in determining the most appropriate level of instruction for each child (Betts, 1946; Johnson & Kress, 1965). Instructional level was characterized by fluent oral reading with 95% accuracy in recognition of words and comprehension averaging 75% over oral and silent selections.

The Daniels IWRI test consists of graded lists of words. The ability to immediately recognize isolated words at sight was determined by flashing individual words between two index cards at a rate of 1 per second. Words not recognized at sight were reexposed for the student to apply word analysis skills. Eighty percent was specified as the level of adequate performance. To reflect the standards observed in area schools, a more lenient criterion than that suggested by Johnson and Kress (1965) was selected.

The Temple ISI was used to provide a measure of spelling ability after each word was pronounced and used in a sentence. As suggested by Johnson and Kress (1965), spelling grade level was considered as the highest level at which at least 75% of the words were spelled correctly.

An informal listening inventory was used to determine the level at which each child could best profit from aurally presented classroom instruction. One graded selection from each level of difficulty of the Temple IRI was read to the students, and questions were asked at the end of each selection to determine whether or not the child had adequate listening and conceptual skills to comprehend the passages. Analysis of passages used at each level of difficulty suggested that selections had high content validity as a measure of auditory comprehension expected in traditional grade placements. Testing was begun at the level appropriate to the grade placement of the child and was continued until the highest level, reflecting at least 75% comprehension, was obtained (Kress & Johnson, 1965).

Informal assessment instruments are an important part of the psychoeducational battery described in this study. Kretschmer (1972) has advocated the use of informal instruments rather than standardized tests because of the lack of relationship between the type of cognitive skills measured on standardized tests and those required in a school setting. Additional criticism of standardized tests for overestimating actual levels of functioning has come from Farr and Tuinman (1972). Because standardized tests generally are multiple-choice tests, the potential for correctly answering a question is enhanced with every distractor the examiner can eliminate. In contrast, informal procedures use probed recall rather than multiple-choice questioning; therefore, the generation of a correct answer by chance is minimal.

PROCEDURE

To characterize the functioning of CAP-disordered children, the data were organized into means, standard deviations, and mean deficits for each test variable. Mean deficits were obtained by subtracting mean test scores from a measure of expected performance on that particular test. For subtests of the DTLA the expected level of performance was considered to be in accord with mental age. This assumption was justified because scores on these subtests are obtained from age-appropriate norms. Deficits for the achievement variables were obtained by subtracting each achievement test score from the Horn reading expectancy grade (REG; Torgerson & Adams, 1954). The REG has been shown to be a valid measure of expectancy in reading (Bond & Tinker, 1973; Smith, 1980).

To determine the statistical significance of differences between mean test scores, 10 tests for correlated data were performed: 1) performance IQ versus verbal IQ, 2) auditory attention span versus visual attention span, 3) oral directions versus auditory attention span, 4) oral direction versus visual attention span, 5) REG versus IRI level, 6) REG versus SAT grade equivalency, 7) REG versus word recognition at sight, 8) REG versus word analysis level, 9) REG versus ISI grade

level, and 10) REG versus ILI grade level. The two auditory attention span subtests were averaged, as were the two visual subtests of
the DTLA.

To compare functioning of groups with different degrees of CAP
disorders, mean deficits and standard deviations were calculated for
the mild and severe CAP groups. Differences between the groups were
statistically analyzed using *t*-tests for independent samples and a
0.05 level of significance. To determine whether any particular combination of these deficit scores and full-scale IQ could be used to differentiate between mild and severe CAP disorders, a discriminant function analysis (Veldman, 1967) was utilized. Twenty-four subjects
(15 with severe and nine with mild disorders) for whom complete data
on all variables was available were included in this analysis.

RESULTS AND DISCUSSION

Mean test scores, standard deviations, and mean deficits in expected
performance for the entire CAP group are presented in Table 1. Performance on all learning aptitude subtests, except auditory attention span
for unrelated words and related syllables, was within expected limits.
Performance on all achievement tests was below expected levels.

Intelligence

The mean intelligence of the CAP-disordered sample was above the
average range. Although Lee (1971) reported that CAP dysfunction
and low intelligence are associated, this study indicated that CAP disorders do exist among children with above average and superior intelligence. Performance IQ scores were greater than Verbal IQ scores,
although the difference was not statistically significant. No significant
differences between full-scale IQ of mildly and severely CAP-
disordered groups were observed. More variability in the full-scale IQ
of severely impaired subjects (standard deviation=11.95) was noted
than in that of mildly impaired subjects (standard deviation=6.50).

Learning Aptitude

The oral directions subtest of the DTLA was the least difficult for CAP-
disordered subjects; performance showed an average deficit of four
months compared to norms from nonhandicapped children. The oral
directions subtest measured ability to execute tasks when stimuli were
presented visually and auditorily. No significant differences between
the performance of mildly and severely CAP-disordered subjects were

Table 1. Means and standard deviations obtained on tests administered to all CAP-disordered children.

Measure	Mean	Standard deviation	Mean deficit
Intelligence			
Verbal	108	10.01	
Performance	111	12.76	
Full-scale	110	11.93	
Age			
Chronologic	9;7	2.89	
Mental	10;7		
Learning aptitude (in age-equivalent scores)			
Auditory attention span—words	6;8	2.86	3;1
Auditory attention span—related syllables	7;2	2.72	3;5
Average auditory attention span	6.9	2.54	
Visual attention span—objects	10;0	3.62	0;7
Visual attention span—letters	9;5	2.14	1;2
Average visual attention span	9.7	2.55	
Oral directions	10;3	2.43	0;4
Grade	3.7	2.88	
REG	5.3	3.25	
Achievement (in grade scores)			
IRI	2.4	2.71	2.9
ILI	3.5	2.58	1.8
Sight word recognition	3.0		2.3
Word analysis	3.9		1.4
Spelling	3.0		2.4
SAT	3.7	2.87	1.6

noted. The mean deficit for the visual attention span for letters subtest was 1 year, 2 months. For the visual attention span for objects subtest, the average deficit was 7 months. There was no significant difference between visual subtests and oral directions scores. Comparison of the performance of mildly and severely CAP-impaired groups indicated that severely impaired subjects performed significantly less adequately than their mildly impaired counterparts on the objects subtest but showed no significant differences on the letters subtest. Students with CAP problems had significantly greater difficulty with the auditory subtests of the DTLA than with the visual subtests or oral directions subtest. The mean deficits were 3 years, 1 month, for auditory attention span for words and 3 years, 5 months, for auditory attention span for related syllables. It seems that children with auditory processing deficiencies have difficulty with immediate recall of linguistic auditory stimuli regardless of the nature of the stimuli, but have somewhat greater difficulty when it is necessary to sequence rapidly presented meaningful stimuli involving semantic and syntactic relations.

Achievement

When compared to REG, all achievement test scores were significantly depressed. However, when expectancy was based on actual grade placement of each student, all achievement scores except IRI instructional level were within the span of one grade. Although mean SAT performance and grade placement were identical (3.7), the higher than average mean IQ of the sample suggests that students could be expected to achieve at higher than average levels. The discrepancy between performance on standardized and informal reading measures supports Farr and Tuinman's (1972) observation that pupil performance on standardized tests is significantly better than performance on an individually administered IRI.

Laterality

An analysis of the laterality tests for eye, hand, and foot preference indicated higher than expected frequency of crossed, mixed, and incomplete dominance. Of the 20 subjects for whom complete data were available, 17 failed to show consistent preference for one side of the body.

Discriminant Function Analysis

One discriminant function was generated which accounted for 100% of the variance. There was no significant difference between group centroids. Thus, the combination of all test variables used in the psychoeducational battery did not significantly discriminate between mild and severe CAP disorders, but selected tests did indicate differences.

IMPLICATIONS

Information about the characteristics of CAP-disordered children on a traditional psychoeducational battery has implications for educators who are faced with identifying learning-disabled children who should be referred for audiologic testing. Knowledge of the characteristics associated with CAP disorders may help educators to make proper referrals and thereby obtain information to facilitate learning. Comparison of discrepant scores on auditory and visual subtests of the DTLA can be an indication of CAP disorder. Superiority of oral directions subtest performance over all other DTLA subtests may be an indication that CAP children are using their relatively intact visual modality to compensate for their deficit. The adequate performance of even severely CAP-disordered children on the oral directions subtest suggests that the auditory system may not be assessed independently when visual cues are presented.

Use of the discrepancy between REG and achievement test scores may be a better indicator of a CAP dysfunction than comparison of grade placement and achievement scores. The high incidence of abnormal laterality among CAP-disordered children suggests the possibility of a subtle neurologic disorder (Harris, 1979) that may underlie auditorily based learning disabilities.

The inability of the data to discriminate between mild and severe CAP groups, as defined in this study, suggests that degree of CAP dysfunction is not reflected in psychoeducational testing. What we have determined, however, is that performance on a traditional psychoeducational battery may be used to identify children who should be referred for further audiologic testing. An auditorily based learning problem is suggested by a discrepancy between subtest performance on the auditory and visual subtests of the DTLA, with the visual scores 2 or more years higher than the auditory scores. Deficiencies in spelling ability and sight vocabulary when compared with grade placement and REG also suggest auditory processing problems. The presence of these indicators in a child who seems to be having difficulty in school despite standardized achievement scores that are grade-appropriate warrants referral for central auditory processing testing.

REFERENCES

Abrams, N. 1976. Effectiveness of teaching word recognition to tactile-kinesthetic preferring first graders. Unpublished doctoral dissertation, Fordham University, New York. (Available from ERIC Document Reproduction Service, No. 132540.)

Angelo, R. 1980. Identification of central auditory dysfunction in learning disabled children. Unpublished doctoral dissertation, Lehigh University, Bethlehem, Pa. (Available from Dissertation Abstracts International, No. 8102496.)

Baker, H., and Leland, M. 1967. Detroit Tests of Learning Aptitude. Bobbs-Merrill, Indianapolis.

Banas, N., and Willis, I. H. 1979. Prescriptive teaching from the DTLA. Academic Therapy 14:466–493.

Bateman, B. 1968. A pilot study of mentally retarded children attending summer day camp. Mental Retardation 6:39–44.

Betts, E. A. 1946. Foundations of Reading Instruction with Emphasis on Differentiated Guidance. American Book Company, New York.

Bond, G. L., and Tinker, M. A. 1973. Reading Difficulties: Their Diagnosis and Correction. Prentice-Hall, Englewood Cliffs, N.J.

Bunch, C. 1928. Auditory acuity after removal of the entire right cerebral hemisphere. Journal of the American Medical Association 90:2102.

Dandy, W. E. 1928. Removal of right cerebral hemisphere for certain tumors with hemiplegia. Journal of the American Medical Association 90:823–825.

Daniels, P. 1963. Individual Word Recognition Inventory. The Reading Clinic, Temple University, Philadelphia.

Farr, K., and Tuinman, J. J. 1972. The dependent variable: Measurement issues in reading research. Reading Research Quarterly 7:413–423.

Flowers, A. 1964. Central auditory abilities of normal and lower group readers. State University of New York, Albany, New York. (Available from ERIC Document Reproduction Service, No. ED 003846.)

Harber, J. 1980. Are auditory perceptual skills requisite for reading success?, Reading World 19:272–279.

Harris, A. 1979. Lateral dominance and reading disability. Journal of Learning Disabilities 12:337–343.

Johnson, M. S., and Kress, R. 1965. Informal Reading Inventories. International Reading Associates, Newark, Del.

Katz, J. 1962. The use of staggered spondaic words for assessing the integrity of the central auditory nervous system. Journal of Auditory Research 2:327–337.

Kretschmer, M. C. 1972. Subject matter as a factor in testing comprehension. The Reading World. 11:275–285.

Lee, C. 1971. Relationships between central auditory abilities, IQ and reading achievement in students referred for diagnosis. Unpublished doctoral dissertation, United States International University, San Diego. (Dissertation Abstracts International, order No. 7125396.)

Madden, R., Gardner, E. F., Rudman, H. C., Karlsen, B., and Merwin, J. C. 1972. Stanford Achievement Test. Harcourt, Brace, and Jovanovich, New York.

Myklebust, H. R. 1965. Learning disorders: Psychoneurological disturbances in children. Rehabilitation Literature. 25:354–360.

Orlando, C. 1971. Relationships between language laterality and handedness in eight and ten year old boys. Doctoral dissertation, University of Connecticut, Storrs. (Dissertation Abstracts International, order No. 7129895.)

Orton, S. T. 1937. Reading, Writing and Speech Problems in Children. Norton, New York.

Pekulski, J. 1973. Validity of three brief measures of intelligibility for disabled readers. Journal of Educational Research 67:67–68.

Pinheiro, M. 1977. Neural basis of central auditory diagnosis in children and adults. Paper presented at the Northeast Regional Conference, American Speech and Hearing Association, Boston, April 1977.

Rourke, B. P., Young, G. C., and Flewelling, R. W. 1971. The relationship between WISC verbal-performance discrepancies and selected verbal, auditory-
perceptual, visual perceptual, and problem-solving abilities in children with
learning disabilities. Journal of Clinical Psychology 27:475–279.

Slosson, R. 1974. The Slosson Intelligence Test. Slosson Educational Pub-
lishers, East Aurora, New York.

Smith, L. 1980. Readability formulae. Reading Improvement 17:140–148.

Stubblefield, J., and Young, C. E. 1975. Central auditory dysfunction in learning disabled children. Journal of Learning Disabilities 8:32–37.

Tallal, P. 1976. Auditory perceptual factors in language and learning disabilities. In: R. M. Knights and D. J. Bakker (eds.), The Neurophysiology of
Learning Disorders, pp. 319–320. University Park Press, Baltimore.

Temple University Reading Clinic. 1953. Informal Reading Inventory. Annual
Reading Institute, Philadelphia.

Torgerson, T., and Adams, G. 1954. Measurement and evaluation for the
elementary school teacher. Holt, Rinehart and Winston, New York.

Veldman, D. J. 1967. Fortran programming for the behavioral sciences. Holt,
Rinehart and Winston, New York.

Vernon, M. D. 1971. Reading and its difficulties. Cambridge University Press,
New York.

Wechsler, P. 1974. Wechsler Intelligence Scale for Children. The Psychological
Corporation, New York.

Wellman, M. 1980. Relationships among cerebral laterality hand position while
writing, reading ability, and WISC subtest performance. Doctoral dissertation, University of Connecticut, Storrs. (Available from Dissertation Abstracts International, No. 8103250.)

Willeford, J. 1978. Sentence tests of central auditory function. In: J. Katz (ed.),
Handbook of Clinical Audiology, 2nd Edition, pp. 252–261. Williams &
Wilkins, Baltimore.

Chapter 18

Classroom Acoustical Environments for Children with Central Auditory Processing Disorders

Philmore J. Hart

All physical environments affect our senses and our behavior. Environmental deprivation or excessive stimuli can produce erratic behavior in normal humans (Hall, 1966). Physical settings can affect our senses and our consequent behavior. On entering a cathedral, for example, we walk softly and whisper. Although too much or too little excitement in the physical environment can affect behavior, it cannot override internally motivated behavior. A physical setting can form a support system for people and their activities, either by direct physical support such as a comfortable chair, by appropriate illumination, or by introducing an architectural background that will help avoid overstimulation (Sommer, 1969). The best physical environment provides supportive physical systems and is conducive to positive emotional behavior. Many children with central auditory processing problems are affected by nonrelevant sights and sounds. They have difficulty concentrating on study material or listening to and understanding the teacher. In this chapter, we concentrate on acoustical properties of the environment that affect the learner.

Humans react selectively to auditory and visual stimuli, selecting a figure from the background, that is, the sounds we wish to hear and attend to from the acoustical background. Selection is based on various factors: the loudest, the most active, or the most interesting.

The problem is to design a classroom environment that provides acoustical support for the child with a CAP disorder in selecting and attending to educational messages without distraction from competing, irrelevant noises. We limit the auditory choices open to the child by designing a classroom setting that will 1) limit background sounds and noises and 2) enhance the clarity and intensity of informational messages from the teacher and/or other students. Classrooms in the United States have generally not been designed to meet these criteria either for typical or for distractible students. Classrooms constructed before World War II are generally long and narrow, with high (over 12 feet) ceilings and hard, reflective wall, floor, and ceiling surfaces. This design results in long reverberation times, often over 1 sec in duration. (Reverberation refers to prolongation of sound in a room after the source itself has ceased to vibrate.) High reflectivity of surfaces results in reverberant sound predominating over direct sound and arriving at a listener's ears at various time intervals, interfering with the intelligibility of speech. This classroom design fit the then-prevailing teaching mode: the teacher speaks, the students listen. Such a design allows the teacher's voice to carry throughout the room and for any noise to be heard by the teacher.

Such a design presents a disadvantage for classrooms today, however, where teacher or student may speak from any location in the room, where groups of students talk and work in different areas, and where a profusion of sounds and noises from various activities bounces around the room. Obviously, the pre-World War II classroom does not provide a fitting and supportive environment for the CAP-disordered child. It may instead frustrate and confuse such children by allowing extraneous sounds to bombard them.

Classrooms constructed before World War II were generally walled with solid masonry, with the walls between classrooms covered on both sides with plaster. These walls constituted a thick, solid mass designed to stop sound travel from room to room. Within the room, however, this design created a highly reflective surface with little sound absorption. The result is a flood of sounds from within the room but low transmission of sounds from other classrooms. The latter is a definite advantage for the distractible child. However, typical urban schools built before World War II were located in close proximity to a street, most often at an intersection of two main streets. With a large exterior glass area to provide light and ventilation, street noise flowing into the classroom is great and often distracting. A low signal-to-noise ratio (S/N) results, so that the teacher's voice is often at an equal or less intense level than the exterior noise.

Classrooms built after World War II were designed according to different criteria and constructed of different materials. Typical classrooms are slightly wider than those from before World War II, with a somewhat lower ceiling height of approximately 10–11 feet. Walls are often constructed of exposed concrete block, with asphalt tile floors and a flat, suspended acoustical tile ceiling. This results in a classroom with a reverberation time of approximately 1 sec (0.9 sec was deemed a reasonable standard at the time), making for better speech clarity within the room than its predecessor. Although this was an important improvement, the external sound transmissions through the porous concrete block walls allowed externally generated speech and noise to offset much of the reduction of internally generated message competition.

The typical postwar school is located on a much larger site, usually on a residential street, with trees and space forming a good insulation shield from the offensive exterior noise. Perhaps the greatest acoustical problem associated with the post-World War II classroom is the change of teaching/learning modes from the didactic to a mixture of didactic, group, and individual study methods. These change the locations of the sources of sounds within the room, making good acoustical design more difficult.

Many present classrooms, therefore, do not create an ideal acoustical environment for all students, including the child with CAP problems. As a result, we enter our consideration of sound-tuning existing classrooms without a set of stable constants. Almost every classroom is physically different, the teachers' approaches are dissimilar, the number of students in regular classrooms varies from 20 to 50, and the ratio of learners with CAP problems to other students is unknown. There have been no definitive studies as to the proper acoustical environment for the distractible child, much less actual field testing of designed settings.

Efficient environments for hearing-impaired students have been studied. Testing has defined appropriate criteria for optimum speech intelligibility. We use these data here to suggest criteria for acoustical classroom environments suited to the child who is distractible or who demonstrates difficulty in understanding speech under poor acoustical conditions.

SUGGESTED ACOUSTICAL STANDARDS OF CLASSROOMS FOR DISTRACTIBLE CHILDREN

The following suggested standards are adapted from Ross (1978) and Børrild (1978):

1. *Reverberation time* From 0.6 to 0.9 sec within the 125- to 2000-Hz range, with the lower time considered best for speech clarity.
2. *Empty classroom sound level* Within a range of 30–35 dB on the "A" scale of a sound level meter.
3. *Signal-to-noise ratio* The S/N ratio should be at least +10 dB; that is, the teacher's voice should project at at least 10 dB louder than the ambient classroom background noise level.
4. *Distance between speaker and listener* A distance of 6–8 feet is the best range for speech clarity and intensity. This includes the direct voice sound and close-by reflected sounds.
5. *Reflections* Reflections of a specific direct sound should arrive at the ear of the listener within 50 msec to be completely integrated with the nonreflected direct sound. "The intensity of the direct versus reflected sounds and their relative times of arrival . . . are the most important determiners of speech intelligibility in a room" (Ross, 1978, p. 472).
6. *Sound transmission class* The sound transmission class (STC) of the dividing walls between classrooms and corridors should be class 50 (dB) or more. Particular attention should be given to the complete sealing of all intersections of the wall to floor, ceiling, and openings.
7. *Classroom configuration and size* The objective is to create a relatively diffuse sound field. Classroom shape should approximate a square. Long, narrow rooms, domed ceilings, and irregular or circular rooms should be avoided. Classroom dimensions of 25 × 30 feet, with a ceiling approximately 12 feet high, are optimal. This increases the likelihood of a diffuse sound field, as does increasing and scattering of sound absorption material throughout the room.
8. *Special classrooms* Assuming 10 students in a special classroom for distractible children, and allowing 30 square feet per student, the room should be a square, 18 × 18 feet with a 9-foot ceiling. All of the above standards apply to a smaller classroom, except that reverberation time should be lowered to 0.4 sec for good speech clarity.

Using the above standards, a team of teachers, speech-language clinicians, audiologists, architects, and acousticians could design a classroom that provides a healthy acoustical environment for all students, and in particular the child with CAP disorders. A prototype classroom is proposed based on a set of assumptions stated below. As these vary from the actual needs of an individual classroom or school, so will the actual design.

DESIGN ASSUMPTIONS

Recommendations for the prototype renovated classroom are based on the following assumptions:

1. The design is for conversion of an existing classroom to better fit the acoustical requirements of both normal and CAP-disordered children.
2. There are 24 elementary students in the classroom, four of whom are particularly distractible.
3. Classroom size is 24 × 36 feet, with a 12-foot ceiling, windows along one long side, and an entrance from the passageway along the opposite side near the front of the room (Figure 1).
4. Teaching/learning modes used are a combination of didactic, individual, and small-group study. The didactic sessions involve all of the students at a given time; individual and group study may be concurrent.
5. CAP-disordered students can derive benefit from an acoustically controlled classroom.

DESIGN RECOMMENDATIONS

1. The renovated classroom will be divided into two areas (Figure 2): a) a large central area designed for didactic recitation and group study, and b) two smaller areas along end walls for individual and small-group study.
2. The larger central area will be shaped into a square 24 × 24 feet by dropping two 6-foot-wide ceiling soffits along the end walls. Within the central space, the acoustical design should conform to the suggested acoustical standards.
3. The original classroom was oriented toward one 24-foot end wall, with windows on the left side. The new design orients the class toward the passageway wall, with the chalkboards relocated on this wall. This new configuration allows each student to be closer to the teacher and to receive the full effect of the reflecting chalkboard wall now located on the 36-foot wall behind the normal position of

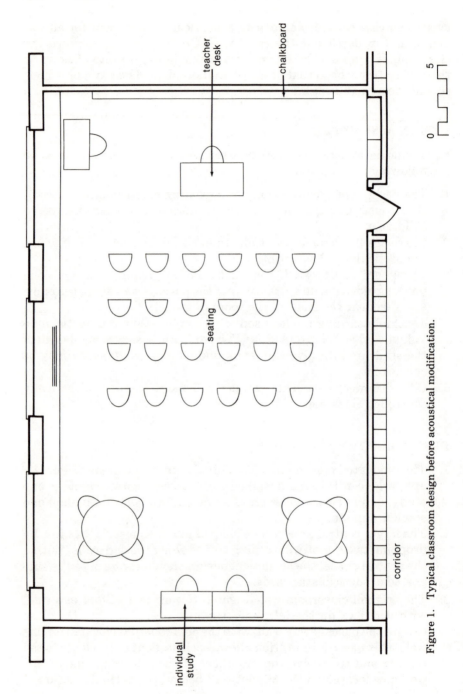

Figure 1. Typical classroom design before acoustical modification.

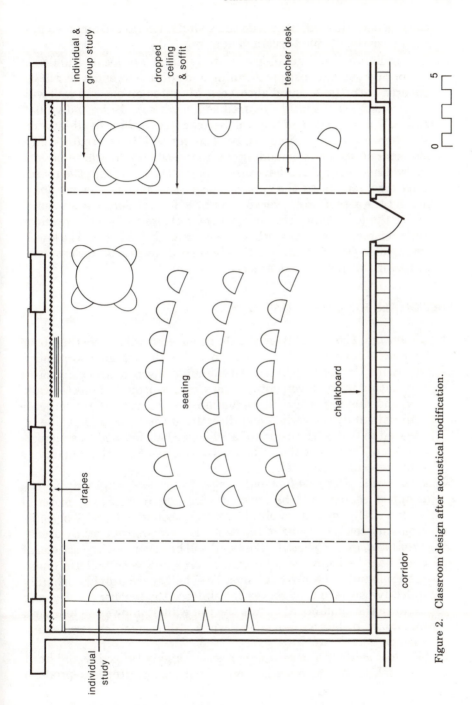

Figure 2.   Classroom design after acoustical modification.

the teacher. This will help keep the sound reflection to direct sound time near the 50-msec recommendation.

4. The individual and small-group study areas are located under a 7-foot-high, sound-absorbent ceiling and soffit. The end wall will be covered with 100% sound absorbers. Mounted on one end wall will be a continuous counter top used as a work surface for individual study. The opposite end wall will be kept free to allow flexibility for small-group or individual study. The concept is to create study areas for all students, including the distractible child, where the latter will not readily overhear other conversations within the room. This area relates to the central space, so that the teacher may attract the attention of everyone for brief instruction. The students under the low ceiling simply turn their chairs to face the teacher and then return to their work without major disturbance. The lower ceiling also creates a more intimate scale to form a better environment for the individual learner.

MATERIALS RECOMMENDATIONS

1. *Flooring*   The entire floor should be covered with carpeting, both to muffle noise at its source and to add to the sound absorption of the room. Carpeting will tend to eliminate sharp, distracting noises emanating from movement of chairs, desks, dropped objects, walking, and running. The noise reduction coefficient (NRC) of carpet is approximately 0.30 when laid directly to the floor, and can be increased to 0.55 with the use of a 40-ounce hair felt pad as an underlayment. The carpet should be rated as a class A finish to qualify as a fire-resistant material.

2. *End walls*   Both 24-foot end walls, from desk height up to the dropped ceiling, will be covered with sound-absorbing material with an NRC of 1.00 to absorb as much sound energy as possible from any conversations in the central or small-group study areas.

3. *Front wall (passageway)*   This wall will be covered with sections of chalkboard within the total central area and with bulletin board material under the lower ceilings. The chalkboard provides a highly reflective surface that serves to reinforce the teacher's voice, and because the chalkboard covers the full wall, it allows the teacher a maximum of lateral movement while still serving as a reflective surface.

4. *Window wall*   The rear wall is glass, a highly reflective and hard material. It will therefore be covered with heavy drapes to produce

an NRC of 0.55. Because heavy drapes do not allow natural daylight through, and it is crucial to good acoustical design to have the rear wall absorptive, the drapes will be treated as a flexible item, with the teacher opening and closing them according to the acoustical needs of the class.

5. *Central ceiling* The existing ceiling is plaster, a highly reflective material. A lay-in acoustical tile system will be suspended to a height of 11 feet. The acoustic tile will be in an NRC range of 0.70–0.80, will have a flame spread of 0–25 (class 25), and will be mounted with hold-down clips to tie each tile to the suspension system. Lighting will be provided by fluorescent fixtures, 2 × 4 feet, wired to provide two levels of illumination: 35-foot candles when two fluorescent tubes per fixture are turned on, and 70-foot candles when all four tubes within the fixture are turned on.

6. *Dropped ceiling and soffit* The dropped ceiling area along each end of the room, which forms the protective sound shield for the individual and small-group study area, will be constructed of a suspended metal grid measuring 2 × 2 feet, and lay-in acoustic tile. The tile is the same as that used in the central ceiling described above. This type of construction can be placed within the existing ceiling and walls without major renovation. For general illumination, fluorescent light fixtures (2 × 2 feet) will be built into the ceiling. Task lights will be mounted on the wall over the built-in work surface to provide 100-foot candles.

7. *Wall attenuation* If the sound transmission through the existing walls is too high for sound comfort and provides distraction for the susceptible children, a double wall should be constructed. Leaving a 1-inch air space from the existing wall, erect another wall constructed with 4-inch steel studs and ⅝-inch gypsum board drywall. Fiberglass sound insulation, 4 inches thick, should be placed within the stud space. All cracks should be sealed, and the stud channel retainers at ceiling and floor should be set in sealant during erection. This should amount to a STC class of over 50 dB and serve as an excellent sound stop.

8. *Corridor noise reduction* If the corridor directly outside the classroom is a noise generator, steps should be taken to reduce its effects. The entry door should be sealed with felt or vinyl sound stripping, the corridor floor carpeted, and the ceiling covered with acoustical tile.

Sound control is both a science and an art. Although the materials can be calculated for their absorption and reflectivity, the location of the source of the sound and the position of the listeners are critical. Teachers need to understand acoustical principles to manipulate the classroom sound environment so as to create the best possible support for the child with CAP problems. Armed with the knowledge that the optimum distance between speaker and listener is 6–8 feet, the teacher can make every effort to seat the child within this range. The room should be tuned for each activity: use the heavy drapes mounted over the rear glass area and placement of the children and their activities as primary tools of control and manipulation. Awareness, changing the physical setting depending on the activity, and thoughtful observation of the results of each configuration constitute the key to good acoustical tuning of the classroom. A good, flexible acoustical environment along with sensitive teachers can serve as practical support systems for CAP-disordered children as they go through the difficult process of increasing their listening, concentration, and attention.

REFERENCES

Børrild, K. 1978. Classroom acoustics. In: M. Ross and T. Giolas (eds.), Auditory Management of Hearing Impaired Children, pp. 145–179. University Park Press, Baltimore.

Hall, E. 1966. The Hidden Dimension. Doubleday, Garden City, N.Y.

Ross, M. 1978. Classroom acoustics and speech intelligibility. In: J. Katz (ed.), Handbook of Clinical Audiology, pp. 469–478. Williams & Wilkins, Baltimore.

Sommer, R. 1969. Personal Space. Prentice-Hall, Englewood Cliffs, N.J.

Index